A: Se

E: Salt Basins F: Rake G: Shovel

BIOLOGICAL AND BEHAVIORAL ASPECTS OF SALT INTAKE

THE NUTRITION FOUNDATION

A Monograph Series

HORACE L. SIPPLE AND KRISTEN W. MCNUTT, EDS.: *Sugars in Nutrition,* 1974

ROBERT E. OLSON, ED.: *Protein-Calorie Malnutrition,* 1975

ANANDA S. PRASAD, ED.: *Trace Elements in Human Health and Disease, Volume I, Zinc and Copper, 1976; Volume II, Essential and Toxic Elements,* 1976

MORLEY R. KARE AND OWEN MALLER, EDS.: *The Chemical Senses and Nutrition,* 1977

JOHN N. HATHCOCK AND JULIUS COON, EDS.: *Nutrition and Drug Interrelations,* 1978

CLIFFORD F. GASTINEAU, WILLIAM J. DARBY, AND THOMAS B. TURNER, EDS.: *Fermented Food Beverages in Nutrition,* 1979

MORLEY R. KARE, MELVIN J. FREGLY, AND RUDY A. BERNARD, EDS.: *Biological and Behavioral Aspects of Salt Intake,* 1980

In Preparation

JENNY T. BOND, L.J. FILER, JR., GILBERT A. LEVEILLE, ANGUS THOMSON, AND WILLIAM B. WEIL, EDS.: *Infant and Child Feeding*

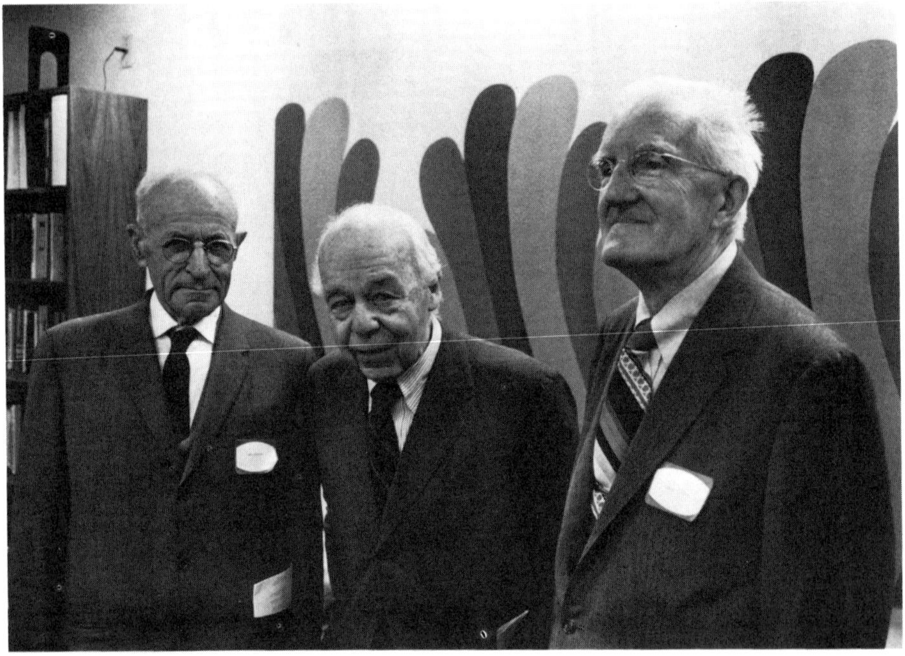

Three pioneer scientists in the area of sodium chloride research: Drs. Samuel Lepkovsky, Curt P. Richter, and Edward F. Adolph.

BIOLOGICAL AND BEHAVIORAL ASPECTS OF SALT INTAKE

EDITED BY

MORLEY R. KARE

Monell Chemical Senses Center
University of Pennsylvania
Philadelphia, Pennsylvania

MELVIN J. FREGLY

Department of Physiology
University of Florida
College of Medicine
Gainesville, Florida

RUDY A. BERNARD

Department of Physiology
Michigan State University
East Lansing, Michigan

1980

ACADEMIC PRESS

A Subsidiary of Harcourt Brace Jovanovich, Publishers

New York London Toronto Sydney San Francisco

ACADEMIC PRESS, INC.
111 Fifth Avenue, New York, New York 10003

United Kingdom Edition published by
ACADEMIC PRESS, INC. (LONDON) LTD.
24/28 Oval Road, London NW1 7DX

Library of Congress Cataloging in Publication Data
Main entry under title:

Biological and behavioral aspects of salt intake.

(Nutrition Foundation series)
Papers presented at a symposium held at Monell Chemical Senses Center, University of Pennsylvania.
Includes bibliographies and index.
1. Salt--Physiological effect--Congresses. 2. Salt in the body--Congresses. 3. Ingestion--Congresses. I. Kare, Morley Richard, Date II. Fregly, Melvin J. III. Bernard, Rudy A. IV. Series: Nutrition Foundation, New York. A monograph series – The Nutrition Foundation.
QP535.N2B56 612'.3926 79–24599
ISBN 0–12–397750–9

PRINTED IN THE UNITED STATES OF AMERICA

80 81 82 83 9 8 7 6 5 4 3 2 1

Contents

PART III
FACTORS AFFECTING SALT PREFERENCE

PART IV
NEUROLOGICAL ASPECTS OF SALT INTAKE

PART V
PHYSIOLOGICAL AND PATHOLOGICAL ASPECTS OF SALT INTAKE

List of Contributors

Numbers in parentheses indicate the pages on which the authors' contributions begin.

E. F. ADOLPH (141), Department of Physiology, University of Rochester, Rochester, New York 12863

JOHN E. ALMAN (113), Harvard School of Dental Medicine, Boston, Massachusetts 02115

LINDA M. BARTOSHUK (83), Department of Epidemiology and Public Health, Yale University Medical School, and John B. Pierce Foundation, New Haven, Connecticut 06510

FREDERIC C. BARTTER (341), Hypertension-Endocrine Branch, National Heart, Lung, and Blood Institute, National Institutes of Health, Bethesda, Maryland 20014, and Research Service, Audie L. Murphy Memorial Veterans Hospital, San Antonio, Texas 78284

DOUGLAS L. BAYLEY (289), Monell Chemical Senses Center, University of Pennsylvania, Philadelphia, Pennsylvania 19104

G. K. BEAUCHAMP (69), Monell Chemical Senses Center, and Department of Otorhinolaryngology and Human Communication, University of Pennsylvania, Philadelphia, Pennsylvania 19104

R. A. BERNARD (397), Department of Physiology, Michigan State University, East Lansing, Michigan 48824

JOSEPH G. BRAND (289), Monell Chemical Senses Center, and Department of Biochemistry, School of Dental Medicine, University of Pennsylvania, Philadelphia, Pennsylvania 19104

R. W. BRYANT (167), Leidy Laboratory, Department of Biology, University of Pennsylvania, Philadelphia, Pennsylvania 19104

HOWARD H. CHAUNCEY (113), Dental Service, Veterans Administration Outpatient Clinic, and Department of Oral Medicine and Oral Pathology, Harvard School of Dental Medicine, Boston, Massachusetts 02115

J. P. C. CHIANG (319), Protein and Biochemistry Research Laboratory, Miles Laboratories, Inc., Elkhart, Indiana 46514

ROBERT J. CONTRERAS (299), Department of Psychology, Yale University, New Haven, Connecticut 06510

D. A. CORNELIUS (319), Protein and Biochemistry Research Laboratory, Miles Laboratories, Inc., Elkhart, Indiana 46514

BEVERLY J. COWART (13), Department of Psychology, George Washington University, Washington, D.C. 20052

PATRICIA A. DANIEL (13), Department of Psychology, Brown University, Providence, Rhode Island 02912

CATHERINE S. DELEA (341), Research Service, Audie L. Murphy Memorial Veterans Hospital, San Antonio, Texas 78284

D. A. DENTON (229), Howard Florey Institute of Experimental Physiology and Medicine, University of Melbourne, Parkville, 3052, Victoria, Australia

V. G. DETHIER (411), Zoology Department, University of Massachusetts, Amherst, Massachusetts 01002

WILLIAM E. DICKINSON (49), Salt Institute, Alexandria, Virginia 22314

R. L. DOTY (397), Department of Physiology, University of Colorado, Colorado Springs, Colorado 80907

N. J. EBERTS (319), Protein and Biochemical Research Laboratory, Miles Laboratories, Inc., Elkhart, Indiana 46514

K. ENGELMAN (397), Hospital of the University of Pennsylvania, Philadelphia, Pennsylvania 19104

A. N. EPSTEIN (167), Department of Biology, University of Pennsylvania, Philadelphia, Pennsylvania 19104

JOHN L. FALK (205), Department of Psychology, Rutgers University, Piscataway, New Jersey 08854

S. J. FLUHARTY (167), Department of Psychology, University of Pennsylvania, Philadelphia, Pennsylvania 19104

RICHARD H. FORSYTHE (221), Campbell Soup Company, Campbell Institute for Research and Technology, Camden, New Jersey 08161

MARILYN S. FREGLY (3), Department of Behavioral Studies, University of Florida, Gainesville, Florida 32611

MELVIN J. FREGLY (55, 145, 247), Department of Physiology, University of Florida, College of Medicine, Gainesville, Florida 32610

TOSHIRO FUJITA (341), Research Service, Audie L. Murphy Memorial Veterans Hospital, San Antonio, Texas 78284

ROBERT I. HENKIN (367), Center for Molecular Nutrition and Sensory Disorders, Georgetown University Medical Center, Washington, D.C. 20007

M. R. KARE (69), Monell Chemical Senses Center, University of Pennsylvania, Philadelphia, Pennsylvania 19104

TERUKAZU KAWASAKI (341), Research Service, Audie L. Murphy Memorial Veterans Hospital, San Antonio, Texas 78284

RALPH A. MILLER (221), Campbell Soup Company, Campbell Institute for Research and Technology, Camden, New Jersey 08101

GREGORY MOOSER (275), School of Dentistry, University of Southern California, Los Angeles, California 90007

G. ROLFE MORRISON (127), Department of Psychology, McMaster University, Hamilton, Ontario, Canada

J. F. NELSON (229), Howard Florey Institute of Experimental Physiology and Medicine, University of Melbourne, Melbourne, Victoria, Australia

DEBORAH G. NEWSOME (247), Department of Physiology, College of Medicine, University of Florida, Gainesville, Florida 32610

CLAUDE PAQUE (31), 15, Rue de Bagdhad, Rabat, Morocco

B. ROBINZON (69), Monell Chemical Senses Center, University of Pennsylvania, Philadelphia, Pennsylvania 19104

SUSAN S. SCHIFFMAN (99), Department of Psychiatry, Duke Medical Center, Durham, North Carolina 27710

JAY SCHULKIN (331) Department of Philosophy, University of Pennsylvania, Philadelphia, Pennsylvania 19174

F. J. SCHWENDE (319), Protein and Biochemistry Research Laboratory, Miles Laboratories, Inc., Elkhart, Indiana 46515

M. STERNBERG (319), Protein and Biochemistry Research Laboratory, Miles Laboratories, Inc., Elkhart, Indiana 46515

EDWARD M. STRICKER (185), Department of Psychology and Biological Sciences, University of Pittsburgh, Pittsburgh, Pennsylvania 15260

MAISY TANG (205), Department of Psychology, Rutgers University, Piscataway, New Jersey 08854

TERRY N. THRASHER (145), Department of Physiology, School of Medicine, University of California, San Francisco, California 94143

KUNIO TORII (345), Monell Chemical Senses Center, University of Pennsylvania, Philadelphia, Pennsylvania 19104

SHARON WALLACE (113), Harvard School of Public Health, Boston, Massachusetts 02115

JAMES M. WEIFFENBACH (13), Oral and Pharyngeal Development, National Institute of Dental Research, National Institutes of Health, Bethesda, Maryland 20014

R. A. WEISS (397) Department of Physiology, Michigan State University, East Lansing, Michigan 48824

GEORGE WOLF (331), Department of Natural Sciences, State University of New York, Purchase, New York 10057

List of Participants

International Conference on Biological and Behavioral Aspects of Sodium Chloride Intake

Monell Chemical Senses Center

January 24-26, 1979

Dr. Edward F. Adolph
Dr. Linda M. Bartoshuk
Dr. Gary K. Beauchamp
Dr. Rudy A. Bernard
Dr. Joseph G. Brand
Dr. Richard W. Bryant
Dr. Howard H. Chauncey
Dr. Carol M. Christensen
Dr. Robert J. Contreras
Dr. William Darby
Dr. Derek A. Denton
Dr. Vincent G. Dethier
Mr. William E. Dickinson
Dr. Alan N. Epstein
Dr. John L. Falk
Dr. Hans Fisher
Dr. Richard H. Forsythe
Dr. Marilyn S. Fregly
Dr. Melvin J. Fregly
Dr. Mark Hegsted
Dr. Robert I. Henkin
Dr. Morley R. Kare
Dr. Lynn A. Larsen
Dr. Samuel Lepkovsky
Dr. Gordon J. Mogenson
Dr. Gregory Mooser
Dr. G. Rolfe Morrison
Dr. Robert P. Multhauf
Dr. Claude Paque
Dr. Curt P. Richter
Dr. Boaz Robinzon
Mr. Jacob Rosenthal
Dr. Susan Schiffman
Dr. Carmel Schrire
Ms. Peggy Smith
Dr. M. Sternberg
Dr. Edward M. Stricker
Dr. Terry N. Thrasher
Dr. Kunio Torii
Ms. Sharon Wallace
Dr. Linda L. Walsh
Dr. James M. Weiffenbach
Mr. R. A. Weiss
Dr. George Wolf
Dr. Irving A. Woods

Foreword

Salt savoureth and seasoneth all things.
John Florio (1553?-1625)
Second Fruits Folio 53

Salt is what makes things taste bad when it isn't in them.
Anonymous

There are six flavors and of them all, salt is the chief.
Sanscrit proverb

The importance that a food commodity assumes in man's experience is reflected in the saga of his quests for it as well as in the richness of his language in allusions to the substance. Salt is near unique on both counts, ranking with or above sugar and spices. For example, the connotations of the word "salt" occupy 3½ pages in the unabridged Oxford English Dictionary, with an additional 2 pages of derivatives, "sugar" occupies 2½ pages with 2 pages of derivatives, and "spice" 1 page plus another of derivatives.

Proverbial and allusive uses or derivatives signify the value of or great importance attached to salt: for labor—salary; necessary adjunct of food, hence hospitality—"to eat a man's salt"; efficient, worthy—"to be worth one's salt"; excellence—"the salt of the earth"; pungency—"salty"; rank of esteem—"beyond the salt," e.g., seated as a guest at a position of honor on the other side of the large, ornate silver or porcelain salt container.

The quest for salt (NaCl) by herbivores is exhibited in their seeking out "salt licks," and is regarded as an expression of physiological need. The social, developmental, and anthropological aspects of salt intake are examined in the first section of this work. Man's quest well may have had similar origins, but early his demands expanded due to the increasing roles of the commodity as a condiment, preservative, and, later, manufacturing and industrial material. Throughout recorded history, there are references to and descriptions of the varied uses of salt and methods of salt production. These were vividly illustrated in Agricola's "De Re Metallica," published in 1556 (examples are portrayed in the end papers of this volume). The drive to obtain salt is evident today in all societies and is greatly accelerated in the industrial world due to the varied uses of this commodity. The fascinating and at times romantic story of the roles of salt in man's social development is authoritatively related in Robert P. Multhauf's scholarly work "Neptune's Gift: A History of Common Salt," published by The Johns Hopkins University Press, Baltimore, 1978.

Of today's enormous production of salt in the United States of 20.3 million tons only 4.4% is of food grade, which is used for all food purposes—processing (baking, cheese manufacturing, meat preservation, etc.) and table salt. Estimates of salt consumption by individuals vary enormously; the best and most recent estimates for the United States are 8–10 gm daily (Chapter 4). These are "average" figures, and considerable variation occurs depending on the individual's appetite for salt, appetite expressing many determinants, biological and behavioral.

This book probes the existing knowledge of those factors that alter man's appetite for salt. It summarizes observations from comparative physiological studies as well as in man. It does so because of the physiological and pathological significance attached to levels of salt intake in health and in disease and the need to modify intakes under differing biological conditions—sometimes to increase, sometimes to decrease salt intake. Many aspects of the physiological and pathological implications of levels of salt intake are examined in the last section. Sweepingly broad generalizations that all persons should drastically curtail salt intake are patently unsound, and the exceedingly low levels of intake advocated by some are clearly unacceptable to the vast majority of the population in the United States. Furthermore, the advocacy of these levels for all persons is not based on sound physiological evidence.

A Select Committee appointed by the Life Sciences Research Office of the Federation of American Societies for Experimental Biology under contract with the U.S. Food and Drug Administration in a report entitled "Evaluation of the Health Aspects of Sodium Chloride and Potassium Chloride as Food Ingredients" (1979) states in part:

> Sodium chloride, an essential constituent of the body and present in many foods, exhibits acute and chronic toxic effects when ingested in excessive amounts. Excess sodium chloride may induce hypertension in rats. There is a strong genetic component in the hypertensive response, and by selective breeding, strains of "spontaneously" hypertensive rats have been developed. Hypertension has been evoked by excess sodium chloride in the food or drinking water of dogs but the effects were reversible and related to osmotic factors.
>
> Salt appetite is an important expression of personal preference in relation to diet, and salt contributes to palatability of foods. For some, salt-containing foods have important cultural values. Foods in which salt is important for preparation or preservation are a prominent component of many diets.
>
> The causes of hypertension in man are related to genetic and environmental factors: race, family history, variations in endocrine and kidney function, degree of obesity, and life-style. Although the findings of epidemiological studies suggest a relationship between salt intake and onset of hypertension, the evidence that salt consumption is a major factor in causing hypertension is not conclusive. However, available data suggest that 10 to 30 percent of the U.S. population is genetically predisposed to hypertension and is exposed to a higher risk by ingestion of sodium

chloride at current levels. The Select Committee believes that a reduction of sodium chloride consumption by the population will reduce the frequency of hypertension.

For man, the daily requirement of sodium chloride is less than 1 g (17 mg per kg), an amount exceeded by that present as a naturally-occurring ingredient of most diets. The daily requirement is subject to considerable fluctuation from such conditions as excessive sweating and diarrhea. It is not possible, on the basis of currently available data, to recommend a level of intake of sodium chloride that could be considered optimal for health. Other dietary sources of sodium, the level of potassium, and the sodium to potassium ratio in the diet need to be considered.

Because of increasing use of processed foods in the diet, individuals who prefer to restrict salt intake find it difficult. The amount of sodium chloride consumed as a result of commercial food processing is about 70 to 100 mg per kg per day. The average daily intake of sodium expressed as sodium chloride from all sources is about 180 mg per kg for an adult (10 to 12 g per day). Such an intake exceeds estimates of the amount (range 2 to 10 g per day) that may elicit hypertension in susceptible individuals. A lower daily consumption of sodium chloride promises health benefits for the proportion of the population susceptible to hypertension.

It is to promote better understanding of the hard scientific information concerning the nature of man's appetite for salt and the variation of that appetite as an expression of biological needs, normal and disturbed physiology, differing environmental conditions, and behavioral patterns, that this work was assembled. The Monell Chemical Senses Center, The Nutrition Foundation, and the National Institutes of Health joined in supporting this effort and invited a group of internationally recognized scientists to examine and summarize critically their long experience in and knowledge of this area. These scientists prepared reviews that were discussed in a small workshop hosted by the Monell Chemical Senses Center. The texts subsequently were revised and edited for this publication.

This work should prove invaluable as a benchmark for all those concerned with research in this area of physiology or behavioral science, in food science and technology, medicine, or, with the utilization of existing knowledge, in the planning of nutritional programs in public health or therapeutic regimens.

This second volume resulting from collaboration between The Monell Chemical Senses Center and The Nutrition Foundation continues the tradition of this Nutrition Foundation Series "to provide systematic coverage of new nutritional knowledge in important areas, to define research needs, and to stimulate more effective application of scientific knowledge in the field of human nutrition." The scientific community at large is indebted to the leadership of The Monell Chemical Senses Center, to the participants, and to the editors for their provision of this useful benchmark in a subject area of much importance, but one not widely appreciated or understood.

William J. Darby
President
The Nutrition Foundation, Inc.
New York and Washington, D.C.

Preface

This book, based on a symposium on the "Biological and Behavioral Aspects of Salt Intake", is the culmination of many discussions on this fascinating subject. It seemed clear that the time had come to bring together from a number of disciplines those investigators who have viewed salt in the many roles it plays for all animals. It was hoped that a broad interdisciplinary symposium would offer a forum for cross-fertilization of the various disciplines represented. Few opportunities have existed for such an exchange of ideas and information on salt intake, probably because this subject area has no single discipline for a home.

Sodium chloride is the most abundant salt of sodium found naturally. It is also the principal mineral component of the circulating blood and tissue fluids of the body. A large variation in the sodium and chloride concentrations in blood may have significant physiological consequences. It may affect the electrical activity of all body cells, the osmotic pressure of plasma, and hence the distribution of body fluids, and acid-base balance. Normal function of the cells of the body requires close regulation of the sodium concentration of extracellular fluid.

Regulation of the sodium concentration and/or salt content of the body involves two main processes: the control of sodium intake and the control of sodium loss. A great deal of information is available regarding the physiological control of sodium loss from the body and the hemodynamic, hormonal and other factors that influence it. Physiologists, particularly, have concentrated their efforts in this area. Much less concrete information is available regarding control of sodium intake. In fact, it is unknown in most species whether sodium intake is controlled or whether it is fickle and independent of control. There is, however, evidence in sheep and rabbits that sodium intake may be as closely controlled as output. Additional evidence exists that the rat may control its sodium intake, but only if the sodium is in solution. This interesting observation suggests that *dietary* sodium intake may not be controlled in this species, or, at least, controlled secondarily to dietary caloric intake. The time is propitious to consider this aspect since there may be wide species variations in this regard. Some species may maintain control over both output and intake of sodium; others may control sodium output and only that portion of sodium intake ingested with fluid. Still others may control only sodium output. It is possible experimentally to produce the remaining example, that is, an animal that can only control its sodium intake; an example of such an animal would be the adrenalectomized rat. Because salt intake and the factors affecting it may have important medical implications, basic information of this type will be required for the various animal species to place the factors affecting their sodium intakes in the proper physiological context.

The existence of a salt appetite in humans and other animals is widespread and has been well documented. Yet current nutritional knowledge suggests that salt intake may exceed the established need for it. Since salt has become a cheap and abundant commodity in our civilization, it is now an important issue whether the excessive intake of salt evident in the diets of many Americans is a primary factor in the high incidence of high blood pressure in this country. Perhaps the appetite for salt which served animals and man so well when salt was in scarce supply has become a liability during a time when salt is so readily obtainable.

A great deal of basic information is needed in virtually every aspect of salt intake. For example, we may question whether control of salt intake is essential, or even important, in most animal species that are capable of controlling their sodium excretion. Information is incomplete regarding the physiological, social, and behavioral factors that influence salt appetite in most animal species. Whether the salt appetite is genetically innate or environmentally and culturally acquired is also unsettled for most species. Some of these issues are discussed in this volume.

The symposium offered the opportunity to honor three of the pioneer investigators in the area of sodium intake and sodium exchange. Dr. Edward F. Adolph of the University of Rochester, Dr. Samuel Lepkovsky of the University of California at Berkeley, and Dr. Curt P. Richter of the Johns Hopkins University, all octogenarians , attended the conference and contributed to its success.

The availability of space and funds limited the number of participants to forty individuals. It is unfortunate that all those who have contributed to our understanding of the mechanisms underlying the initiation of a salt appetite could not be invited to attend. It is my hope that the contributions to this book will capture some of the excitement and flavor of the symposium for those who did not attend.

A symposium such as this could not have been planned and executed without financial support. We are grateful to The Nutrition Foundation and the National Institute of Neurological and Communicative Disorders and Stroke (Grant 1-R13-NS-14736-01) for providing the major support. Thanks are also due to staff of the Monell Chemical Senses Center for assistance and cooperation in hosting the symposium and the many functions associated with it.

Melvin J. Fregly

PART I
SOCIAL, DEVELOPMENTAL, AND ANTHROPOLOGICAL ASPECTS OF SALT INTAKE

Chapter 1

Salt and Social Behavior

MARILYN S. FREGLY

I. INTRODUCTION

Billions of years ago oceans covered this planet, and salt deposits remain as the residues of these long-vanished seas. In Antarctica tons of salt lie frozen on the floor of a dry valley. In fact, on every continent subterranean deposits, briny wells, and salt domes remain as scattered remnants of this epoch.

Most scientists believe that life began in a salty marine environment, and it is a matter of continual speculation why this highly diffusible substance (sodium chloride) should have become a basic constituent of our unicellular ancestors and an essential component of all protoplasmic systems. When the briny seas were ultimately abandoned, salt remained as the principal inorganic constituent of the extracellular fluid in which the cells of the organism were now immersed.

According to geochemists the first oceans were less briny than they are now, but the salt which surrounds every cell of the human body links us with this era of our remote ancestors. We spend our first months of life in a ''sea'' of saline solution; the fetus even passes through an early stage with gill-like ridges and tail. By weight we are approximately 70% fluid—the same percentage of the

BIOLOGICAL AND BEHAVIORAL
ASPECTS OF SALT INTAKE

ISBN 0-12-397750-9

earth's surface that is covered by ocean—but the concentration of sodium in extracellular fluid is less than that of the present oceans.

It was A. B. Macallum (1926) who speculated from measurements of the inorganic elements in plasma of a wide range of animals that the "sea" within us may be the same salinity as the seawater of the period in geologic time at which each species evolved. He called these paleoratios.

II. SODIUM AND THE PALEORATIOS

If one compares the percentage composition of the salt constituents of seawater of today with that of the salt constituents of human plasma, the major cation in both is sodium. The other cations are potassium, calcium, and magnesium (Table I). The major anion present in both seawater and blood is chloride. Carbonate, bromide, and sulfate are also present. In blood, plasma protein also contributes to the ionic composition.

In spite of certain similarities in the percentage composition of seawater and serum, the concentration of all anions and cations in seawater is nearly double that of human plasma. Macallum (1926) noticed this disparity. He chose to compare the inorganic constituents of seawater with plasma by setting the sodium concentrations of both plasma and seawater equal to 100. The concentration of the other inorganic constituents were then expressed as a percentage of the sodium concentration. Here seawater and plasma from a number of species have approximately the same composition, with sodium chloride being the major constituent of both (Table II).

The greatest discrepancy occurs in the case of magnesium for which the

TABLE I

Comparison of the Percentage Composition of the Salts of Seawater and Blood Serum[a]

	Seawater	Blood serum
Sodium	30.59	36.3
Magnesium	3.79	0.23
Calcium	1.20	1.1
Potassium	1.11	1.8
Chlorine	55.27	41.2
Sulfate	7.66	0.4
Carbonate	0.21	12
Bromide	0.19	0.000001

[a] Modified from Henderson (1913) and Altman and Dittmer (1961).

TABLE II

Comparison of Inorganic Composition of the Blood Plasma of Certain Elasmobranchs, Teleosts, and Mammals (Na = 100)[a]

	Na	K	Ca	Mg	Cl	Total salts (%)
Dogfish (*Acanthis vulgaris*)	100	4.61	2.71	2.46	165.7	1.77
Cod (*Gadus callarias)*	100	9.51	3.93	1.41	149.7	1.28
Pollock (*Pollachicis virens*)	100	4.33	3.10	1.46	137.8	1.29
Dog	100	6.86	2.52	0.81	128.5	0.95
Mammal (average)	100	6.69	2.58	0.80	118.3	0.90
Ocean water	100	3.61	3.91	12.11	180.9	2.60–3.17

[a] From Macallum (1910).

plasma concentration is lower than seawater by an order of magnitude. Macallum (1910) explained this exception in the following way:

> The resemblances are very close except in the case of magnesium but this exception and the minor differences in the case of potassium and calcium are explained as due to the alteration in composition which the ocean has undergone since the Protovertebrate form appeared, for not only has there been an increase since then in the saline concentration of the ocean water but there has obtained a change in the proportions of its basic constituents. This has been brought by the continual elimintion of the calcium and potassium and the retention of the sodium and, in large part, of the magnesium derived from the river discharge from the land areas of the globe.

The ratios listed in Table II were called ''paleoratios'' which to Macallum (1926) represented the inorganic composition of the sea at the time a particular species evolved. Although the salt concentration of plasma increased during geologic time as the oceans became more briny, the ratios of the inorganic constituents remained unchanged. Macallum (1926) believed the earliest and primary function of the kidney was to maintain this paleoratio and secondarily to act as an excretory organ.

An intriguing example of the separation of the excretory function and of the maintenance of the paleoratio is in the shark. Its ancestors probably arose about 500 million years ago in the Cambrian period, but the kidneys of the present-day shark busily maintain the Cambrian paleoratio.

The shark makes up for its evolutionary backwardness by retaining urea. Its blood urea concentration is at least tenfold higher than that of man. The high urea level is necessary to help the shark balance the osmotic pressure of its plasma against the present-day ocean water. Without the high blood concentration of urea, water would be pulled from the shark into the ocean with the consequence that the shark would become dehydrated . . . in the ocean!

By these and other studies on the lower vertebrates, Macallum (1910) suggested why protoplasmic organisms contain various levels of sodium as well as how each species maintains its physiological balance in relation to other inorganic elements. The fact that the concentration of sodium in extracellular fluid is the highest of all the inorganic constituents reflects its importance physiologically. Sodium is important in the maintenance of the electrical activity of all cells and in the regulation of extracellular fluid volume. Hence it is important that mechanisms have evolved to assure a relatively constant plasma sodium concentration.

A great deal of information is now available regarding the physiological mechanisms that affect the loss of sodium from the body. Much less information is available regarding the physiological and other mechanisms affecting its intake. It is this aspect that I should like to consider now.

III. VARIABILITY OF SALT INTAKE

The desire for salt in some species of animals (herbivores) more than others (carnivores) has been noted by countless observers throughout history. It has also been exploited by both hunters and husbandmen. The ruminants and hoofed animals supplement their forage with salt whenever it is available. Nomadic hunters watched for them at natural salt licks and used salt as bait when salt licks could not be found. The herbivora, whose potassium intake is very high and sodium intake is low, will show a marked deficiency in growth and milk output, even serious illness, if their diet is not supplemented with sodium chloride. The carnivores need no added salt and show no craving for it.

The German physiologist Bunge (1902) wondered why humans desire salt if carnivores show no craving for it. He measured the potassium and sodium contents of a wide variety of diets from human milk to cereals, grains, and blood and postulated that the herbivore's longing for salt was an attempt to balance the high potassium content of its diet. He suggested that man's desire for salt must have come late in his million-year hunting phase when he switched to the use of grain foodstuffs. Thus Bunge's famous hypothesis was that extra dietary salt is needed by populations consuming predominantly vegetable products. The excess salt was presumed to be necessary for the more effective excretion of potassium.

Bunge (1902) supported his conclusion on the basis of anthropological studies which he thought indicated that nomadic societies mainly subsisting on meats do not add salt to their food; whereas, once agriculture developed, salting became necessary. He linked this with his observation that intake of salt is accompanied by the rapid onset of potassium excretion. Moreover, he emphasized that the large amounts of salt usually consumed are out of proportion to what he thought were biological needs.

However, Bunge's anthropological data bear scrutiny. Some African tribes, subsisting mainly on a vegetarian diet, use potassium-rich plant ashes rather than salt as a condiment. In East and South Africa salt intake comes from the consumption of animal blood and from cattle urine. In other areas such as in sub-Saharan Africa, salt was an item of trade and barter, but was not necessarily consumed by the trader inhabitants. In fact, the sub-Saharan people show a lack of salt appetite both in zones of sweet water and in hypersaline areas, as Paque (1977) points out. The historical reputation of Timbuktu with its great desert caravans of camels plying the 450-mile journey back and forth from the Taodeni salt swamp has led travellers and other observers to a misguided notion about local salt consumption. The transport or trade of salt does not necessarily imply its heavy use by the carriers or the indigenous populations.

In fact, a considerable number of human groups do not add salt to their food even though salt is readily available. Kroeber (1942) compiled a list of food and salt habits of North American Indians on the Pacific coast. Important in this respect is that salt was used in the southern half, but the northern half was saltless. The boundary of demarcation is sinuous, but there were virtually no exceptions. The line begins at the Columbia River and follows the Cascade Mountains south, then cuts across the northeast corner of California into Nevada, then turns south a distance. Salt was eaten everywhere to the south and not eaten anywhere to the north of this line.

Kroeber (1942) asks what do the two contrasting areas mean?

> The following have been or might be suggested as causes of nonuse of salt: prevalence of sea food; of a meat diet; of warmer climate. The first will not hold; salt users extend farther north on the coast than inland. As to animal as against plant food, there is no very clear preponderance of either in either part of the region considered. Temperature fits the distribution better, but not exactly: The coast of northern California and Oregon is cool and foggy. A climate causing loss of body salt through sweating might be thought of as causing an increased physiological craving for salt. The strongest attachment to salt, as indicated by the number of deprivation taboos, ritual journeys, and salt ceremonies, evidently exists in southern California and Arizona, an area generally of long hot summers and heavy evaporation. However, this region constitutes only a small core of the distribution of salt use as shown by the Survey; the peripheral areas are several times as large. It must therefore be concluded that whatever underlying urge there may be in physiology as influenced by diet and climate, the specific determinant of salt use or nonuse in most instances is social custom, in other words culture.

Also Kaunitz (1956) cites studies in the Melville Islands in Australia, the Kalahari Desert in South Africa, and Tierra del Fuego in South America which lead to the same conclusion that the use or nonuse of salt by various tribes is irrespective of the amount of agricultural products they consume. Thus, one might have expected that Bunge's (1902) theory could never have achieved importance; but curiously enough, this has not been the case, and the concept is still being cited without equivocation by current textbooks of nutrition and anthropology (Newman, 1975).

Last, the observation is probably of significance that the Siriono Indians of eastern Bolivia, a hunting people, were ignorant of salt until it was introduced to them by an American cattle rancher (Holmberg, 1950). At first, they found it distasteful, but they later developed a craving for it. This would seem to indicate that once some people are conditioned to salt they cling to its use stubbornly and may go to great lengths to fulfill an appetite beyond physiological necessity.

Even present day anthropologists are still divided in opinion (Neuman, 1977) on whether the salt taboos surrounding menstruation, pregnancy, puberty/initiation rites, warfare, and mourning among the Southeastern Indians of the United States serve a physiological or a magical function, as dietary regulators, or as superstitious protective rituals without other rationale.

A comparative study from language and folklore of the ceremonial uses of salt unearths a variety of conflicting symbolic meanings. Salt betokens wit, wisdom, virility, fertility, barrenness, friendship, and food for good and evil spirits. "Ye are the salt of the earth," the Bible tells us. Jews sealed covenants by exchanging salt. Bedouins traditionally will not attack a man whose salt they have eaten. In Slavic lands bread and salt, gifts of welcome, signal life-long health and happiness to a bride and groom. Hebrews, Greeks, and Romans salted sacrifices to their gods.

Salt was not only an additive and preservative of human and animal food, but also became elevated in ritual importance as a "curative." It was one of the first medicines for man and beast. In Biblical times newborn babies were washed and rubbed with salt to ward off evil spirits. In the Roman Catholic Church to this day, salt, as a symbol of purity and incorruptibility, is placed in the mouth at baptism. However, to spill salt is considered unlucky—although one can counteract the ill effect by tossing a pinch of it over the left shoulder.

And salt became a determinant of social status. The word "salary" and presumably the expression "not worth his salt" are derived from the Roman soldier's salt allowance (*salarius*), just as another expression "to put salt on its tail" takes us back to feudal times when every lord of the manor made special provision of salt for his dove and pigeon cotes. The size of a medieval salt-cellar and the arranging of the guests "above" or "below the salt" are reminders that some of our forebears came off worse than the lord's pigeons.

IV. SALT AND SOCIAL ORGANIZATION

Whatever gustatory or spiritual properties salt possessed, there is no question that this once precious substance had economic value and played an important role in the development (and downfall) of civilizations.

In addition to its use as a condiment, medicine, and preservative, salt was found to serve as flux in glass-making and metal smelting and, of course, the first pottery glaze. In the process of glass-making, the brine which drained off the mounds of sand was collected and then boiled down in earthen pots. Fragments of these boiling pots belong to the pre-Christian era and were used by the Aztecs of Central America. Yet in many places in Africa they were still used during Livingstone's day.

Foul salt was used as a fertilizer in the reign of the Emperor Vespasian until it was superseded during the last century by chemical compounds, the bulk of which are still manufactured at or near sites of the old salt industry. These sources of supply and the earliest centers of production are enshrined in the place names of many lands which remind us where the brine springs, rock deposits, or sea evaporation pans were and, in many places, are located still. One thinks of the Yens of China, of Salamis in Cyprus, of Salinae and the Via Salaria in Central Italy, of Salins in Burgundy, of the Halles of Central Europe, of Pwllheli in North Wales, and of Saltcoats and Prestonpans in Scotland. And it is no coincidence that the region of Hallein and Hallstadt in the Tyrol has yielded the most extensive finds of the prehistoric age in Europe.

Other vestiges of the salt trade are still with us. Salt was once worth its weight in gold, traded ounce for ounce, where it was scarce. Marco Polo reported the high value in Himalayan regions of salt coins bearing the seal of the Great Khan of Cathay, and semi-nomadic chieftains still exact tolls on the great caravan routes. In the early twentieth century Ethiopia used salt disks as money.

V. SALT AND POLITICAL PATTERNS

M. R. Bloch (1963) suggests that salt and its trade determined political patterns and forms of government: where salt was plentiful, the society tended to be free, independent and democratic; where it was scarce, he who controlled the salt, controlled the people. In Africa the scarcity of salt made it more precious than human freedom; it was, in fact, a most powerful factor in the slave trade. As recently as 1882 a traveller in British East Africa reported that he was offered a young girl for four loaves of salt. And Sir Harry Johnston (1905–1906) was so impressed by the fierce craving for salt among some of the tribes of Liberia that he saw in it a fundamental factor underlying race migration and speculated on whether the craving might be responsible for the strange perversion to cannibalism among the Bele.

In contrast, along the shores of the Mediterranean and the North Sea, farmers and fishermen built free societies and small independent communities without fortifications. But in the ancient river-valley civilizations of the Nile, Babylon, India, China, Mexico, and Peru, the kings maintained their rule and obtained their income through their monopoly of salt, on which the population was helplessly dependent. By their control of the military forces that guarded the stores of salt, these rulers exercised a power of life and death over their people.

To perceive this we need only remember the sites of ancient civilizations. We think at once of the Dead Sea, the world's saltiest body of water. Near its shores is a hill of salt (Mount Sodom) where salt has been quarried since the Bronze Age. It is no coincidence that some of the earliest known agricultural settlements arose in this area, at Jericho and near the mouth of the Jordan.

It is known that the Phoenicians quarried salt in Spain, and prehistoric salt quarries containing stone axes have been found in Asia Minor (Armenia), in South America, at Hallstatt in the Austrian Alps, and at Camp Verde in Arizona, which made possible the Salt River valley civilization of pre-Columbian times. In China, in a salt-water swamp at the great bend of the Yellow River, ancient solar pans are still in operation. Elsewhere early settlements grew up around salty springs and the salt-boiling civilizations go back to Neolithic time such as in the Tyrol region of the Alps, the Moselle and Franche-Comte areas of France, the Saale and Luneburg area in Germany, and Droitwich in England. The solar evaporation pans of seawater apparently go back at least to Mycenaean times.

But what of the areas where salt had to be hauled by camel, river barge, or ship? The salt trade, particularly the overland traffic, inevitably had military, social, and political consequences. These trade routes had to be protected against bandits and marauders with convoys, fortifications and way stations, shipping ports and trading posts. In short, the system of "protection" came into existence.

In the ancient river-valley civilizations such as the Nile, kings laid down the systems of government policies, monopolies, taxes, tolls and levies which are with us today. The Ptolemies in Egypt, the Seleucids in Syria and ancient Rome developed government monopolies of the commodity, just as medieval successors, the Papacy and the Italian city states, did later (Bridbury, 1955). Eventually, these governmental forms and taxes profoundly influenced the fiscal systems of England, Holland, Prussia, and Russia and indeed most of Europe. Similarly, it is possible to prove that there exists a direct link between the Arab tolls under the great Mogul empire and the British government's monopoly in India as organized by Warren Hastings (Hughes, 1934). Marco Polo's account of the tolls levied by the Great Khan points to an even longer tradition which continues in the fiscal system of modern China (Adshead, 1970).

Students of recent history will also recall that the salt monopoly and salt tax was the rallying point of populist movements: Gandhi's treatise (1930) protesting the British salt tax bears a striking similarity to that of Benjamin Franklin's complaint against the salt tax in the reign of George III and to the French revolutionist's outcry against the *gabelle*.

It is not surprising then that a commodity of such multiple uses and in such fundamental demand should have been a coveted object which changed history and played a role in altering the balance of power among nations.

Even though salt is no longer the precious substance it once was, man's "appetite" for sodium chloride to fulfill biological and other needs invites our continued speculation.

REFERENCES

Adshead, S. A. M. (1970). "The Modernization of the Chinese Salt Administration." Harvard Univ. Press, Cambridge, Massachusetts.

Altman, P. L., and Dittmer, D. S. (Eds.) (1961). "Blood and Other Body Fluids." CH. 2. Fed. Am. Soc. Exp. Biol., Washington, D. C.

Bloch, M. R. (1963). The social influence of salt. *Sci. Am.* **209,** 89–98.

Bridbury, A. R. (1955). "England and the Salt Trade in the Later Middle Ages." Oxford Univ. Press (Clarendon), London and New York.

Bunge, G. (1902). "Textbook of Physiological and Pathological Chemistry." McGraw-Hill (Blakiston), New York.

Gandhi, M. P. (1930). "Monograph on Common Salt." Federation of Indian Chambers of Commerce and Industry, Calcutta.

Henderson, L. J. (1913). "The Fitness of the Environment." Beacon Press, Boston, Massachusetts.

Holmberg, A. R. (1950). "Nomads of the Long Bow." No. **10,** p. 35. Smithson. Inst. Soc. Anthropol., Washington, D. C.

Hughes, E. (1934). "Studies in Administration and Finance 1558–1825 with Special Reference to the History of Salt Taxation in England." Manchester Univ. Press, Manchester.

Johnston, H. (1905–1906). Liberia. *In* "Annual Report of the Board of Regents of the Smithsonian Institution," House Doc. No. 113, pp. 247–264. US Govt. Printing Office, Washington, D. C.

Kaunitz, H. (1956). Causes and consequences of salt consumption. *Nature (London)* **178,** 1141–1144.

Kroeber, A. L. (1942). Cultural element distribution. XV. Salt, dogs, tobacco. *Univ. Calif., Berkeley, Anthropol. Rec.* **6,** 1–20.

Macallum, A. B. (1910). The inorganic composition of the blood in vertebrates and invertebrates. *Proc. R. Soc. London, Ser. B* **82,** 602–624.

Macallum, A. B. (1926). The paleochemistry of the body fluids and tissues. *Physiol. Rev.* **6,** 316–357.

Neuman, T. W. (1977). A biocultural approach to salt taboos: The case of Southeastern United States. *Curr. Anthropol.* **18,** 289–308.

Newman, M. T. (1975). Nutritional adaptation in man. *In* "Physiological Anthropology" (A. Damon, ed.), pp. 210–259. Oxford Univ. Press, London and New York.

Paque, C. (1977). Comments. *Curr. Anthropol.* **18,** 302–303.

Chapter 2

Saltiness in Developmental Perspective

JAMES M. WEIFFENBACH, PATRICIA A. DANIEL, and BEVERLY J. COWART

Organisms undergo orderly change throughout their lives. This is the essential phenomenon of development. The study of developmental change offers a uniquely promising strategy for understanding the anatomy, physiology, and behavior of mature organisms. Significantly, a developmental approach speaks directly to the possibility of intervening to modify adult functioning. The developmental study of sweet taste perception has been advocated in relation to the public health problems arising from the overingestion of sugar (Weiffenbach,

BIOLOGICAL AND BEHAVIORAL
ASPECTS OF SALT INTAKE

ISBN 0-12-397750-9

1978). Similarly, adult overingestion, or abuse, of salt may be approached through examining the relevant taste modality. We will review salt sensitivity and preference in early life and offer a catalogue of potentially controllable sources of influence which might affect the development of saltiness perception.

I. DEVELOPMENTAL CHANGE

A. The Role of Stimulation

Stimulation from the environment plays a highly significant role in the development of sensory and perceptual functioning. Sensory stimulation is a determinant in the morphological development of receptors and is essential for the physiological development of peripheral and central nervous system mechanisms. Much of the developing organism's interaction with its environment can be described in terms of learning. Lipsitt *et al.* (1977) have suggested that learning which occurs during the early stages of development may be more skillful than that exhibited at any subsequent time. Exclusive reliance on a learning model may, however, cut off profitable ways of looking at developmental change (Weiffenbach, 1978). Greenberg *et al.* (1968) have pointed to a class of stimulation effects not easily encompassed by learning concepts. Gottlieb (1976) has proposed that stimulation has its influence on development through the induction, maintenance or facilitation of functioning.

The developmental calendar on which an organism is exposed to environmental events may play an important role in determining how that exposure affects subsequent perceptual functioning. If, as was once thought, the newborn's sense of taste were dormant, then fetal and neonatal exposure to taste substances would have no direct effect on perceptual development. The study of behavioral development suggests that during certain time periods, generally early in life, environmental influences are particularly effective: these are the so-called critical periods (Scott, 1962). Regardless of whether there are critical periods for exposure to the salty taste, it is clear that the schedule on which foods high in salt are introduced is particularly worthy of attention. Early introduction means not only that the stimuli act on a less mature and perhaps more malleable organism but that cumulative exposure at all subsequent periods is increased.

Substances that stimulate the taste system may directly stimulate and affect the development of other organismic systems. Specifically, after saline is tasted it may be swallowed and activate the physiological mechanism of the alimentary route controlling mineral utilization and excretion. It is clear that these mechanisms themselves undergo developmental change since the healthy term or preterm infant exhibits a precariousness of sodium balance that would be pathological in an adult (Aperia *et al.*, 1972, 1975). The development of these mechanisms may be influenced by exposure to dietary salt, but will be considered only in relation to our primary concern: the perception of saltiness.

B. A Developmental Ecological Framework

A model is required in order to conceptualize how the influences which shape the developing taste system generate the stimuli which directly impinge upon the appropriate receptor surfaces. To be useful the model must also represent the dynamic interaction of the sensory system with its changing environment. The model we propose for the special case of saltiness perception reflects the general developmental ecological approach of Bronfenbrenner (1977).

Visualize a circle surrounded by a series of concentric rings. The central circle contains the taste system per se. Within this central circle the salivary system and the sodium regulatory mechanisms of the body interact with the developing taste system. Whether, and to what extent, stimuli for the salty taste are effective depends both on the developmental status of the taste system and on the electrolyte milieu that surrounds its receptors. The circle can be thought of as encompassing sensory and physiological mechanisms relevant to the perception of saltiness.

The individual's psychological functioning is represented by the first ring surrounding the essentially physiological systems of the central circle. Here are represented individual differences in taste preferences, appetite, and general patterns of choice. The interaction of these variables with bodily mechanisms for sensing and utilizing salt is clearly of significance for development.

The proximate social environment, represented by the next ring, impinges directly on the individual's psychological functioning and through it influences the individual's exposure to salt. Initially, the proximate social environment is limited to the family, its dietary patterns and eating habits determining completely the individual's dietary exposure to salt. Later, the influence of the peer group may become critical.

Cultural and historical influences (Rozin, 1976) are conceptualized as occupying the outermost concentric ring. Stabilizing influences at this level include racial or ethnic food traditions. Variation is introduced by changes in food processing practices, secular trends in eating away from home, and changes in the advice given by health professionals.

The elements represented in the model are in continuous dynamic interaction. The interrelations among elements change as the individual grows and develops. Thus, we may wish to think not of a two-dimensional disk but of a solid cylinder extending through ontogenetic time. Developmental change is reflected by variation in the relative widths of the concentric rings observed in cross-sectional cuts through the cylinder at different points along its length.

II. DEVELOPMENT OF THE TASTE SENSE

A. The Fetus

An examination of the development of the taste sense rightfully begins prenatally. The oral area is precocious in sensory development, with the earliest fetal responses to externally applied sensory stimuli being elicited by touching around the mouth (Humphrey, 1972). Specialized cells of the peripheral taste apparatus of the human fetus are identifiable at 7 weeks and reach morphological maturity at 13–15 weeks (Bradley and Stern, 1967). Suggestive evidence that the gustatory system is functional in the later part of gestation comes from observations by DeSnoo (1937) and by Liley (1972) to the effect that tastants injected into the amniotic fluid elicit changes in swallowing. The fluid environment of the human fetus is adequately supplied with stimuli for the salty taste. However, what is known of the responses of the fetal taste system to saltiness comes primarily through analogy with the fetal lamb (Mistretta and Bradley, 1977, 1978; Johnson and Salisbury, 1977).

B. The Newborn

Attempts to define the sensory capacities and to understand the perceptual functioning of the human newborn present the classic problems associated with making inferences from behavior. Differential ingestion, like differential visual fixation, implies both discrimination and preference, but equivalent ingestion, or fixation, may indicate either that the baby cannot tell the difference between the stimuli or that he, in some sense, "doesn't care." The student of babies is deprived of the electrophysiological evidence that investigators of animal behavior can employ. Exposed to the strong temptation to think of babies as "little adults," investigators may become frustrated with the babies' inability to make verbal reports and attempt to introspect for the infants.

Studies bearing upon the newborn's response to salty tasting fluids are found along with the much more extensive literature on the neonate's response to sweet tasting fluids in the usually cited sources on the general topic of neonatal taste (Peiper, 1963; Pratt *et al.*, 1930). A modern chronology of the study of the newborn's response to sapid solutions has been supplied by Lipsitt (1977). The overview presented below is organized by method and deals specifically with responses to salt stimuli.

1. Facial Gestures

The earliest reported attempts to determine if the infant's taste sense was functioning at birth involved the observation of facial gestures (Peiper, 1963). Subsequent studies which have employed facial gestures generally agree that the newborn responds to saline solutions. The facial gestures are characterized as rejecting or suggestive of negative affect and may be accompanied by vomiting and retching. Similar facial gestures can be demonstrated in preterm infants (Aiyar and Agarwal, 1969; Peterson and Rainey, 1910) and in infants born without a cerebral cortex (Sternberg, 1901). Some investigators have failed to elicit facial gestures (Shinn, 1909) or have argued that the data are insufficient to demonstrate that the basis for the elicitation of different facial gestures is taste quality (Stirniman, 1935; Peiper, 1963). Others emphasize the high levels of stimulation required to elicit consistent response (Flasarova, 1959).

2. *Tongue Movements*

With a specially designed nipple Nowlis (1973) separately measured anterior and posterior tongue motion components of sucking. He characterized these as reflexes of acceptance and rejection, respectively. Sugar elicits acceptance, quinine hydrochloride rejection. Preliminary results indicate that physiological saline can elicit a mild version of the response to quinine and that even saline one-quarter to one-tenth this strength elicits mild rejection or nonvigorous acceptance.

Weiffenbach (1977) employed a reflexlike lateral tongue movement elicited by micro drops of fluid to study responses to saline. He found that adaptation of the response to drops of water or glucose solution leaves residual responding to saline intact in much the same way that adaptation to water leaves residual responding to glucose. This suggests that postadaptation stimulation with saline is effective because it activates receptors insensitive to, and thus not subject to adaptation by, previous water or glucose stimulation. It is significant that all the fluids elicit tongue movement in the same direction, toward the side of stimulation. Thus the adaptation paradigm is critical for the demonstrations of differential responding which suggest that different sensory mechanisms underlie responses to water, to glucose, and to saline.

3. *Modification of Sucking Pattern*

Jensen (1932) observed parametric variation in the degree to which suckle feeding was disrupted as a function of the concentration of saline introduced. It is probably significant that the saline was introduced as a change in the fluid being delivered and that the response measure was disruption of pattern. Subsequent studies that contrast intake during separate bouts of feeding from bottles differing in saline content failed to demonstrate discrimination (see intake section below).

Crook (1978) presented his subjects with a nipple that initially did not deliver any fluid. When the expected burst–pause pattern of suckling was well established, he introduced small quantities of fluid (0.04 ml) into the infant's mouth during specified pauses in sucking. Relative to drops of water, sugar drops lengthen and saline drops shorten subsequent bursts of sucking. This elegant study is the first to show truly opposite responses to sugar and salt. It encourages the tentative identification of these responses as positive and negative affective reactions.

4. Physiological Responses

Canestrini (1913) appears to have been the first to have used cardiovascular and respiratory indicators of taste discrimination. In modern times, Lipsitt (1977) has analyzed heart rate and respiration rate along with sucking in response to increments in sugar concentration. His results are somewhat in conflict with those of Canestrini. One of us (P. A. D.), in collaboration with Lipsitt, extended the use of heart rate to studies of saltiness but employed the stimulus presentation schedule of Crook (1978). Her preliminary results for sucking conform to Crook's and indicate heart rate changes for salt distinct from those for sugar. These results lend credence to the proposition that salt is hedonically negative for the newborn.

5. Intake Measures

Desor and her associates devised a technique capable of demonstrating discriminative intake for various sugars versus water. These discriminations are probably taste based since they are concentration dependent (Desor *et al.*, 1973), of different magnitude for sugars of different sweetnesses (Desor *et al.*, 1973), and evident for Similac 13 versus an isocaloric sugar solution (Desor *et al.*, 1977). Newborns can modify their ingestive behavior on the basis of sweetness, higher intake being associated with increased sweetness. Evidence was also obtained suggesting that these phenomena are relatively stable over the first six months of life.

The successful methodology of the sweetness studies was then applied to the study of the newborns' ingestion of NaCl solutions (Desor *et al.*, 1977). Intake of 0.05 to 0.20 *M* NaCl in 0.07 *M* sucrose was compared with intake of a 0.07 *M* sucrose control. No significant differences were demonstrated. The study is flawed because the role of the 0.07 *M* sucrose is unclear, because the control baseline is unstable, and because acceptance of its results would require accepting the null hypothesis. However, combined with other evidence, it makes a crucial point about the ability of the newborn to inhibit suckling on the basis of a salty taste.

Evidence concerning the newborn's ingestion of salt in formula comes from the report of an accidental mass poisoning that occurred when NaCl was substituted for sugar in a nursery formula (Finberg *et al.*, 1963). Until they became quite ill, all the infants drank avidly. In one instance a breast-fed infant received the formula as a supplement. This infant continued to ingest it until he convulsed and became comatose. All of the bottle-fed infants ingesting the fatal salt formula responded with retching and vomiting on at least one occasion. Newborns do not inhibit suckle feeding of even relatively high concentrations of NaCl.

These observations are not inconsistent with the conclusions reached on the basis of other methods of study, i.e., NaCl is detected by newborns and elicits negative affective responses from them. It would appear that both detection of NaCl and hedonic response to it can be separated from the ability to inhibit suckle feeding.

C. The Child

Few taste studies have included child subjects, and only some of these have investigated saltiness. Moreover, since studies have differed extensively in method, it is difficult to compare their findings and to extract a coherent picture from the data. Studies that measure sensitivity will be reviewed before considering investigations of preference.

1. Sensitivity

Threshold sensitivity for the salty taste has been examined developmentally in three studies. Canciullo (1958) tested more than 500 children and found that reaction time to a threshold level stimulus (0.008 *M* NaCl) increased across the ages of 5 to 10 years. At the same time, however, "negative" responses (defined as a failure to respond within 5 seconds) decreased across this age range, at least among females. These apparently contradictory findings render the study difficult to interpret. Hermel *et al.* (1970) obtained crude recognition thresholds for the saltiness of NaCl from 118 subjects representing 5 age groups (4-6, 7-11, 12-14, 20-25, and 48-60 years). What is reported of their data and analysis suggests that recognition thresholds for the salty taste do not change dramatically between the ages of 4 and 25. Murphy (1977), employing the ascending method of limits (1 or 2 runs), determined more exact detection thresholds for 98 subjects between the ages of 5.5 and 83.6 years. However, she considered the data from the children in her two youngest groups (5.5-6.5 years and 11.3-12.5 years) to be too variable and eliminated it from her report. Richter and Campbell (1940) expressed similar concern about sucrose thresholds they obtained from children 7-10 years of age. The high variability in children's responses may reflect attentional difficulties, a failure to understand the nature of the task, or frequent guessing.

Salt thresholds of normal children (ranging in age from 5 to 17 years) have also been obtained to provide control data in studies of children with cystic fibrosis (Wotman *et al.*, 1964; Hertz *et al.*, 1975)* and low zinc levels (Hambidge *et al.*, 1972). These thresholds are all roughly comparable to those obtained from

*Studies by Henkin and Powell (1962) and Desor and Maller (1975) also investigated salt thresholds in children with cystic fibrosis. They are not considered in the present context because the control group of the former included both children and adults, while normative adult data obtained with the technique employed in the latter study have not been published.

adults with similar measurement techniques (see Wotman *et al.*, 1964; Wolf *et al.*, 1978; Henkin *et al.*, 1963, respectively).

Significantly, in all of these studies forced choice procedures were used, and none found the high variability reported by Richter and Campbell (1940) and Murphy (1979), both of whom employed "yes/no" formats. Thus it is clear that one can obtain acceptable threshold measures from children if consideration is given to attentional and motivational difficultues when setting task requirements (cf. Rovee *et al.*, 1975).

Most of the above studies indicate that the salt thresholds of children and young adults do not differ. Working at suprathreshold levels of stimulation, however, Lumia (1960) found a developmental increase in sensitivity to salt. He measured differential sensitivity about 5 reference solutions (0.04, 0.08, 0.16, 0.24, and 0.32 *M* NaCl) using the methods of limits. The difference thresholds of his youngest subjects (7–11 years) were significantly greater than those of the adults (20–30 years), although differences between adult and elderly subjects (70–90 years) were not significant. Unfortunately it is unclear whether he required yes/no or forced choice responses, or whether he encountered greater variability within his younger group than within the older ones which might have contributed to the higher mean threshold of the former.

Given the diverse findings, no general statement concerning salt sensitivity in childhood can be made. Obviously measurement technique can play a critical role in determining the nature of the results. Since the salty tasting stimuli encountered in the environment are substantially above threshold, further investigation of the possibility of developmental changes in suprathreshold sensitivity would be of particular interest.

2. *Preference*

Using an intake measure similar to that employed with newborns, Beauchamp (cited in Beauchamp and Maller, 1977) has demonstrated that 6-month-old infants ingest as much saline (0.15, 0.10, and 0.20 *M* NaCl) as deionized water, while children between 1.5 and 3 years drink less saline than water. This change in response to saline might be due to an insensitivity to salt at 6 months or to a change in preference for saline between the ages of 6 months and 1.5 years. Either explanation seems unlikely since it has been demonstrated that newborns both discriminate saline solutions from water and react negatively to them; although they, like the 6-month-old infants, do not inhibit saline intake. It is more probable that the emergence of differential intake depends upon the development of the ability to inhibit ingestive behaviors, which may in turn be tied to the graduation from suckling to drinking from a cup.

The fact that the toddlers in Beauchamp's study rejected saline does not necessarily mean that young children find salt distasteful or reject it in all contexts. Davis (1928, p. 670) found that weanlings would occasionally choose to eat salt, unmixed with other foods, even though it often caused them to choke and "splutter." Filer (1978) presented children between 2 and 6 years of age with identical jars of salted and unsalted beef stew and found that the salted stew was selected for consumption with significantly greater frequency than the unsalted variety. Similarly, when G. K. Beauchamp (personal communication) presented 4- to 8-year-olds with a choice between salted and unsalted pretzels, they chose to eat the salted snack significantly more often.

Desor *et al.* (1975) measured taste preferences for NaCl in 618 subjects between the ages of 9 and 15 years and in 140 adults. Subjects tasted each of four saline concentrations (0.05, 0.10, 0.20 and 0.40 *M* NaCl) and ranked them from most to least preferred. Only the first-choice preference data were analyzed. The results indicate that while the largest percentage of subjects in both age groups preferred the lowest concentration of salt, the younger subjects differed from the adults in that more of the children selected the saltiest solution as their most preferred. Only the younger black subjects, however, showed a marked tendency to prefer the saltiest sample.

In a study designed to determine the relationship between blood pressure, salt preference, salt threshold, and body weight, Lauer *et al.* (1976) measured the preference for salt in tomato juice and beef broth. Ninety-five children between the ages of 11 and 16 years were asked to salt samples of juice and broth to their desired level of preference. They also rated a series of broths and juices, varying in salt concentration, on a 9 point hedonic scale. While neither preference measure was related to blood pressure, taste threshold, or relative weight, both generally indicated that children prefer these foods with salt added. The amounts of salt added by subjects to broth and to tomato juice were highly correlated. Whether this consistency in expressed preference extended to the rating measure was not reported.

In sum, the available data indicate that children as young as 2 years of age prefer salted to unsalted foods and that this preference continues throughout childhood. There are no clear measures of the amount of salt preferred or of whether that amount changes with age. Although there is some suggestion of a change in hedonic response to salt (from negative to positive) during the first few years of life, this may be a function of the context in which salt is presented or of the preference measure employed. A better understanding of the early development of salt preference depends upon a clarification of the relationships among various measurement techniques and between those techniques and eating behavior.

III. PATTERNS OF ENVIRONMENTAL EXPOSURE TO SALT

Several papers (American Academy of Pediatrics, 1974; Dahl, 1968; Filer, 1971; Fomon *et al.*, 1970; Guthrie, 1968; Kerr *et al.*, 1978; Puyau and

Hampton, 1966) have focused specifically on salt in the diets of infants and children, reviewing dietary sources and patterns of consumption at different ages in development. Our selective review of environmental exposure to stimuli eliciting the salty taste will begin with the fetus and proceed ontogenetically.

A. During Prenatal Life

The fetal taste system develops in an electrolyte milieu, amniotic fluid, which is perceived as slightly to strongly salty by adults (J. Bosma; P. A. Daniel and B. Reilly, personal communications). On the average the concentration of sodium in amniotic fluid is 1.26×10^{-1} *M*, while that of chloride is 1.03×10^{-1} *M* (Dittmer, 1961). There are gradual shifts in concentration of salts over the course of gestation. More abrupt changes in composition occur as a result of fetal urination. After the 12th week of gestation, fetal swallowing circulates amniotic fluid across oral* receptors (cf. Mistretta and Bradley, 1977). Near term, the fetus swallows about 450 milliliters of amniotic fluid every 24 hours, a volume similar to that ingested by the breast feeding infant (Hellman and Pritchard, 1971). Wolf and Taussig's (1973) demonstration that amniotic fluid contains salivary isoamylase suggests that the fetal salivary system is functional and may contribute to the saltiness of the taste environment in which the fetus develops. Fetal saliva would provide important increments in the level of salty stimulation reaching oral receptors, particularly if its sodium content is as high as that of newborn saliva (Prader *et al.*, 1955).

B. In Infancy

During the neonatal period salt exposure is dependent on parents' decision to feed by breast or by bottle. Prior to 1900 almost all infants in the United States were breast fed for the first 6 to 9 months of life (American Academy of Pediatrics, 1974). Recent estimates (Fomon, 1975), however, indicate that only 20% of the infants in the United States are breast fed as newborns and that by 3 to 4 months the percentage declines to 10%. By 6 to 9 months only 2% are being breast fed. The increasing use of artificial formula has implications for salt intake. Over the first few months of life the daily sodium intake of the nursing infant is 5 to 10 mEq, whereas the formula-fed infant receives 2 to 3 times that amount (American Academy of Pediatrics, 1974). The advisable daily intake of

*Nonoral receptors sensitive to salt may be present in the human fetus. Based on observations made on sheep, Johnson and Salisbury (1977) suggest that fetal laryngeal receptors are salt sensitive. Fetal breathing would provide variation in prenatal salt stimulation at this site. One could reasonably infer from the observations made on a single newborn by LaLonde and Eglitis (1961) that the fetus also has pharyngeal, uvular, and soft palate taste buds. The salt sensitivity of such extralingual taste buds is, of course, speculative.

sodium, allowing for growth needs and for losses through skin and urine, is in the range of 6 to 8 mEq for children from birth to age 3 years (Ziegler and Fomon, 1974). Taitz and Byers (1972) report a widespread tendency for mothers in Britain to use too little water in preparing dried milk formula and thereby expose their infants to dangerously high concentrations of salt. It would appear that while the breast-fed infant gets adequate sodium, the formula-fed infant may be exposed to an excess.

Beyond the newborn period the diet becomes increasingly mixed. Cow's milk (whole, skim, 2%, or evaporated) and semi-solid food or "beikost" are introduced. Anderson and Fomon (1974) report that commercially prepared, strained and junior foods are fed to most infants before the end of the first month. A recent study (Auerbach, 1978) found that bottle-fed infants tend to be started on solid food about 8 weeks earlier than breast-fed infants and are more likely to be fed commercial rather than home-made baby food. Given the typical mixture of milk and "beikost," the sodium composition of the infant's diet rises considerably over what it was during the newborn period. Cow's milk itself has three times the concentration of sodium, potassium, and chloride of human milk (Fomon and Filer, 1974); and baby food contributes similar amounts of electrolytes to the diet (American Academy of Pediatrics, 1974). A 1972 survey found that 2-month-old infants on a mixed diet ingested 13.5 mEq, 6-month olds, 29 mEq, and 12-month olds 63 mEq of sodium per day (American Academy of Pediatrics, 1974). Prompted by concern over evidence linking high salt intake to the development of hypertension (Dahl, 1968), a National Academy of Sciences Committee recommended that the infant food industry greatly reduce the amount of salt that had been added to strained and junior foods (Filer, 1971). This change was introduced by two of the three major manufacturers in January, 1977, and by the third about a year later (Kerr *et al.*, 1978). However, Kerr *et al.* found that 61% of the 3- to 14-month-old infants in their survey were routinely being fed home-made foods which, more often than not, had been seasoned for the family before the infant's portion was separated. Under these conditions babies ingest more than they would have had they been fed salted commercial baby food and 64% over the maximum recommended by the National Academy of Sciences. The weanling is increasingly at risk for overexposure to sodium.

C. In Childhood

Beyond infancy, food choices become more varied and it becomes more difficult to determine the exact salt composition of the diet. Exposure to saltiness is difficult to measure as salt is added both in food processing (Freis, 1976) and as table salt. Dietary surveys of children (Guthrie *et al.*, 1973; Owen and Lippman, 1977) have focused on the intake of protein, calories, vitamins, and some minerals and have failed to examine specifically the issue of salt consumption. The American Academy of Pediatrics (1974) reports that salt intake tends to be consistently high for all children since they adopt the eating habits of their parents and are influenced by peers, media advertising, and other factors outside the home. Recent estimates of average adult intake of NaCl are 6–18 grams per day (U. S. Senate, Select Committee on Nutrition and Human Needs, 1977).

Exposure to dietary salt may, in fact, be greater for children. Data from the Health and Nutrition Examination Survey (National Center for Health Statistics, 1978) suggest that they eat more of some high salt food than adults. Specifically, children age 1 to 17 years consume far more salty snacks than adults, with an average of only 16% reporting that these foods are seldom or never eaten. Blacks consume more salty foods than do whites. The salt exposure mediated by snack foods may well have been increased as a result of the Child Nutrition Act of 1972 which allows vending machines to be placed in school rooms in competition with school lunch programs (Moyer, 1977).

Some trends in food processing and in the food consumption patterns of the general population contribute to the high level of salt consumption in children. Meneely and Battarbee (1976) report that salt intake from processed foods has risen while use of table salt has declined slightly. Chemical additives in processed foods also lead to higher sodium intake, as described for monosodium glutamate by Bartoshuk *et al.* (1974). Some canned soups which are advertised to appeal specifically to children are high in both salt and monosodium glutamate.

The trend toward eating more meals outside of the home has increased the child's exposure to salt. McEnery and Davis (1978) report that one-third of the money spent on food in this country is spent in restaurants or fast food chains. McDonald's, the largest of the fast food chains (Kottak, 1978), appeals specifically to the child consumer through media advertising and various promotional schemes. One cheeseburger quarter-pounder alone will give the child over 3 g of salt (Jacobson, 1978).

The impact of television advertising on children's dietary habits has received a great deal of publicity recently. Although the Federal Trade Commission is specifically concerned with the promotion of sweetened food products to children, foods that increase exposure to salt are also advertised on television.

Besides the obvious impact of dietary choices on consumption of salt, there is an unexpected influence of modern living which deserves mention. The salt used to melt snow and ice on roads and highways appears to be entering the public water supply. In the State of Massachusetts a 1977 survey found that the salt content of the water supplies of 106 towns had surpassed the level recommended by the American Heart Association and the limit for persons on a low salt diet (Howard, 1977). There is concern that these levels will continue to rise. The public health significance of this trend already can be inferred from a study

(Calabrese and Tuthill, 1977) which compared the blood pressure of high school students in two towns, one with a high and one with a low level of sodium in the water supply. Those students in the high sodium community had a blood pressure distribution several years older (i.e., higher) than their peers in the town with the lower sodium water supply.

Not only could long-term consumption of water with a high salt concentration have direct health effects, but it could also provide a background adaptation level for salt taste. It might be speculated that such continuous background exposure would cause a decline in taste sensitivity and a shift in preference to higher concentrations.

These problems with salt in the water supply are further exacerbated if the family uses an artificial water softening device in the home. According to Robertson (1975), excess sodium is produced by these devices and is consumed through tap water.

IV. SUMMARY

Humans begin life in the salty environment of amniotic fluid. After birth, most infants are fed artificial milk formulae which provide two to three times as much salt as human milk. Early introduction of solid foods leads to a dramatic rise in salt consumption over the first year of life. The gains made through reducing the salt in processed infant foods may be overshadowed by a trend toward early introduction of homemade foods which have been salted for the family taste. Beyond infancy salt consumption increasingly resembles the high intakes of the adult population. This is due to the child's adopting the family eating pattern, which includes heavy use of salted, processed foods. In addition, commercial promotions of salted snack foods are often specifically directed at children. Elevated levels of salt in local water supplies is a new and unexpected factor in salt exposure.

V. PROSPECTS

Success in understanding saltiness perception depends on an adequate conceptualization of development to guide the collection of clearly defined measures of functioning and the meaningful characterization of sensory experience. Numerous models based on exploration of other perceptual modalities are available. Explorations of developmental dietary patterns offer one opportunity to assess exposure history. The recent success in applying sophisticated psychophysical methods to infants and young children encourages further research efforts directed at characterizing the saltiness perception of the human in ontogenetic perspective. Relating the development of saltiness perception to strategies for modifying salt ingestion patterns requires further parametric exploration of the relation of suprathreshold intensity to the perception of saltiness.

ACKNOWLEDGMENTS

Author Daniel's contribution was supported by United States Public Health Service Fellowship 1 F32 HD 05339-02. Author Weiffenbach's investigations were supported in part by project CIC 7-06-1054 from the Bureau of Medicine and Surgery, Navy Department, Washington, D.C.

REFERENCES

Aiyar, R., and Agarwal, J. (1969). Observations on the newborn: A study of 10,000 consecutive live births. *Indian Pediatr.* **6,** 729–742.

American Academy of Pediatrics, Committee on Nutrition (1974). Salt intake and eating patterns of infants and children in relation to blood pressure. *Pediatrics* **53,** 115–121.

Anderson, T. A., and Fomon, S. J. (1974). Beikost. *In* "Infant Nutrition" (S. J. Fomon, ed.), 2nd ed., pp. 408–434. Saunders, Philadelphia, Pennsylvania.

Aperia, A., Broberger, O., Thodenius, K., and Zetterström, R. (1972). Renal response to an oral sodium load in newborn full term infants. *Acta Paediatr. Scand.* **61,** 670–676.

Aperia, A., Broberger, O., Thodenius, K., and Zetterström, R. (1975). Development of renal control of salt and fluid hemostasis during the first year of life. *Acta Paediatr. Scand.* **64,** 393–398.

Auerbach, K. G. (1978). A study of timing of first solid foods: Comparison of breast and bottle feeding mothers. *Birth Fam. J.* **5,** 27–31.

Bartoshuk, L. M., Cain, W. S., Cleveland, C. T., Grossman, L. S., Marks, L. E., Stevens, J. C., and Stolwijk, J. A. J. (1974). Saltiness of monosodium glutamate and sodium intake. Letter to the Editor. *J. Am. Med. Assoc.* **230,** 670.

Beauchamp, G. K., and Maller, O. (1977). The development of flavor preferences in humans: A review. *In* "The Chemical Senses and Nutrition" (M. K. Kare and O. Maller, eds.), pp. 291–311. Academic Press, New York.

Bradley, R. M., and Stern, I. B. (1967). The development of the human taste bud during the foetal period. *J. Anat.* **101,** 743–752.

Bronfenbrenner, U. (1977). Toward an experimental ecology of human development. *Am. Psychol.* **32,** 513–531.

Calabrese, E. J., and Tuthill, E. W. (1977). Elevated blood pressure and high sodium levels in the public drinking water. Preliminary results of a study of high school students. *Arch. Environ. Health* **32,** 200–202.

Canciullo, D. (1958). Sensibilita gustativa nei bambini. *Minerva Otorinolaringol.* **8,** 245–264.

Canestrini, S. (1913). Ueber das Sinnesleben des Neugeborenen. *Monogr. Gesamtgeb. Neurol. Psychiatr.* p. 104.

Crook, C. K. (1978). Taste perception in the newborn infant. *Infant Behav. Dev.* **1,** 52–69.

Dahl, L. K. (1968). Salt in processed baby foods. *Am. J. Clin. Nutr.* **21,** 787–792.

Davis, C. M. (1928). Self selection of diet by newly weaned infants. *Am. J. Dis. Child.* **36,** 651–679.

DeSnoo, K. (1937). Das trinkende Kind im Uterus. *Monatsschr. Geburtshilfe Gynaekol.* **105,** 88–97.

Desor, J. A., and Maller, O. (1975). Taste correlates of disease states: Cystic fibrosis. *J. Pediatr.* **87,** 93-96.

Desor, J. A., Maller, O., and Turner, R. (1973). Taste in acceptance of sugars by human infants. *J. Comp. Physiol. Psychol.* **84,** 496-501.

Desor, J. A., Green, L. S., and Maller, O. (1975). Preference for sweet and salty in 9- to 15-year old and adult humans. *Science* **190,** 686-687.

Desor, J. A., Maller, O., and Greene, L. S. (1977). Preference for sweet in humans: Infants, children and adults. *In* "Taste and Development: The Genesis of Sweet Preference" (J. M. Weiffenbach, ed.), pp. 161-172. US Govt. Printing Office, Washington, D.C.

Dittmer, D. S., ed. (1961). "Blood and Other Body Fluids," p. 448. Fed. Am. Soc. Exp. Biol., Washington, D.C.

Filer, L. J. (1971). Salt in infant foods. *Nutr. Rev.* **29,** 27-30.

Filer, L. J. (1978). Studies of taste preference in infancy and childhood. *Pediatr. Basics* **12,** 5-9.

Finberg, L., Kiley, J., and Luttrell, C. N. (1963). Mass accidental salt poisoning in infancy. *J. Am. Med. Assoc.* **184,** 121-124.

Flasarova, B. (1959). Chutove Citi u Novorozencu. *Cesk. Pediatr.* **14,** 526-529.

Fomon, S. J. (1975). What are infants fed in the United States? *Pediatrics* **56,** 350-354.

Fomon, S. J., and Filer, L. J., Jr. (1974). Milks and formulas. *In* "Infant Nutrition" (S. J. Fomon, ed.), 2nd ed., pp. 359-407. Saunders, Philadelphia, Pennsylvania.

Fomon, S. J., Thomas, L. N., and Filer, L. J., Jr. (1970). Acceptance of unsalted strained foods by normal infants. *J. Pediatr.* **76,** 242-246.

Freis, E. D. (1976). Salt, volume, and prevention of hypertension. *Circulation* **53,** 589-595.

Gottlieb, G. (1976). Conceptions of prenatal development: Behavioral embryology. *Psychol. Rev.* **83,** 215-234.

Greenberg, D., Uzgiris, I. C., and Hunt, J. McV. (1968). Hastening the development of the blink-response with looking. *J. Genet. Psychol.* **113,** 167-176.

Guthrie, H. A. (1968). Infant feeding practices. A predisposing factor in hypertension. *Am. J. Clin. Nutr.* **21,** 863-867.

Guthrie, H. A., Owen, G. M., and Guthrie, G. M. (1973). Factor analysis of measures of nutritional status of preschool children. *Am. J. Clin. Nutr.* **26,** 497-502.

Hambidge, K. M., Hambidge, C., Jacobs, M., and Baum, J. D. (1972). Low levels of zinc in hair, anorexia, poor growth, and hypogeusia in children. *Pediatr. Res.* **6,** 868-874.

Hellman, L. M., and Pritchard, J. A. (1971). "Williams Obstetrics," 14th ed., p. 220. Appleton, New York.

Henkin, R. I., and Powell, G. F. (1962). Increased sensitivity of taste and smell in cystic fibrosis. *Science* **138,** 1107-1108.

Henkin, R. I., Gill, J. R., and Bartter, F. C. (1963). Studies on taste thresholds in normal man and in patients with adrenal cortical insufficiency: The role of adrenal cortical steroids and of serum sodium concentration. *J. Clin. Invest.* **42,** 727-735.

Hermel, J., Schonwetter, S., and Samueloff, S. (1970). Taste sensation and age in man. *J. Oral Med.* **25,** 39-42.

Hertz, J., Cain, W. S., Bartoshuk, L. M., and Dolan, T. F. (1975). Olfactory and taste sensitivity in children with cystic fibrosis. *Physiol. Behav.* **14,** 89-94.

Howard, D. V. (1977). Framing water policy. *Mass. Aud. News.* **16** (9), 3-4.

Humphrey, T. (1972). Central representation of the oral and facial areas of human fetuses. *In* "Third Symposium on Oral Sensation and Perception" (J. Bosma, ed.), pp. 98-136. Thomas, Springfield, Illinois.

Jacobson, M. (1978). Shaking out the truth about salt. *Nutr. Action* **5** (3), 3-7.

Jensen, K. (1932). Differential reactions to taste and temperature stimuli in newborn infants. *Genet. Psychol. Monogr.* **12,** 363-479.

Johnson, P., and Salisbury, D. M. (1977). Preliminary studies on feeding and breathing in the newborn. *In* "Taste and Development: The Genesis of Sweet Preference" (J. M. Weiffenbach, ed.), pp. 111-123. US Govt. Printing Office, Washington, D.C.

Kerr, C. M., Reisinger, K. S., and Plankey, F. W. (1978). Sodium concentration of homemade baby foods. *Pediatrics* **62,** 331-335.

Kottak, C. P. (1978). Rituals at McDonald's. *Nat. Hist.*, **87** (1), 75-83.

LaLonde, E. R., and Eglitis, J. A. (1961). Number and distribution of taste buds on the epiglottis, larynx, soft palate and uvula in a human newborn. *Anat. Rec.* **140,** 91-93.

Lauer, R. M., Filer, L. J., Reiter, M. A., and Clarke, W. R. (1976). Blood pressure, salt preferences, salt threshold, and relative weight. *Am. J. Dis. Child.* **130,** 493-497.

Liley, A. W. (1972). Disorders of amniotic fluid. *In* "The Pathophysiology of Gestation" (N. S. Assali, ed.), Vol. 2, pp. 157-206. Academic Press, New York.

Lipsitt, L. P. (1977). Taste in human neonates: Its effect on sucking and heart rate. *In* "Taste and Development: The Genesis of Sweet Preference" (J. M. Weiffenbach, ed.), pp. 125-140. US Govt. Printing Office, Washington, D.C.

Lipsitt, L. P., Mustaine, M. G., and Zeigler, B. (1977). Effects of experience on the behavior of the young infant. *Neuropaediatrie* **8,** 107-133.

Lumia, V. (1960). Richerche sulla sensibilita gustativa differenziale per il sapore salato in soggetti di diversa eta. *Arch. Fisiol.* **59,** 279-287.

McBurney, D. H. (1966). Magnitude estimation of the taste of sodium chloride after adaptation to sodium chloride. *J. Exp. Psychol.* **32,** 869-873.

McEnery, P. T., and Davis, C. A. (1978). Nonpharmacologic interventions in hypertension. *Pediatr. Clin. North Am.* **25,** 127-136.

Meneely, G. R., and Battarbee, H. D. (1976). High sodium-low potassium environment and hypertension. *Am. J. Cardiol.* **38,** 768-785.

Mistretta, C. M., and Bradley, R. M. (1977). Taste in utero: Theoretical considerations. *In* "Taste and Development: The Genesis of Sweet Preference" (J. M. Weiffenbach, ed.), pp. 51-64. US Govt. Printing Office, Washington, D.C.

Mistretta, C. M., and Bradley, R. M. (1978). Taste responses in sheep medulla: Changes during development. *Science* **202,** 535-537.

Moyer, A. (1977). "Better Food for Public Places: A Guide for Improving Institutional Food." Rodale Press, Emmaus, Pennsylvania.

Murphy, C. (1977). The effect of age on taste sensitivity. *In* "Special Senses in Aging" (S. S. Han and D. H. Coons, eds.), pp. 21-33. Inst. Gerontol., Ann Arbor, Michigan.

National Center for Health Statistics (1978). "Selected Findings: Food Consumption Profiles of White and Black Persons Aged 1-74," Vital and Health Statistics, No. 210. U.S. Department of Health, Education and Welfare, Washington, D.C.

Nowlis, G. (1973). Taste elicited tongue movements in human newborn infants: An approach to palatability. *In* "Fourth Symposium on Oral Sensation and Perception: Development in the Fetus and Infant" (J. F. Bosma, ed.), pp. 292-303. US Govt. Printing Office, Washington, D.C.

Owen, G., and Lippman, B. S. (1977). Nutritional status of infants and children, U.S.A. *Pediatr. Clin. North Am.* **24,** 211-227.

Peiper, A. (1963). "Cerebral Function in Infancy and Childhood." Consultants Bureau, New York.

Peterson, F., and Rainey, L. H. (1910). The beginnings of mind in the newborn. *Bull. Lying-In Hosp. N.Y.* **7,** 99-122.

Prader, A., Gautier, E., Gautier, R., Naf, D., Semer, J. M., and Rothschild, E. J. (1955). The Na and K concentration in mixed saliva: Influences of secretion rate, stimulation, method of collection, age, sex, time of day, and adrenocortical activity. *In* "The Human Adrenal Cortex" (G. E. W. Wolstenholm and M. P. Cameron, eds.), pp. 382-395. Little, Brown, Boston, Massachusetts.

Pratt, K. C., Nelson, A. K., and Sun, K. H. (1930). The behavior of the newborn infant. *Ohio State Univ. Stud. Contrib. Psychol.* **10.**

Puyau, F. A., and Hampton, L. P. (1966). Infant feeding practices, 1966: Salt content of the modern diet. *Am. J. Dis. Child.* **111,** 370-373.

Richter, C. P., and Campbell, K. H. (1940). Sucrose taste thresholds of rats and humans. *Am. J. Physiol.* **128,** 291-297.

Robertson, J. S. (1975). Letter: Surfeit of sodium in softened water. *Lancet* **1,** 1246.

Rovee, C. K., Cohen, R. Y., and Shlapack, W. (1975). Life-span stability in olfactory sensitivity. *Dev. Psychol.* **11,** 311-318.

Rozin, P. (1976). Psychobiological and cultural determinants of food choice. *In* "Appetite and Food Intake" (T. Silverstone, ed.), pp. 285-312. Abakon Verlagsgesellschaft, Berlin.

Scott, J. P. (1962). Critical periods in behavioral development. *Science* **138,** 949-958.

Shinn, M. W. (1909). Notes on the development of a child. *Univ. Calif. Publ. Educ.* **1,** The University Press, Berkeley, California.

Sternberg, W. (1901). Geschmacksempfindung eines Auencephalus. *Z. Psychol. Physiol. Sinnesorg.* **27,** 77-79.

Stirniman, F. (1935). Versuche uber Geschmack und Geruch am ersten Lebenstag. *Jahr. Kinderhk.* **146,** 211-227.

Taitz, L. S., and Byers, H. D. (1972). High calorie/osmolar feeding and hypertonic dehydration. *Arch. Dis. Child.* **47,** 257-260.

U.S. Senate, Select Committee on Nutrition and Human Needs (1977). "Dietary Goals for the United States." US Govt. Printing Office, Washington, D.C.

Weiffenbach, J. M. (1977). Sensory mechanisms of the newborn's tongue. *In* "Taste and Development: The Genesis of Sweet Preference" (J. M. Weiffenbach, ed.), pp. 205-217. US Govt. Printing Office, Washington, D.C.

Weiffenbach, J. M. (1978). The development of sweet preference. *In* "Sweeteners and Dental Caries" (J. H. Shaw and G. G. Roussos, eds.), Spec. Suppl., *Feeding, Weight and Obesity Abstracts,* pp. 75-87.

Wolf, R. O., and Taussig, L. M. (1973). Human amniotic fluid isoamylases: Functional development of fetal pancreas and salivary glands. *Obstet. Gynecol.* **41,** 337-342.

Wolf, R. O., Weiffenbach, J. M., Folio, C. J., and Benheim, A. G. (1978). Saliva and sweet or salty taste. *J. Dent. Res.* **57** (A) 91.

Wotman, S., Mandel, I. D., Khotim, S., Thompson, R. H., Jr., Kutscher, A. H., Zegarelli, E. V., and Denning, C. R. (1964). Salt taste thresholds and cystic fibrosis. *Am. J. Dis. Child.* **108,** 372-374.

Ziegler, E. E., and Fomon, S. J. (1974). Major minerals. *In* "Infant Nutrition" (S. J. Fomon, ed.), 2nd ed., pp. 267-297. Saunders, Philadelphia, Pennsylvania.

Chapter 3

Saharan Bedouins and the Salt Water of the Sahara: A Model for Salt Intake

CLAUDE PAQUE

I. INTRODUCTION

Salty water is a basic part of the environment both in the Sahara and in Morocco. In fact, J. G. Jackson (1830) noted that as early as the 1790's a hole

BIOLOGICAL AND BEHAVIORAL
ASPECTS OF SALT INTAKE

ISBN 0-12-397750-9

dug a foot deep in the Tafilalt region yielded brackish water. At the other edge of the Desert, Du Bois-Aymé also noted in his "Description of Egypt" (1809) that the wells "are mere shallow holes dug in the sand, whose water, although drinkable, is nearly always salted." At about the same time, R. Caillé (1830) made the same point both about the Western and the Central areas of the Sahara.

Although it has been known for a long time that the peoples of the Sahara are destined to use salty water for the whole of their existence, very few investigations have been carried out on the consequences and problems of such usage.

In 1961, at the onset of the first scientific expedition to Tarfaya (Cape Juby), three fundamental questions arose. The first was to determine, as far as possible, the quantity of salt added to food by a people required to use salty water as drinking fluid. The second was to evaluate, as far as possible, the level of sodium excreted by these people. The third question was to obtain information regarding the food and fluid given to infants. These infants apparently tolerate heat without obvious disorders. The notion that such infants suffer a high mortality rate is not correct.

II. METHODS

This work is the result of a series of expeditions which I have carried out: Tafilalt and Jebel Bani (in 1958); missions of the Institut Scientifique Chérifien to the Western Sahara (in 1961 and 1964); and Maïder and Jebel Sarho (in 1965). The objectives of these expeditions were as follows: (1) to analyze the mineral concentrations of the water *actually* consumed; (2) to subsist on the local food and water personally, or at least to taste them; (3) to partake of and/or note exactly the foodstuffs used for subsistence; (4) to analyze samples of urine. These analyses were undertaken by the Laboratoire du Service d'Hydrogéologie du Maroc (M. A. Bertrand) and by the Laboratoire de Chimie-Physique of the Institut National d'Hygiène du Maroc (M. J. Lévèque).

I will not describe in detail any materials or methods used in these studies since they are, above all, observations of behavior. It was necessary in each case to fulfill the contradictory requirements of becoming accepted by the group being studied, *without disturbing its routine*. This also required having at least the rudiments of the spoken language, if only to be able to bypass the interpreter or at the very least, to be able to verify questions put to the subjects by the interpreter.

III. RESULTS

A. Salt Intake of a Population Entirely Dependent on Heavily Salted Water

Among the peoples of the Sahara who live near the Tarfaya well at Cape Juby, no salt is added to any foodstuff since the water supplies the sodium (Paque,

1963a). Water from these wells had a sodium concentration of 1104 mg/liter (Table I). Thus, in this region one finds habitually no salt in the tents of the natives. When questioned, the inhabitants (Teknas, R'Guilbat, etc.) frequently told me that the salt in drinking water was more than sufficient for their needs. Others indicated by gestures that the salted water of the wells gave them headaches (Paque, 1964b).

Inhabitants explained that the salt water used for cooking, baking of bread, cakes or gruels of cereals, provided enough salt without any need for additional salt.

However, in a few tents, I sometimes found salt, most often a reddish rock-salt which is preferred to any other salt if it is used at all. It may also be used for the camels who seem to need much more salt than men (cf., Paque, 1963b). When the inhabitants of a salted area move toward one where the water is sweet, they generally bring with them some cooking salt (Paque, 1964b).

B. Salt Intake of Saharan Peoples Using Sweet Water or Only Slightly Salty Water

In a zone of sweet water, it is interesting to note that salt is still used sparingly. Thus, in 1961, a Tekna living far from the coast in a country where the water was sweet said once: "I only take salt when I need it," i.e., usually not at all (Paque, 1964b).

In the same Western Sahara in 1964, a group of R'Guibat women using relatively sweet water [228 mg/liter of Na (Table I)] had no cooking salt in their tents and stated *that they detested salt*. One of them even burst out, "Salt, I never take it." Children nearby gesticulated to show that salt gave them headaches (Paque, 1974a, 1977a).

C. Urinary Sodium Concentration of a Population Entirely Dependent on High Saline Water as Drinking Fluid

In 1961, the well of Tarfaya appeared to be the best place to study the urinary sodium concentration of a population subjected to heavily salted water. For complicated reasons, sweet water from the Canary Islands was no longer imported, and the road from Tantan, which was the nearest well containing sweet water, was almost impassable even for a four-wheel drive vehicle. Thus, of necessity, the brackish and very disagreeable water of Tarfaya's well was the only drinking fluid that one could find in the little town.

Therefore, nineteen samples were obtained at dawn near the well from individuals of the Teknas, R'Guibat, and Laroussiynes groups. The samples were sealed and the analysis of sodium performed later at Rabat by flame photometry.

The results may be summarized as follows: (1) 4 samples exhibited a sodium concentration slightly below 5 g/liter; (2) 8, a concentration below 4 g/liter; (3) 6

TABLE I

Salt Water Electrolyte Composition (Southern Morocco and Western Sahara)

Localities	Composition (mg/liter)										Dry residue (g/liter)
	Na	K	Ca	Mg	Cl	CO_3	P_2	SO_4	NO_3	F	
Goulimine 1959	69	—	—	—	—	—	—	—	—	—	
1961	69	3	117	137	127	181	0.5	39	23	0	0.6
(Khettara)[a] 1964	72	—	—	—	—	—	—	—	—	—	
Tarjich 1959 (Seguia)[b]	117	6	189	109	185	118	0.6	697	—	1.2	1.4
Agadir-Tissint 1959 (Seguia)[b]	1121	26	189	180	1704	240	0.4	848	—	0.6	4.3
Tantan 1961 (Well)	266	23	88	73	418	107	0.5	129	36	0.6	1.2
Abattih 1961 (Well)	217	14	84	38	355	127	0.5	83	14	—	—
Tarfaya 1961 (Well)	1104	19	133	119	1732	111	0.7	331	36	—	3.8
Hassi R'Guibat 1964	228	19	60	60	255	301	0.8	69	0	—	0.6
Hassi Zehar 1961 (Wells for camels)[c]	4025	105	311	146	5650	146	0.8	1300	7.2	2.7	12.6

[a] Khettara: Underground galerie to collect water.
[b] Seguia: Canal for irrigation equally used by the population.
[c] Camels which are ruminants need heavy salted waters.

samples, below 3 g/liter; and (4) 1 sample revealed a high concentration of 9 g/liter, a figure which was not checked again (Paque, 1963a).

Despite the relative salinity of the water (see Table I), 14 concentrations appeared to be relatively low. This may, of course, not correctly reflect the concentrations over a 24-hour period (cf., Paque, 1974b, 1975).

D. Water Intake in Western Sahara

Daily water intake among Bedouins in the Sahara appears to fall into three categories: (1) that observed during drought conditions; that is, no camel's milk and more or less water available. Under these conditions, *Saharans drink water*; (2) the grazing periods after rainfalls when camel's milk is available. At these times, Saharans drink milk almost exclusively; (3) that observed during the desert "hazards." This is a time when neither water nor milk is available (Paque, 1976a).

The year 1961 came during a period of severe drought which had lasted 5–7 years. I was able at this time to make some observations and perform approximate calculations about water intake both in the little town of Tarfaya and in the tents of the country.

At Tarfaya, Bedouins appeared to drink only at meals, a general habit which appears to have very few exceptions. Three traditional glasses of tea (prepared with the brackish water from the well) are consumed at each meal. These consisted of 50–70 ml of liquid each. Meals consisted of cereals, oil, dates, and dried or boiled camel's meat served without salt. Tarfayans usually eat three times a day. Therefore, the daily water intake appeared to be approximately 600–700 ml (Paque and Levêque, 1962).

However, the situation was somewhat different for the nomadic Bedouin. Only women appeared to have regular meals, men being outside with the camels or traveling through the Sahara. Thus, an approximate calculation of daily water intake could only be performed by way of the amount of water transported *from the wells to the tents*, together with the number of inhabitants living in them. In the Sahara, water is used almost exclusively for drinking and cooking. Hence, two cans of water containing 50 liters each were used per week, for a tent of 7 persons; it gave 1.5 to 2 liters per person per day (Paque, 1976a).

The two values of water intake observed in our study, i.e., 600–700 ml for drinking and 1.5–2.0 liters for the day, are consistent with those given later by Th. Monod for himself and his Bedouin companions during his crossing of the Sahara, i.e., three glasses of 70 ml, three times a day (630 total) and an average of 2 liters a day per person (Monod, 1964).

Finally, during the periods after rainfall, when the sleeping vegetation quickly resuscitates, things are quite different. During these weeks or months, camel's milk is the only food and is drunk almost exclusively, although more or less salted water is sometimes added to it. Thus, Monteil (1940) stated that the camels of the R'Guibat-el-Gwasen (cf., Hart, 1962) grazed 4 months without going to the wells. At these times, as I witnessed in April, 1964, there was plenty of curdling milk in big wooden pans outside tents (curdled milk is called "*leben,*" the chief Desert nourishment). Consequently, water intake during this period is related to the intake of curdled milk.

Thus, in sum, the daily water intake did not appear (with the exception of the desert hazards) the great problem that one might easily imagine for Saharan Bedouins. The only problem is the rainfall . . . *for the camels* and their milk (Paque, 1974b, 1975).

E. Salt Waters Appear Better for Saharan Thirst than Pure Water

In May, 1958, after a long and thirsty journey through the Bani region of Southern Morocco, I experienced for the first time the heavily salted water of Agadir-Tissint (word for word: the cellar for salt) containing 1.2 g of sodium/liter (Table I). This was the only water we could find. It seemed to me that this water, cool and salted, quenched thirst more rapidly and more definitively than pure water. Under similar circumstances, I was accustomed to drinking pure water for hours to quench my thirst completely. During this trip I continued to drink salted water. It seemed to me that I was then less thirsty, and sweated less (Paque, 1960).

Thus, after experiencing water with salt concentrations ranging from 1.2 to 12.6 g/liter during the expedition through Western Sahara, in 1961, I arrived at the following conclusions which I have described in an earlier publication (Paque, 1964b):

> When one has . . . drunk salt water for a certain period it seems that one is less thirsty and one perspires less. In other words, 'water conservation' appears to be better and thermolysis (cooling) more economic. One steps out of the role of the traveller streaming with sweat to approach that of the drier and more efficient native of the region.
>
> This is an observation which would perhaps merit extensive investigations, more especially as the diminution of thirst seems to occur with less salted water (i.e., less than 4 g/liter of *total* salts) which is more palatable like that of Tantan in 1961 (1.2 g/liter of dry residue; 260 mg Na/liter.

The fact that hypotonic saline concentrations appeared to quench *Saharan* thirst better than pure water was also confirmed for animals (see Discussion).

F. Desert Infant Feeding and Salt Waters

Since water and electrolyte imbalance (heat disorders, diarrheas, vomiting) appear to be some of the main problems of infants living in hot, dry climates, the question was whether saline waters were given to infants in the Sahara. If they were, did salty water contribute to infant homeostasis (and nutrition) under desert conditions, and how (Paque, 1958, 1960)? Hence, the following survey was carried out.

1. Infant Feeding

All the infants are breast-fed until the age of 2 (a precept of the Koran), and then weaned abruptly.

However, at approximately 8–12 months of age, the parents start to feed the baby with the *same foods* they eat, i.e., bread, tea, gruels, oil and of course, when available, curdled camel's milk or occasionally goat's milk. The baby passes an important milestone when it begins to eat. Thus, the baby progressively learns to eat during the last months of suckling, *but an adult food without salt* (a custom whose consequences elsewhere than the Sahara will be discussed below).

2. Drinking

In the tents, water and tea prepared with the saline water available appeared to be the main drinks for infants. In 1961, the water of Tantan (Table I) was used most, except in Tarfaya where tea was prepared with the brackish water of the well.

Thus, when infants were given water and tea and sugar to drink they ingested not only water but the sodium, magnesium, calcium, and phosphorus contained in it.

3. Hot Weather: Tea and Breast Feeding on Demand

The most striking observation I have made appears to be that during the hottest part of the day, in the tents, where it can sometimes get very hot, babies from 1 to 2 years incessantly suckle their mothers and drink tea. Thus, in these circumstances (40°C inside the tent) mothers sit on carpets, their breasts easily available under their saharan blue gowns (i.e., like Roman veils); glasses of tea lie on the trays and the baby goes *incessantly* from one source of fluid to the other. Consequently, the child is provided with minerals and sugar from the tea and proteins from her mother's milk.

G. Nutritional State, Health, and Diseases

All the infants I saw in 1961 were in perfect health. I saw no cases of undernutrition and still less of edema. The babies are habitually strong and plump until they are 2 years old. Upon inquiry as to the diseases a baby might contract, I was advised by both a physician and by nurses and hospital attendants that "there are no visits to the doctor before the age of 2 years" (Tarfaya, in 1961) and that "here the infants are never ill" (L'Msied, in 1961, on the road to Tindouf) (Paque, 1964a).

However, I observed during the two surveys (1961 and 1964) one case of "blue" measles (so called because of the dye on the skin from the traditional blue veils); one case of "king's evil" (a young lady); and one case of marasmus (1964), the baby's mother having died when he was 2 or 3 months old and having been poorly fed on a little camel's milk.

Although the country is totally arid, very hot, and has a scarcity of food, no real medical problems resulted from the heat and, on average, a fairly good nutritional state was maintained (Paque, 1964a).

IV. DISCUSSION

Although the facts that have been observed until now appear to be perfectly integrated (i.e., salt and water intakes, water and salt expenditures) they will be discussed separately.

A. Behavior of Saharan Bedouins toward Salt

The lack of a salt appetite among Saharans using notoriously salted water appears to be a purely physiological phenomenon (Paque, 1974a). Thus, wild rabbits living in the salt desert of Australia having a urinary concentration of sodium equal to 100 mEq/liter (i.e., more or less equivalent to the figures given on p. 33) exhibit a narrow zonation of the adrenal cortex, low blood aldosterone, *and no appetite for salt* (Denton, 1967). Thus, lack of salt appetite in these circumstances has nothing to do with taste or customs.

However, lack of salt appetite in sweet water regions, and the very sparing use of salt which persists, appear to be a much more complex phenomenon, depending on many factors. The first factor is apparently the persistence among the Bedouins of the very subtle and discriminating salt appetite of mammals which, at the same time, permits them to take some salt when they need it—*but only in case of need*—thus avoiding all risk of sodium depletion as well as all risk of sodium excess (Paque, 1974a).

The second factor is undoubtedly the remarkable efficiency of the Bedouins for sodium conservation. In fact, I have neither heard nor read (cf., Du Bois-Aymé, Jackson, Caillé, Du Puigaudeau, Thesiger) of a Bedouin suffering from muscle cramps, and I doubt if any Bedouin has ever taken a salt tablet in his life while crossing the desert. On the other hand, populations acclimatized to heat show a considerable diminution of sodium in the sweat, with exchanges of sodium at a very low level (Kirmiz, 1962). Consequently, in the Sahara, the sodium in camel's milk and/or that of the water available appear to be habitually more than sufficient. Therefore, there is no need to add salt during cooking (Paque, 1974a).

Another natural necessity of desert life is the conservation of water by consuming a minimum of salt. On this point, Jackson (1830), in discussing the Sahara, stated that "the peoples, whose interest induces them to cross the desert (for there are no travellers from curiosity in this country), obviate the objection to salt provisions which increase the propensity to drink water by taking with them melted butter, called *smin*; this prepared *without salt* . . ." Thus, the meat there was, and still is, dried in the sun and not salted, and the butter is always absolutely rancid. Hence, cereals, sugar, *smin,* and dates are still the true provisions of the desert (of course, with camel's milk, when available).

Finally, since the life of the desert is essentially characterized by fasting, cold, heat, thirst, and/or warfare, it seems also hardly compatible with even a relative adrenal insufficiency. Consequently, the last factor, and maybe the most important, is also the very probable necessity of conserving intact the corticoadrenal function at its most efficient level, to which an intake of salt always reduced to the minimum would properly contribute; in other words, with an aldosterone secretion entirely able to adjust to the necessary rebound of the survival mechanisms (Paque, 1974a). In fact, Denton has also shown that rabbits who live in an environment devoid of sodium have an enlarged adrenal cortex, together with an elevated circulating aldosterone concentration (Denton, 1967).

In sum, the very sparing use of salt by the Bedouins appears to be linked (1) to the activity of an ever efficient salt appetite, (2) to sodium conservation, (3) to the necessity of saving water, and (4) by the cultural (and/or instinctive) maintenance of a high adrenal efficiency probably linked, at least in part, to a very sparing use of salt (a perfect integration of factors).

B. The Bedouin's Water Economy and Resistance to Thirst: Behavioral or Genetic Factors?

The obvious capacity of Bedouins to save water and their extraordinary resistance to thirst have been already summarized. Behavior, dietary (limiting salt and proteins), and probable genetic factors appear to be the main causes (Paque, 1976a). I shall therefore mention here only a few facets of this most complicated and fascinating problem.

The first factor in saving water, as we have already observed, is obviously as low a salt intake as possible since 60 ml of water are needed to excrete 1 g of salt (Richter, 1956). Hence, foods of the desert devoid of salt are a sound basis for saving water.

Another factor could also be an apparent training to resist thirst. Although there appears to be no way to train the human body to economize water (Adolph, 1947), I must point out that after spending several months both in Southern Morocco and the Western Sahara, I have never yet seen a Bedouin drinking outside his tent (Paque, 1964b). This restraint, even when water is available, appears to be due more to a deliberate attitude rather than to lack of thirst.* Thus, Thesiger (1964) reports that his Bedu companions who had finished their water a long time before arriving at last at Bir Halu, i.e., "the sweet well," waited 5 hours before drinking until the "others" joined the company. They then drank the water of this *sweet* well which was cold, clear and tasted like a strong dose of Epsom salts!†

The general behavior is to drink as little as possible. This deliberate attitude, perhaps learned, probably originated several thousand years ago at the beginning of the "Egyptian Sahara." This training has even become a religious practice for, during the fasting month of Ramadan, one cannot neither drink nor swallow his own saliva from dawn to sunset, even in the worst long days of the desert summer.

Thus, if the body cannot truly be trained to economize water, it may be possible to train it to drink as little as possible in order to expend as little as possible on cooling by avoiding sweating and excessive moisture of the skin. A link between drinking and water expenditure was described by Du Bois-Aymé (1809): "Arabs are extremely sober (. . .); they drink very little, *and endure thirst for days on end.* This extreme sobriety doubtless explains the small amount of all their secretions."

In so far as the following facts can be interpreted, there may also be some genetic factors in the capacity of man to spare salt and water. Thus, as I observed myself, when Black people and Berbers or Saharans are doing the same thing at the same time, the former may be sweating heavily, just like unacclimatized Europeans, whereas the latter are practically dry. Caillé (1830) when first crossing the Sahara in May, 1828, observed that his "negro slave" companions apparently suffered more from thirst, as he did, than the Moors. The slaves also added salt regularly to their food while the Moors never did. Odette du Puigaudeau (1940) (an ethnologist who lived for many years in the tents of Western Sahara) said that when she traveled through the Sahara with the French Army, the daily water rations were as follows: 2 liters for the Moors, 4 liters for Europeans, and 6 liters for the Blacks (tirailleurs), *who were sweating the most.*

"Salt is one of the bases of economic life, I would say even of Saharan social life. The Blacks proceed to extract and *consume* it. Arabs and Berbers get

*"We were tormented with thirst, for we only drank once in the course of the day (. . .) I would fain have drunk oftener, and a smaller quantity at a time, but the Moors who presided over the distribution of the water would not hear of this arrangement, and adhered to the old practice." (Caillé, 1830, Vol. II, pp. 108–109). "These wells, which afford plenty of brackish water, are not more than three or four feet deep. When the water was fit to drink, I went and thrust my head amongst the camels to drink with them. . ." (Caillé, 1830, Wells of Tellig, Vol. II, p. 118).

†In fact, "Bir Halu" had been a sweet well in the past. Due to lack of rainfall and/or overutilization, it became more and more salty. Another example, in Western Sahara, the Hassi-el-Khoui well become unfit for consumption between 1961 to 1964 both for men *and camels*! (cf. Paque 1974b).

enough from the meat and the milk of their herds fed on salted grasses, but they are the ones who transport it through immense deserts'' (du Puigaudeau, 1940).

Thus, translated into terms of ecology and genetics, the above facts and statements appear to mean: (1) it is likely that some people need less salt than others, (2) that those people who need less salt are those who need least water (in desert life), (3) that Arabs and Berbers economize salt and water even if these are readily available (behavior), and (4) that these are the people who have finally taken control of the desert (the successful ''desert dwellers'' of Kirmiz, 1962).

C. Salt Waters of the Sahara and Thirst (The Problems of Salt Tablets)

The Sahara is perhaps one of the best areas of the world to experience the double depletion mechanism of thirst, both cellular and extracellular described by Epstein *et al.* (1973). Thus, in the Sahara, one does not sweat (i.e., by sensible perspiration); ''one simply evaporates'' both through the skin and the respiratory tract (Paque, 1964b, 1974b). The result is a cellular loss of water which rapidly becomes very important without one being aware of it (Adolph, 1947). At the same time, the natural process of cooling through active sweating starts, which leads to a depletion of extracellular volume, the amount of which depends on activity, acclimatization, and perhaps genetics.

On the other hand, Stricker and Jalowiec (1970) have shown that adult rats rendered hypovolemic by means of subcutaneous hyperoncotic solution and offered either isotonic or hypertonic saline as well as water, drink until plasma volume deficits are completely restored. Conversely, when offered only pure water, the rats stopped drinking before matching their deficits because further intake of water was not possible in the face of the increasing dilution of body fluids (Stricker, 1969; Peters *et al.*, 1975).

Thus, the fact that a hypotonic saline solution such as the salt water of the Sahara (see Table I) appears to quench Saharan thirsts better than pure water (Paque, 1964b) seems to find a physiological basis here.

However, many questions remain, particularly the roles of calcium and magnesium in Saharan waters, and the role of salt tablets against Saharan thirst, both cellular and hypovolemic. In light of what has been observed, the use of salt tablets in dry, hot areas may be of concern for many reasons. The first is that they could be taken without any water (Knochel, 1975a,b). The second is that they could be taken without a sufficient amount of water, the result of which would be to pull the water from the cells into the stomach in order to absorb the tablet (as in the first case), thus adding an additional cellular deficit to a previous cellular depletion. Further, salt tablets are generally taken at meals *already* heavily salted and containing proteins. This augments still further ''the propensity to drink water,'' which appears not to be absolutely necessary in desert conditions.

Finally, another reason would also be that such a constant intake of salt would interfere with the natural process of adaptation, both to heat and desert conditions, by impairing adrenal cortical secretion and the renin-angiotensin-aldosterone system (Paque, 1974a), thus making people more and more salt and water dependent.

Thus, salt tablets should be dissolved in the proper amount of water before drinking, thereby avoiding any errors in matching water intake with thirst. Since more water than salt may have been lost by dryness, salt solutions within the range of 0.5 to 1.0 g NaCl per liter should be considered for replacement. Since ingestion of salt cannot prevent a future salt deficit, *but simply augments either plasma volume or thirst,* salt tablets should be taken with the proper amount of water either after or during the deficit but *not* before it.

When crossing the Sahara, Bedouins (1) do not use salt tablets since salt is included in desert water, and (2) thirst is usually quenched only once or twice a day (Caillé, 1830, etc.), and only after emergence of deficits. It would be better to investigate a specific desert water balance as such, rather than with British Army "compo" rations and "salt added liberally to the food" (see Beighton, 1971; Paque, 1976a).

D. Infant Nutrition and Thirst in Hot, Dry Climates

Many years ago it was suggested in Morocco that the cause of compulsive thirst, anorexia, and malnutrition in infants after weaning during the hot season, and almost only in the hot season, was ingestion of too much tap water or sweet tea, without proper *salt* (and protein) intake (Paque, 1956, 1957). Later, clinical and ecological investigations suggested that this polydipsia was mainly a *salt* deficiency polydipsia, accompanied by an extracellular dehydration. In Morocco, as in the Sahara, salt is never added to infants' food (Paque, 1958, 1959). In fact, it was demonstrated later by means of hospital investigations that only an adequate oral supply of salt solution (2.3 g Na/liter) could stop the thirst and incessant polydipsia, and thus allow ingestion of food by the children again (Paque, 1964a).

If hypovolemic and cellular thirsts are the main mechanisms inducing the polydipsia (since hypotonic saline can stop the thirst), ontogenic factors are probably also present and contribute to the polydipsia, in contrast to the adult animal (Paque, 1977b). However, carbohydrates from the sweet tea may also be responsible for the anorexia (Houpt and Houpt, 1976).

Consequently, the Saharan utilization of light saline waters for infants (and children) should not be considered here as a mere anthropological fact, but as a natural prevention of hypovolemic deficits (and possible polydipsia) and perhaps as a possible clue concerning the basic physiological needs of infants in dry, hot climates (Paque, 1958, 1960).

A well balanced fluid intake is important for infants to maintain their necessary nitrogen ingestion. Hypovolemic and cellular thirsts appear to be the main problems when infants lose water and sodium in hot, dry climates. Therefore, the continual attempt to associate prevention to mere maintenance of standards of protein, caloric and vitamin intakes (Jeliffe, 1970), and dismissing heat and water balance, may be one of the principal mistakes of the last thirty years of tropical infant nutrition (Paque, 1967; Paque and Dubois, 1962).

E. A Model for Salt Intake?

Grivetti has recently complained about twentieth century researchers who "continue to seek explanations for cultural behavior using modern analytical models, rather than attempting to understand the mind of ancient man and the factors that molded the cultural and environmental determinants of diet" (Grivetti, 1977, Comment on Neumann's paper 1977). Nurge also complained "a subject not addressed is sodium in drinking water" (Comment on Neumann's paper, 1977). (See Neuman, 1977.)

In fact, the subject of sodium in drinking water has been discussed as much in arid areas (Shotton, 1954; Schoeller, 1955; Paque, 1958, 1960; Margat, 1961) as in Western urban towns (Paque, 1964b). The question which appears to be raised is whether the general behavior of Saharan Bedouins toward salt (i.e., as low an intake as possible except in case of need) could be considered a model whose main characteristic is a large utilization of salt water [i.e., a full free choice of salt intake including the salt of the Saharan Salt Caravans (see Paque, 1977a)] in conjunction with the extreme severity of the milieu. The model raises many questions.

First, the possibility exists that the exclusion of salt from infant food contributes to the full future activity of the corticoadrenal system and prevents future Western salt addiction. This, in turn, raises the question whether the apparent capacity of Saharan Bedouins to economize sodium, as observed above, is learned or genetic.

Second, the possibility exists that drinking lightly salted water (or light saline solutions: 100–200 mg/liter Na) during hot, dry conditions, is a physiological and practical means of preventing infant thirst disorders, such as salt deficiency polydipsia, and their nutritional or pathologic consequences, such as anorexia, diarrhea, or even acute diarrhea (Paque, 1978).

Finally, all this has induced speculation on whether a high aldosterone secretory capacity would be one of the fundamental keys in adaptation to the innumerable stresses of life, and one of the important elements in the prevention of certain forms of arterial hypertension (Paque, 1974a, 1977a; see also Paque, 1976b).

In addition, the behavior of Saharan Bedouins toward salt offers a model in which salt intake appears not to be regulated by the modalities of taste, as in most modern societies (Denton *et al.*, 1976), but by the simple physiological need for maintenance of extracellular volume. In this model salt intake increases when extracellular volume decreases (the salt drive). On the other hand, when extracellular volume is normal and when extra salt may be ingested for whatever the reason (heavily salted water for instance), an internal "stop" signal in the form of a headache appears to occur. This leads one to wonder whether Richter's wild rats, when ingesting hypertonic salt solutions (Richter, 1956), also had headaches. The internal signal could be linked to a high rate of secretion of aldosterone (Paque, 1974a, 1977b).

In conclusion, the selection pressure in the Sahara appears to have been the lack of water, the oversalinity of the milieu, a vestige of ancient seas: in contrast to large areas of the world where selection pressure has occurred as a result of a lack of salt (Denton *et al.*, 1976). Therefore, the behavioral strategy of Saharan Bedouins in protecting their "internal homeostatic environment" (Garcia *et al.*, 1974), as well as to ensure their income, appears to have differentiated a model for salt intake where the role of salt has been maintained in its two primary functions: its physiological role in maintenance of the extracellular volume and as a valuable trade product for people lacking salt (Paque, 1977a).

V. CONCLUSIONS

Instinct has always been, and still is, the best computer. It has solved ecological and alimentary problems which could not even be programmed. Saharan Bedouins' behavioral strategy towards salt appears to be a living "model" which has stood the test of time, a model whose interest perhaps extends the edges of the desert.

In summary, observation, experience, and the above analyses seem to reveal the following facts: Saharan Bedouins appear to offer a model in which salt intake: (1) is directly linked to the salinity of the water, (2) is generally kept, from infancy to adulthood, at the lowest possible level, and (3) appears to be regulated at *two* levels: at low levels, by means of a mammalian salt appetite; at high levels, by means of internal "stop" signals such as headaches. The origins of this model are older than the desert itself, lying in the very roots of mammalian homeostatic behavior.

Water intake of Bedouins appears to be both very low and constant. Extreme sparing of salt (genetic or learned), limited frequency of water intake, careful dietary practices, and particular customs (the veil, clothing) appear to provide a basis for the maintenance of their economy. However, genetic factors may also play a role.

In adults, lightly salted water appears to quench Saharan thirsts (cellular and hypovolemic) better than pure water. In infants, lightly salted water together with breast feeding on demand appears also to make good the possible cellular and hypovolemic deficits, thus preventing climatic infant thirst disorders—and their paramount nutritional consequences.

REFERENCES

Adolph, E. F. (1947). "Physiology of Man in the Desert." (Interscience), Wiley, New York.

Andre, A., Bons, J., Bryssine, G., Bryssine, I., Delannoy, H., Girot, B., Mathez, J., Paque, C., and Sauvage, C. (1975). "Contribution à l'Etude Scientifique de la Province de Tarfaya," pp. 227-252. Edit. Marocaines et Internationales, Tanger.

Beighton, P. (1971). Fluid balance in the Sahara. *Nature (London)* **233,** 275-277.

Caillé, R. (1830). "Travels through Central Africa to Timbuctoo and across the Great Desert to Morocco, performed in the years 1824-1828," 1st ed. (Vol. II, pp. 108-130. Cass, London, 1968).

Denton, D. A. (1967). Salt appetite. *In* "Handbook of Physiology" (Am. Physiol. Soc., J. Field, ed.), Sect. 6, Vol. I, pp. 433-459. Williams & Wilkins, Baltimore, Maryland.

Denton, D. A. *et al.* (1976). "Central Nervous Control of Na Balance—Relations to the Renin-Angiotensin System: Some General Biological Aspects of Salt Appetite," pp. 103-110. Thieme, Stuttgart.

Du Bois-Aymé, M. (1809). "Description de l'Egypte. Mémoire sur les Tribus Arabes des Déserts de l'Egypte, Imprimerie Impériale," Vol. I, pp. 577-594.

du Puigaudeau, O. (1940). "Le Sel du Désert," p. 26. Pierre Tisné, Paris.

Epstein, A. N., Kissileff, H. R., and Stellar, E. (1973). "The Neuropsychology of Thirst: New Findings and Advances in Concepts," pp. 319-320. Holt, New York.

Garcia, J., Hankins, W. G., and Rusiniak, K. W. (1974). Behavioral regulation of the milieu interne in man and rat. *Science* **185,** 824-831.

Hart, D. M. (1962). The social structure of the R'Gibat Bedouins of the Western Sahara. *Anthropol. Rev., Middle East J.* Autumn 1962, pp. 515-527.

Houpt, K. A., and Houpt, T. R. (1976). Comparative aspects of the ontogeny of taste. *Chem. Senses Flavor* **2,** 219-228.

Jackson, J. G. (1830). "An account of Timbuctoo and Housa to which is added Letters descriptive of Travels through West and South Barbary," 1st ed. (p. 349. Cass, London, 1967).

Jeliffe, D. B. (1970). "L'alimentation du Nourrisson dans les Regions Tropicales et Subtropicales." p. 304. O.M.S., Gėneva.

Kirmiz, J. P. (1962). "Adaptation to Desert Environment, a Study on Jerboa, Rat and Man." Butterworth, London.

Knochel, J. P. (1975a). Sept moyens pour tuer un joueur de football américain en période de canicule. *Nouv. Presse Med.* **4,** 2908.

Knochel, J. P. (1975b). *J. Am. Med. Assoc.* **233,** 513-514.

Margat, J. (1961). Les Eaux Salées au Maroc.-Notes at Mémoires du Service Géologique No. 151. Edit. Service Géologique du Maroc, Rabat.

Monod, T. (1964). "Navigation chamelière," Les cahiers de l'Ecole Alsacienne, No. 6, ler trimestre, 1963-1964, pp. 25-26. Paris.

Neumann, T. W. (1977). A biocultural approach to salt taboos: The case of the southeastern United States. *Curr. Anthropol.* **18,** 289-307.

Paque, C. (1956). Le syndrome de malhydratation au cours des dystrophies nutritionnelles marocaines de l'enfance (Note préliminaire). *Maroc Med.* **35,** 791.

Paque, C. (1957). Soif et maladie de l'eau de l'enfant Marocain. (Syndrome d'hyperhydration.) *Maroc Med.* **36,** 171.

Paque, C. (1958). Carence alimentaire en sel après sevrage et facteurs climatiques au cours des malnutritions type kwashiorkor à Rabat. *Presse Med.* **66,** 1572–1575.

Paque, C. (1959). Diète totale par suppression des ingesta et diurèse au cours des malnutritions sévères infantiles. La désintoxication d'eau. *Presse Med.* **67,** 1289–1292.

Paque, C. (1960). Composition électrilytique des eaux salées servant à l'alimentation humaine, prélevées dans le Bâni; intérêt biologique. *C.R. Seances Mens. Soc. Sci. Nat. Phys. Maroc* **26,** 59–61.

Paque, C. (1963a). Alimentation sans sel dans une population nomade sahariienne utilisant des eaux exclusivement salées; approche de l'excrétion urinaire (Na, K). *C.R. Hebd. Seances Acad. Sci.* **256,** 331–332.

Paque, C. (1963b). Un puits sahariien à chameaux: Hassi Zehar. *Mammalia* **27,** 310–311.

Paque, C. (1964a). Absence de malnutrition infantile et de kwashiorkor chez les nomades du Sahara occidental utilisant des eaux salées. *Arch. Fr. Pediatr.* **21,** 367–374.

Paque, C. (1964b). Adaptation des nomades du Sahara occidental aux eaux salées. Une mission scientifique au Cap Juby. *Presse Med.* **72,** 2417–2420.

Paque, C. (1967). Heat as a factor in protein calorie malnutrition. Chronic dehydration and nutritional disorders. *Proc. Int. Congr. Nutr., 7th, 1966* Vol. I, pp. 102–107.

Paque, C. (1971). Mode d'utilisation des eaux salées pour l'alimentation humaine au Maroc et dans les régions arides (Sahara). *C.R. Seances Mens. Soc. Sci. Nat. Phys. Maroc* **37,** 69–90.

Paque, C. (1973). *C.R. Seances Mens. Soc. Sci. Nat. Phys. Maroc* **53,** 312–322.

Paque, C. (1974a). Les eaux salées du Sahara: Incidences surrenaliennes et tensionnelles. *Bull. Acad. Natl. Med., Paris* **158,** 297–302.

Paque, C. (1974b). Sahariiens et eaux salées Sahariiennes. Introduction à une physiologie de l'homme du desert. *Cah. Rech. Agron. (Rabat), Cah.* **33,** 227–352.

Paque, C. (1975). Sahariiens et eaux salées Sahariiennes. Introduction à une physiologie de l'homme du désert. *In* "Contribution à l'Etude Scientifique de la Province de Tarfaya" (A. André *et al.*, eds.), pp. 227–252. Edit. Marocaines et Internationales, Tanger.

Paque, C. (1976a). La consommation d'eau chez les Sahariiens (water balance in the western Sahara). *Nouv. Presse Med.* **5,** 2087–2090.

Paque, C. (1976b). De la nécessité physiologique et préventive des périodes de désodation. *Ann. Hyg. Lang. Fr.—Med. Nutr.* **12,** 393–396.

Paque, C. (1977a). Comment to Neumann's paper on "A Biocultural Approach to Salt Taboos." *Curr. Anthropol.* **18,** 302–303.

Paque, C. (1977b). Polydipsic syndromes in infant malnutrition. *Abstr., Int. Conf. Physiol. Food Fluid Intake, 6th, 1977,* Paris-collège de France, 1977.

Paque, C. (1978). Soif hypovolémique et traitement du cholera infantile par voie orale. (Hypovolaemic thirst and oral treatment of infant cholera—acute diarrhea. *Nouv. Presse Med.* **7,** 2404.

Paque, C., and Dubois, P. (1962). Relations entre la malnutrition sévère (Kwashiorkor) et l'aridité des mois secs à forte évaporation. *Nutr. Dieta* **4,** 272–282.

Paque, C., and Levêque, J. (1962). Approche de l'excrétion urinaire d'une population saharïenne nomade campée dans une zone d'eaux exclusivement salées. *Maroc Med.* **41,** 933–934.

Paque, C., and Veylon, R. (1974). L'Homme, l'eau et le sel. *Nouv. Presse Med.* **3,** 1617–1627.

Peters, G., Fitzsimons, J. T., and Peters-Haefeli, L. (1975). "Control Mechanisms of Drinking," p. 4. Springer-Verlag, Berlin and New York.

Richter, C. P. (1956). "L'Instinct dans le Comportement des Animaux et de l'Homme. Salt Appetite of Mammals: Its Dependence on Instinct and Metabolism," p. 623. Masson, Paris.

Schoeller, H. (1955). "Essai sur la qualité de l'eau destinée à l'alimentation de l'Homme dans les pays arides," Terres et Eaux, Suppl. Sci. No. 4, pp. 4–11. Service Hydraulique, Gouvern. Gén. Algérie.

Shotton, F. W. (1954). "Biology of Deserts. The Availability of Underground Water in Hot Deserts." Cloudlsy-Thompson, London.

Stricker, E. M. (1969). Osmoregulation and volume regulation in rats: Inhibition of hypovolemic thirst by water. *Am. J. Physiol.* **217,** 98–105.

Stricker, E. M., and Jalowiec, J. E. (1970). Restoration of intravascular fluid volume following acute hypovolemia in rats. *Am. J. Physiol.* **218,** 191–196.

Thesiger, W. (1964). "Arabian Sands," p. 65. Penguin Books, London.

Trocme, C. (1960). Le sel et la régulation circulatoire. *Arch. Mal. Coeur Vaiss.* No. 3, 250–290.

Chapter 4

Salt Sources and Markets

WILLIAM E. DICKINSON

I. INTRODUCTION

Salt has been referred to as the *fifth element,* as vital as air, water, fire, and earth. The Bible, which contains 30 references to salt, calls it "the essence of life." Salt has played an important role in our history and the progress of man for centuries. The lack of salt helped defeat Napoleon, and civil war battles raged over salt deposits. Gandhi used the British salt tax as a means of gaining support for the struggle for independence of India.

In the United States we are fortunate to be blessed with an abundant supply of salt. Large salt deposits underlie parts of Michigan, Ohio, New York, and Pennsylvania. Louisiana and Texas are major salt producers. The state of Kansas is also underlain by a bed of salt that extends into parts of Oklahoma and northern Texas. The Texas and Louisiana formations are in the form of salt domes that extend to unknown depths, while the other formations are in bedded deposits. Other sources of salt in the United States include the Great Salt Lake and the San Francisco and San Diego areas of California.

BIOLOGICAL AND BEHAVIORAL
ASPECTS OF SALT INTAKE

ISBN 0-12-397750-9

II. SALT PRODUCTION

Approximately 22 million tons of dry salt is produced annually in the United States. There are three principal methods of production.

A. Mining

Much like coal mining, salt mining involves the sinking of a shaft to the necessary depth, usually some 600 to 2000 feet below the surface. Miners dig into a wall of the mine, and explosives are used to loosen the embedded rock salt. Cars, trucks, or conveyor belts transport the salt to a hoist, where it is carried to the surface.

B. Brine Wells

A brine well operation involves the use of one pipe to introduce water to a salt deposit and a larger pipe, around the first pipe, to remove the brine. Wells may also be joined so that water is introduced into the first well and brine removed from a second well some distance away. No workers are used below ground for brine well operations. After the brine reaches the surface, it is used for production of evaporated salt. The water from the brine is removed by heat processing that leaves granular salt, or flake-type salt, depending upon the method of re-crystallization.

C. Solar Salt

Solar salt is produced through a process of solar evaporation of water from natural brines, such as seawater. Because this process requires specific atmospheric conditions—abundant sunshine, little rainfall, and ample air movement—it is used in only three sections of the United States, namely Great Salt Lake, the San Francisco Bay area, and near San Diego, California.

Solar salt production involves a series of concentrating ponds, where the brine is increased in concentration to the point where salt is about to crystallize. The brine is then transferred to crystallizing ponds where further evaporation causes salt to crystallize and form a salt bed. The salt is removed with special "harvesters," washed, and screened.

III. USES OF SALT

The end uses of salt are as many as they are varied. A statistical report compiled by the Salt Institute lists nine major categories, which are further divided into 28 subcategories. Classification of users ranges from the chemical industry to food processing, with such diverse applications as textile manufacturing and dyeing (see Table I).

The total sales by members of the Salt Institute in the United States, either from domestic production or imports, totalled 24.5 million tons last year, with a value of 487 million dollars.

A major user of salt is the water conditioning industry (see Table I). "Hard water" is found in approximately two-thirds of the United States and the use of salt is vital to the softening process. Softener products include rock and solar salt in the natural form or special tabs and pellets pressed from evaporated salt.

Highway use demands 44.4% of the tonnage sold. Salt is essential for winter mobility and is still the most effective, most economical, and safest method of ice removal known. A report by The Institute for Safety Analysis estimated that the impact of snow- and ice-impeded highways for just 20 snow days per winter would cost the United States $18.4 billion in wages lost in lateness to work, absenteeism, production losses, losses in goods shipments, and additional fuel costs. This does not take into consideration the lives saved by reducing the incidence of traffic accidents or by reducing response time to medical emergencies.

Uses in agriculture center around animal feeding. Vital trace minerals are added to supplement diets and the familiar salt blocks are used in range feeding where they also aid in grazing distribution.

Food-grade salt, the most familiar to the general public, is used not only at the table but is essential in food processing, baking, the manufacture of cheese, and curing of meat. The addition of iodine to salt has been used for many years to prevent certain types of goiter.

Salt is vital to the chemical industry by providing the starting point for caustic and soda ash and chlorine from which many man-made products are derived.

TABLE I

Total Salt Sales by Major End Uses

Use	Amount in dollars ($)	Percentage (%)	Tons	Percentage (%)
Water conditioning	78,947,000	16.2	2,304,800	9.4
Highway	97,779,600	20.1	10,927,000	44.4
Agriculture	73,944,300	15.0	1,980,000	8.1
Food-grade	98,302,900	20.2	1,002,800	4.1
Chemical	37,450,000	7.7	4,114,200	16.7
Totals	386,423,800	79.2	20,328,800	82.7

Thus, these five major categories account for approximately 80% of the total tons and dollar sales of salt.

Of particular interest currently is the consumption of food-grade salt. Our estimates indicate that the American public consumes an average of approximately 8–10 g of salt per day, either from salt added by food processors or salt consumed in cooking and at the table. The sale of the ''round can'' of table salt has not kept up with the increasing population, due to the increased consumption of processed foods and the fact that people are eating out more.

There has been a considerable amount of discussion lately about the role of salt in human health. Various organizations are studying the issue and there is much consideration being given to the optimal amount of salt that is desirable in the human diet. Excretion studies indicate that the average intake of sodium expressed as sodium chloride is about 10 g per day. The Senate Select Committee on Nutrition and Human Needs, chaired by Senator George McGovern, in establishing dietary goals, originally recommended limiting the intake of sodium by reducing the intake of salt to about 3 g per day. This recommendation was later changed to 5 g. In a recent letter from Senator McGovern to the Salt Institute this was clarified to indicate that while the dietary goal calls for reducing intake of salt to about 5 g per day, the Committee recognized the nondiscretionary intake of approximately 3 g per day of sodium chloride (sodium occurring naturally in foods and expressed as sodium chloride). A total consumption of 8 g of salt per day is not a drastic reduction from the present 10 g per day average.

The jury is still out on the role of sodium and health, and it is hoped that the many studies now underway and the various symposia being held will resolve these questions. The salt industry is aware of and concerned about these questions and is cooperating in every way possible. The industry heartily supports the proposed labeling of sodium in processed foods in support of the public's right to know. The industry does, however, oppose such ideas as ''crepe'' labeling with warning words or symbols and limiting additions of salt to processed foods by government regulation. The industry also feels that placing salt in the category of a regulated food additive would not serve a useful purpose in view of the fact that salt is readily available at the table.

Part II
Comparative and Psychophysical Aspects of Salt Intake

Chapter 5

On the Spontaneous Intake of NaCl Solution by Dogs

MELVIN J. FREGLY

I. INTRODUCTION

Of the many mammalian species, the rat, a rodent, and the sheep, a herbivore, seem to have been most thoroughly studied with respect to their spontaneous appetites for NaCl solutions (Denton, 1967; Richter, 1942–1943). Of these two species, the rat has probably been studied to the greater extent. A large variety of physiological and pharmacological factors have been shown to interact in in-

BIOLOGICAL AND BEHAVIORAL
ASPECTS OF SALT INTAKE

ISBN 0-12-397750-9

fluencing the spontaneous NaCl intake of this species. A few of these factors would include the hormonal secretions of the adrenal cortex, thyroid gland, and gonads, as well as pregnancy and the renin-angiotensin system (Braun-Menendez and Brandt, 1952; Denton, 1967; Denton and Nelson, 1970; Fregly, 1967, 1972; Fregly and Newsome, 1974; Fregly and Waters, 1967; Richter, 1942–1943; Shulkes *et al.*, 1972; Wolf and Handal, 1966). Further, a variety of pharmacologic agents, including diuretics, has been shown to influence the appetite of the rat for NaCl solution (Fregly and Kim, 1970; Jalowiec, 1974).

The dog has apparently been overlooked with respect to its spontaneous intake of NaCl solution. It seemed particularly important to study the dog because of the fact that carnivores have long been believed to have no special desire for NaCl owing to the large amount of NaCl ingested in their predominately protein diet (Bunge, 1902). It was the objective of these studies to determine whether purebred Beagle dogs have a spontaneous appetite for NaCl solution when given a choice between it and water to drink and whether certain factors known to increase the spontaneous NaCl intake of the rat also influence the spontaneous NaCl intake of the dog.

II. METHODS

A. Experiment 1. Effect of Graded Concentrations of NaCl Solution on Spontaneous NaCl Intake by Dogs

Five purebred female Beagle dogs 4 to 6 years old were used in these studies. They were kept in large cages (8 × 10 ft) in a temperature-controlled room (25° ± 1°C) which was illuminated from 6 AM to 6 PM. Each dog was given 175 g meat (Hill Packing Co., Topeka, KA) and 200 g commercial dry dog food (Purina Dog Chow, St. Louis, MO) daily. Two identical aluminum buckets were kept in each cage to provide fluid for the animals. All dogs were offered a choice between a NaCl solution and distilled water during 4-day periods throughout the study. During the first period, both buckets contained distilled water. Thereafter the concentration of NaCl solution in one bucket was increased during each period in the following chronological sequence: 0.05, 0.10, 0.15, 0.20, 0.25, and 0.30 moles/liter. Intakes of water and NaCl solution were measured daily at 9 AM at which time all cages were also cleaned and food provided. Fresh water and NaCl solution were also provided daily. All solutions were made up from a concentrated stock solution by serial dilution. All concentrations were checked by flame photometry. The experiment was terminated on the twenty-eighth day.

An additional study was performed on a female purebred Dalmatian couchhound 5 years of age. This animal was the author's pet. She was placed outdoors at 9 AM without food or water in a fenced yard. At 3 PM each day she was brought indoors and allowed to choose between two identical buckets from which to drink. The animal was allowed to drink until satisfied. This generally occurred within one-half hour and was never longer than 1 hour. Ambient outdoor temperatures during this study varied from 20° to 32°C. After completing seven sessions during which both buckets contained distilled water, the following NaCl concentrations were offered as choice with distilled water: 0.005, 0.01, 0.05, and 0.10 moles/liter. The number of drinking sessions for each concentration were 10, 13, 13 and 2, respectively. This animal received dry Purina Dog Chow daily (approximately 350 g) as food during the study.

B. Experiment 2. Effect of the Diuretic Agent, Hydrochlorothiazide, on Spontaneous NaCl Intake by Dogs

1. Study 1

This study was carried out on two purebred female Beagle dogs 4 to 6 years old. It was conducted in a similar manner to that described in Experiment 1 except that different concentrations of NaCl solution were used and the concentrations were generally offered for 2, instead of 4, days. The concentrations of NaCl offered in chronological sequence were: distilled water (4 days), 0.010, 0.020, 0.040, 0.060, 0.080, 0.100, and 0.125 moles/liter (2 days each). Daily measurements of intakes were carried out as described.

On the nineteenth day of the experiment the two dogs were given choice between 0.080 *M* NaCl solution and distilled water daily for 4 days. During the next 4 days each animal received 5 mg hydrochlorothiazide/kg twice daily by mouth (9 AM and 5 PM). Intakes of water and 0.080 *M* NaCl solution continued to be measured daily during this period and for 4 additional days after the treatment ended.

2. Study 2

The two female dogs used above were also used in this study. It was carried out 1 month after the previous study ended. This study was designed primarily to test the effect of hydrochlorothiazide on intakes of water and 0.080 *M* NaCl solution. Daily intakes of water and 0.080 *M* NaCl solution were measured for 6 days, as was body weight. During the next 4 days, each animal was administered 5 mg hydrochlorothiazide/kg twice daily by mouth as in Study 1. Intakes were measured for an additional 2 days after treatment with hydrochlorothiazide.

Two additional female Beagle dogs were used. The differences between this study and that described above were that choice was offered between 0.150 *M* NaCl solution and water, and hydrochlorothiazide was given for 4 days beginning on the third day of the study. In all other respects the conditions were identical.

C. Experiment 3. Effect of the Diuretic Agent, Ethacrynic Acid, and the Hormone, Deoxycorticosterone Acetate, on Spontaneous NaCl Intake by Dogs

1. Study 1

Two female Beagle dogs weighing approximately 10 kg were used. They were maintained under conditions identical to those described in Experiment 1. The dogs were given a choice of distilled water and 0.15 *M* NaCl solution to drink for 9 days. During this time daily measurements of food and water intakes and body weight were made. During the following 3 days each dog was given 10 mg ethacrynic acid (1 mg/kg body weight) twice daily (9 AM and 5 PM) by mouth. Measurement of fluid intakes and body weights continued daily during treatment and for 3 days after treatment.

2. Study 2

This study began in the same fashion as that described in Experiment 1 in which graded concentrations of NaCl solution were offered to the dogs in combination with distilled water. Each concentration was offered for 2 days excepting only the first 4 days when both buckets contained distilled water. The concentrations of NaCl solution offered in chronological sequence were: 0.010, 0.020, 0.040, 0.060, 0.080, 0.100, 0.125, 0.150, 0.200, and 0.250 moles/liter. This portion of the experiment required 24 days to complete. At this time each dog was allowed choice between distilled water and 0.080 *M* NaCl solution for 4 days at which time daily administration of ethacrynic acid (5 mg/animal or 0.5 mg/kg twice daily by mouth) began. The diuretic was administered at 9 AM and 5 PM. After treatment, an additional 10-day recovery period was allowed during which the animals had choice between distilled water and 0.080 *M* NaCl solution. At the end of the recovery period, deoxycorticosterone acetate (Percorten, Ciba Pharmaceuticals Co., Summit, New Jersey) was administered subcutaneously for 4 days at a dose of 25 mg/animal or 2.5 mg/kg of body weight. Measurement of intakes continued daily during treatment and for 10 days thereafter. At this time (day 52 of the study) choice was offered between 0.150 *M* NaCl solution and distilled water for 8 days and between 0.150 *M* $NaHCO_3$ solution and distilled water for an additional 4 days. Daily intakes were measured during these periods.

III. RESULTS

A. Experiment 1

The results of this experiment failed to reveal a preference–aversion curve for intake of NaCl solution by dogs that is so typical of rats (Fig. 1) (Fregly, 1973).

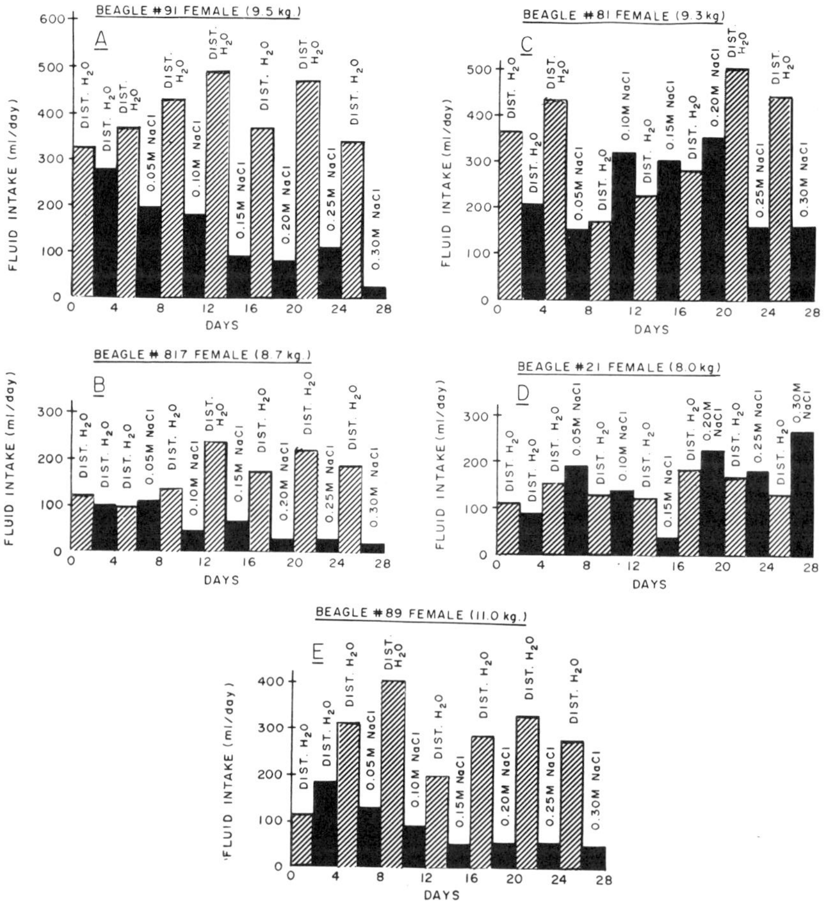

Fig. 1. Simultaneous intakes of water and a NaCl solution are shown for five female Beagle dogs. Choice between distilled water (shaded column) and each NaCl solution (black column) was offered for 4 days. The mean daily fluid intake during each period is shown for the 28 days of the experiment. The conc--tration of NaCl solution offered with distilled water was the same for each period, and each dog is shown in the figure.

When the ratio of NaCl solution ingested to the total fluid (water and NaCl solution) ingested was calculated for each NaCl solution offered and for each dog, it would appear that the dogs used in these studies showed little or no preference for NaCl solution (Fig. 2). In fact, the ratio of NaCl ingested to total fluid ingested decreased as the concentration of NaCl solution increased. With the exception of one dog, all of the animals appeared to have an aversion, rather than a preference, for NaCl solution (Fig. 2).

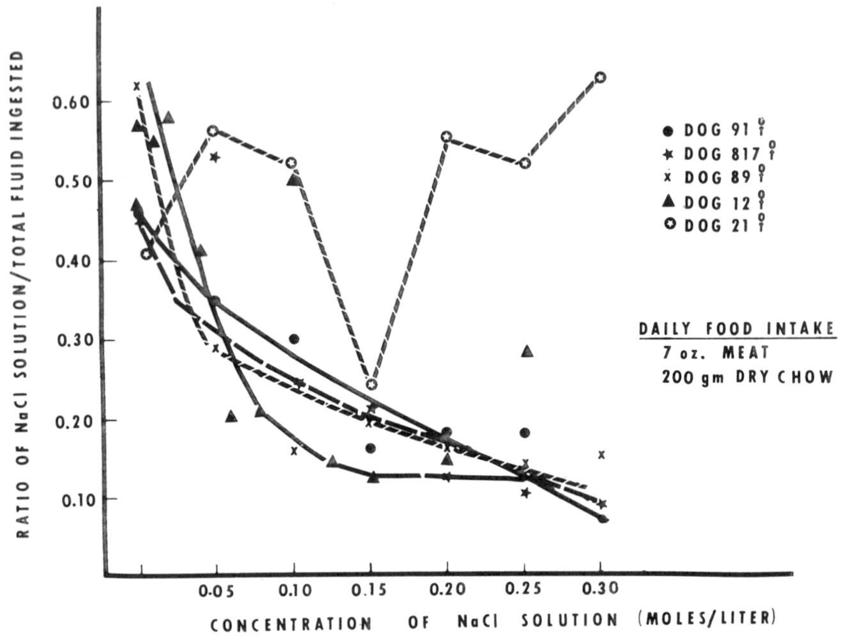

Fig. 2. The ratio of NaCl solution to total fluid (water plus NaCl solution) ingested is shown for each dog in Fig. 1 as a function of the concentration of NaCl solution offered simultaneously with water.

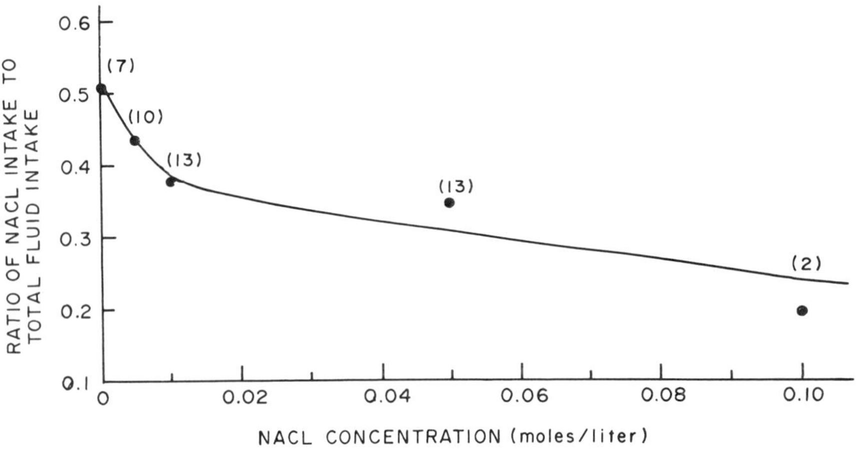

Fig. 3. The ratio of NaCl solution to total fluid ingested is shown for a female Dalmatian dog as a function of the concentration of NaCl solution offered simultaneously with water.

Similar results were observed in one female Dalmatian dog on the basis of "session" testing as opposed to the daily fluid intakes measured in the Beagles. This animal also showed a decrease in the ratio of NaCl solution ingested to total fluid ingested as the concentration of NaCl solution increased (Fig. 3).

B. Experiment 2

The spontaneous NaCl intakes of two additional animals were tested. There was again no consistent evidence of a NaCl appetite in these two animals (Fig. 4). When the diuretic agent, hydrochlorothiazide, was administered daily for 4 days, there was no consistent change in intake of 0.080 *M* NaCl solution but intake of distilled water appeared to increase in both animals. During the recovery from drug treatment, water intake decreased in both animals compared to both pretreatment and treatment periods while intake of NaCl solution decreased in one dog and increased in the second (Fig. 4).

Repetition of this experiment using the same dogs failed again to show any significant effects of administration of hydrochlorothiazide (Fig. 5). The concentration of NaCl solution used was 0.080 *M* because this concentration appeared to be ingested to a lesser extent than water in a more or less consistent fashion in the earlier study. It was reasoned that an appetite for NaCl solution could more easily manifest itself under these conditions if induced by the diuretic agent.

An additional experiment was conducted in which choice was offered between 0.15 *M* NaCl solution and distilled water. Under these conditions hydrochlorothiazide at the same dose used in previous studies appeared to depress total fluid intake, including both water and NaCl solution (Fig. 6). Body weight also decreased during treatment. Thus, this study also provided no evidence that hydrochlorothiazide could increase the spontaneous intake of NaCl solution in the dog.

C. Experiment 3

The first study attempted to determine whether the potent diuretic agent, ethacrynic acid, would influence spontaneous NaCl intakes by dogs. This study showed little or no effect of ethacrynic acid on NaCl intake (Fig. 7). However, a decrease in body weight occurred during treatment.

The spontaneous NaCl intakes by 2 additional animals were tested in this final study in the same manner in which it was tested in Experiment 1. Again, no evidence of an appetite for NaCl solution was obtained (Fig. 8). Ethacrynic acid was administered to these animals at half the dose used in the previous study to assure that the large weight loss induced by the higher dose had not influenced the results. Ethacrynic acid, at half the dose used previously, failed to influence NaCl intake.

When deoxycorticosterone acetate was administered to these animals, there

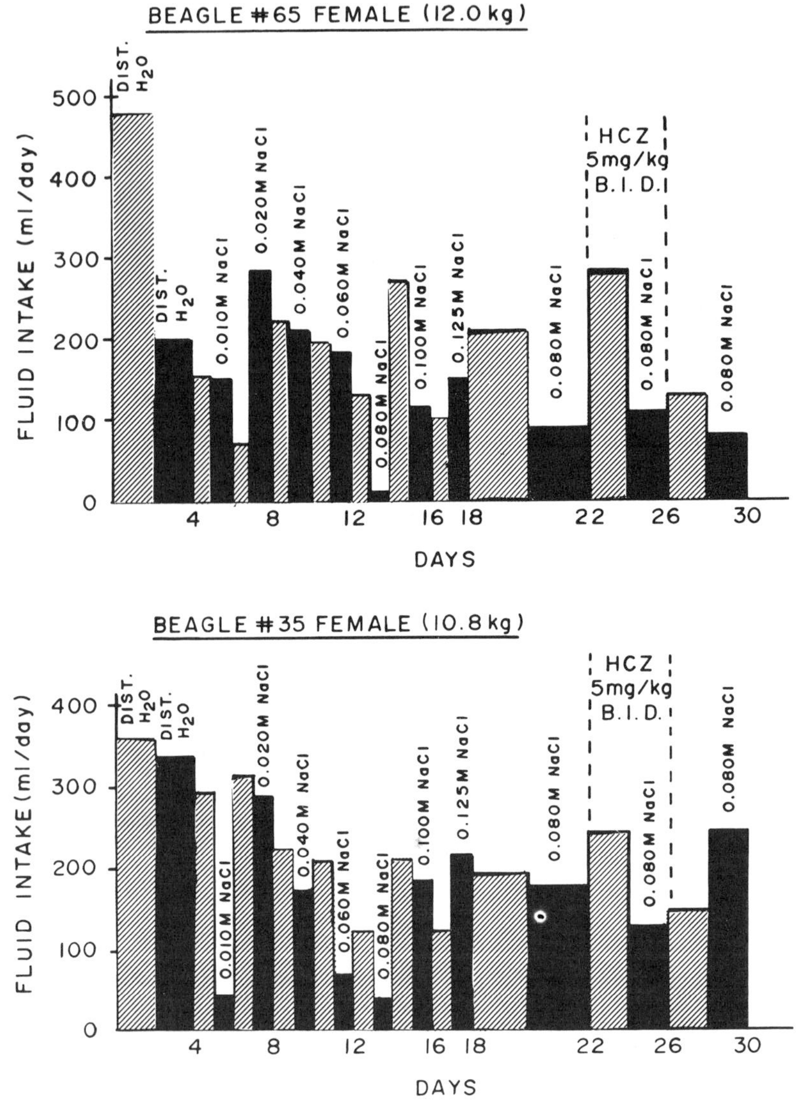

Fig. 4. Simultaneous intakes of distilled water and a NaCl solution are shown for two female Beagle dogs. Choice between distilled water (shaded column) and each NaCl solution (black column) was offered for 2 days. The mean daily intake during each period is shown for the entire experiment. During days 18 to 22, choice was offered between distilled water and 0.08 *M* NaCl solution. Hydrochlorothiazide (HCZ; 5 mg/kg, twice daily) was administered from days 22 to 26. Intakes of distilled water and NaCl solution were measured for an additional 4 days.

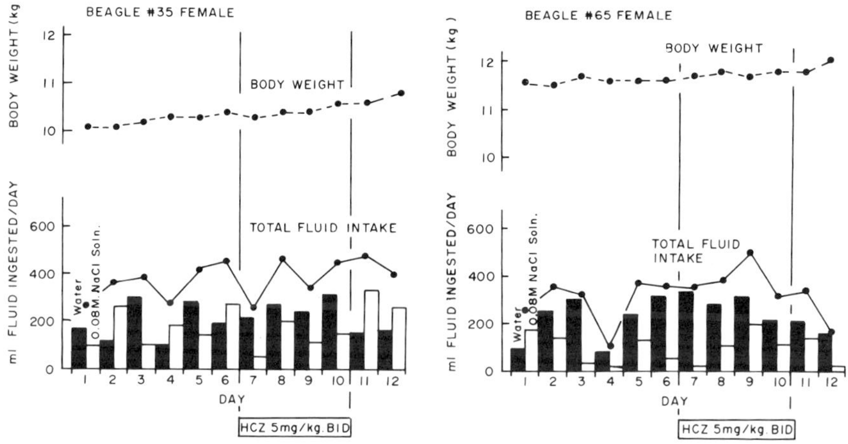

Fig. 5. Simultaneous daily intake of distilled water and 0.08 *M* NaCl solution before, during, and after administration of hydrochlorothiazide (HCZ; 5 mg/kg, twice daily) to two female beagle dogs is shown. The dark column represents water intake while the white column represents intake of NaCl solution. Body weight and total fluid intake are also given in the figure.

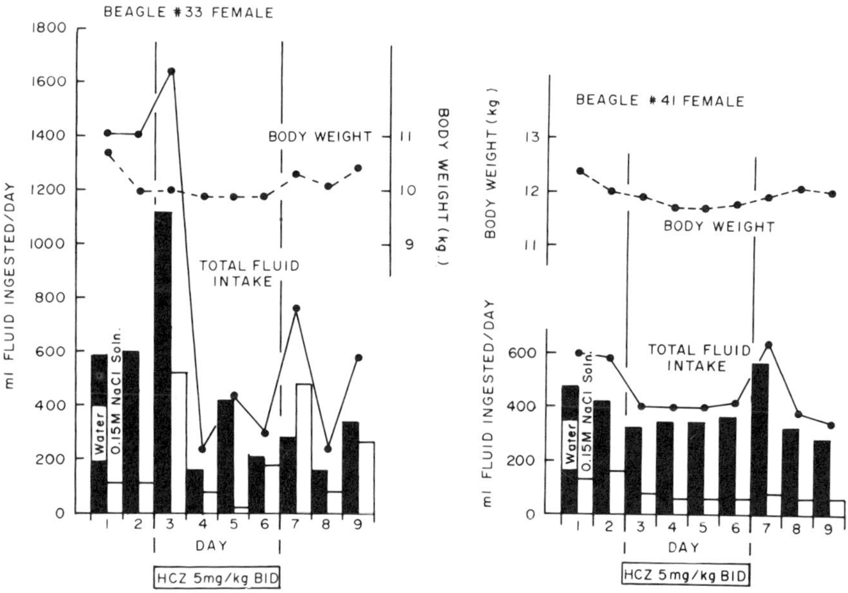

Fig. 6. Simultaneous daily intake of distilled water and 0.15 *M* NaCl solution before, during, and after administration of hydrochlorothiazide (HCZ; 5 mg/kg, twice daily) to two female beagle dogs is shown. The dark column represents water intake while the white column represents intake of NaCl solution. Body weight and total fluid intake are also given in the figure.

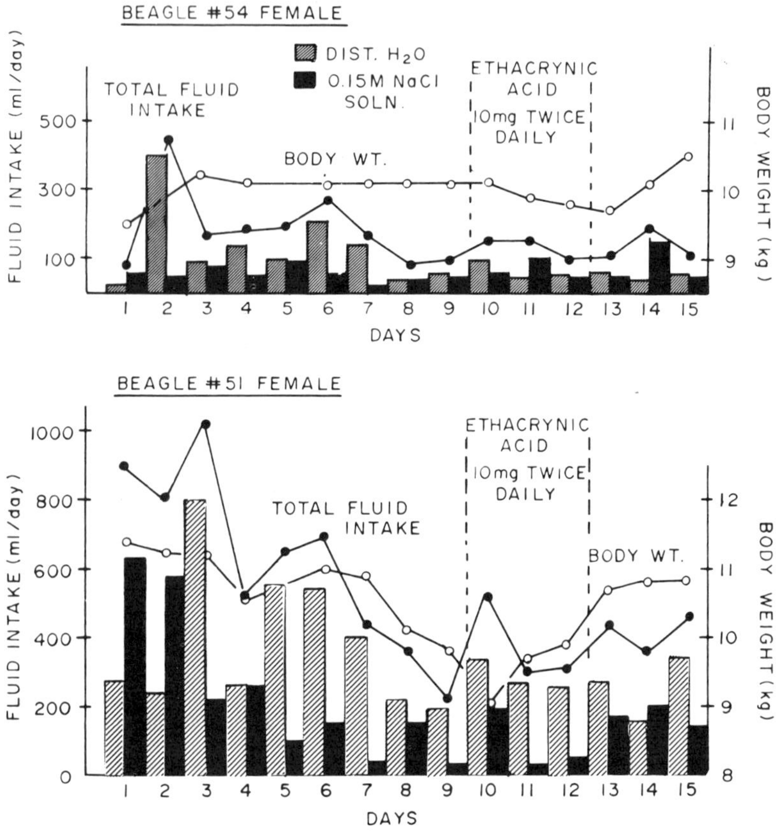

Fig. 7. Simultaneous daily intakes of distilled water and 0.15 *M* NaCl solution before, during, and after administration of ethacrynic acid (10 mg/dog or 1 mg/kg twice daily) to two female beagle dogs. Shaded column represents water intake while the dark column represents intake of NaCl solution. Body weight and total fluid intake are also given in the figure.

was no significant effect on intakes of either water or NaCl solution (Fig. 8). However, during the 10-day period after administration of deoxycorticosterone acetate, a doubling of water intake occurred. Substitution of $NaHCO_3$ for NaCl had no effect on intakes of either water or salt solution.

IV. DISCUSSION

The female dog appears to differ strikingly from the rat with respect to its spontaneous intake of NaCl solution and the factors that affect it. The female dog appears to be more like the cat and chicken, which are reported to have no

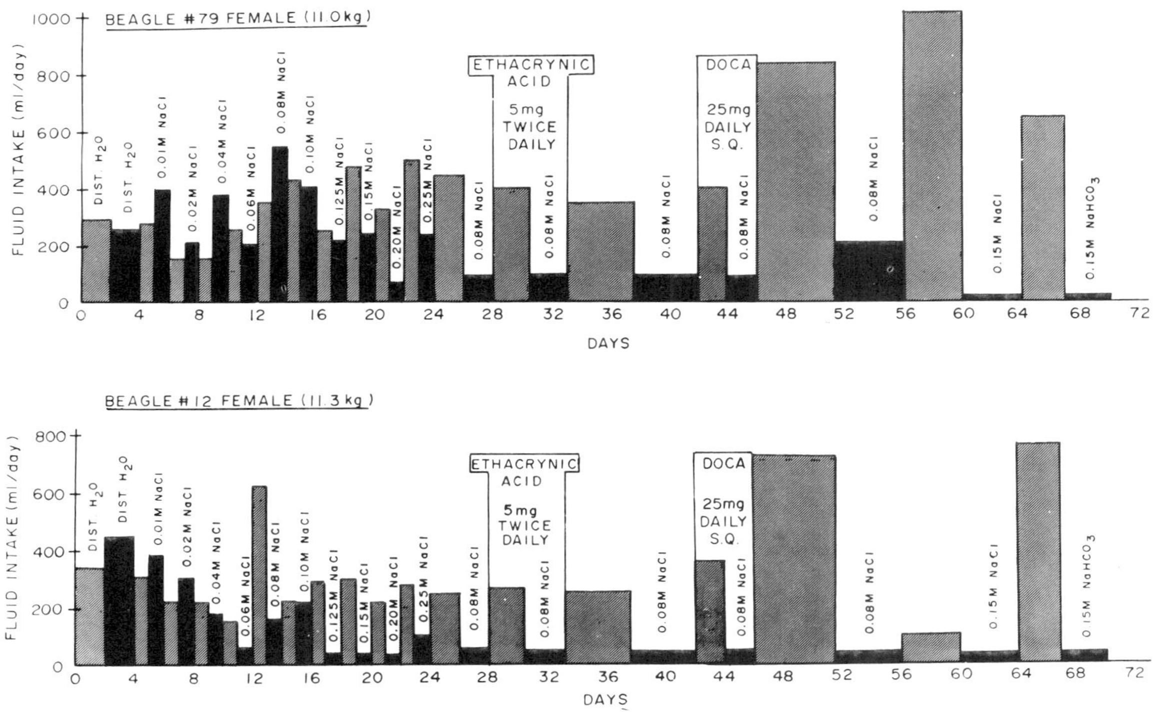

Fig. 8. Simultaneous intakes of distilled water and a NaCl solution are shown for two female beagle dogs. Choice between distilled water (shaded colum) and each NaCl solution (dark column) was offered for 2 days. The mean daily intake during each period is shown for the entire study. During days 24 to 28, choice was offered between distilled water and 0.080 *M* NaCl solution. Ethacrynic acid (5 mg/dog or 0.5 mg/kg body weight twice daily) was administered during the 4 days of drug treatment. Deoxycorticosterone acetate (DOCA, 25 mg/dog or 2.5 mg/kg body weight) was administered from days 42 to 46. During days 56 to 64, intakes of water and 0.15 *M* NaCl solution were measured. During days 64 to 70, choice was offered between water and 0.15 *M* $NaHCO_3$ solution.

preference for NaCl solution (Kare, 1961). The dog differs from these two species, however, in that virtually all concentrations of NaCl solution were ingested to a lesser extent than water (Figs. 2 and 3). Reasons both for the failure to observe a NaCl appetite and for the observation of a relative NaCl aversion in dogs are not clearly understood. Bunge (1902) hypothesized nearly 80 years ago that herbivores prefer NaCl because of their high potassium and low sodium diet while carnivores, with their relatively higher sodium and lower potassium intake, were stated to lack this preference. Anecdotal observations on the salt appetite of subcultures of humans who were predominantly vegetarian, as compared to those who were primarily carnivorous, were said to support the role of dietary sodium and potassium intakes in sodium appetite.

There can be little doubt that the dietary sodium intake of the dogs used here was adequte. Depletion of body sodium by either of two diuretic agents, hydrochlorothiazide or ethacrynic acid, had no consistent effect on spontaneous intake of NaCl solution (Figs. 4–8). Although urine was not collected in these studies, the dose of each of the diuretic agents used has been shown to induce both a diuresis and a natriuresis in dogs (McCarthy *et al.*, 1967). While it would have been desirable to have an analysis of the sodium and potassium balances of the animals during these studies, such an analysis must await additional experimentation. It was felt that drinking behavior would be less affected if the animals were housed in their large home cages rather than confined to small metabolic cages.

Administration of the mineralocorticoid hormone, deoxycorticosterone acetate, to the dog also failed to induce an appetite for NaCl solution as it does characteristically in the rat and rabbit (Braun-Menendez and Brandt, 1952; Denton, 1967; Fregly, 1972; Fregly and Waters, 1967; Wolf and Handal, 1966). Thus, the conditions under which these experiments were performed did not reveal an appetite for NaCl solution in the dog. The dogs also failed to manifest an appetite for $NaHCO_3$ solution. Whether other conditions, such as a low sodium diet, a change of dietary constituents, can uncover an appetite for NaCl solution in the dog remains for further study.

V. SUMMARY

Five purebred female Beagle dogs were offered a choice between distilled water and increasing concentrations of NaCl solution to drink. Concentrations were changed every 4 days. None of the dogs showed a clear-cut preference for any concentration of NaCl solution above that of the water offered simultaneously. In contrast, all dogs except one decreased the volume of NaCl solution ingested, compared to the total volume ingested, as the concentration of NaCl solution increased. Under conditions of a short-term (1 hour) test situation, one female Dalmatian dog also decreased her intake of NaCl solution. Since the diuretic agent, hydrochlorothiazide (HCZ), is known to increase the spontaneous intake of NaCl solution in rats, it was administered per os at 5 mg/kg body weight B.I.D. to six female Beagle dogs for 4 days. In the case of four dogs, choice was offered between 0.08 *M* NaCl solution and distilled water; two other dogs were offered choice between 0.15 *M* NaCl solution and distilled water. HCZ failed to stimulate an increase in intake of either concentration of NaCl solution over that observed prior to administration of the drug. In four other female Beagle dogs the diuretic agent, ethacrynic acid, was administered at a dose of 1 mg/kg B.I.D. for 4 days. Two dogs were offered a choice between 0.08 *M* NaCl solution and distilled water while the other two dogs were offered a choice between 0.15 *M* NaCl solution and distilled water. In no case did ethacrynic acid induce an increase in intake of NaCl solution above that observed prior to administration of the drug. Two of the dogs used in this study were also administered 2.5 mg deoxycorticosterone acetate (DOCA)/kg/day sc for 4 days. During this time they were offered choice between 0.08 *M* NaCl solution and distilled water. DOCA also failed to affect the spontaneous intake of NaCl solution. When choice was offered between 0.15 *M* $NaHCO_3$ solution and water, two beagle dogs drank more water than $NaHCO_3$ solution. It is concluded that dogs do not appear to have a spontaneous appetite for either NaCl or $NaHCO_3$ solutions as is so commonly observed in rats. Experimental conditions known to stimulate salt intake in rats, i.e., administration of either diuretic agents or DOCA, fail to effect the salt intake of dogs. The factors responsible for this difference between rats and dogs remain to be elucidated.

ACKNOWLEDGMENTS

I wish to thank Dr. T. H. Maren, Department of Pharmacology, for the opportunity to use his Beagle colony. I thank Miss Charlotte Wright for drawing the illustrations. Supported by Grant HL solution on their first exposure. The dashed line represents indifference.

REFERENCES

Braun-Menendez, E., and Brandt, P. (1952). Aumento del apetito especifico para la sal provocado por la deoxycorticosterone: Caracteristicas. *Rev. Soc. Argent. Biol.* **28,** 15-23.

Bunge, G. (1902). "Textbook of Physiological and Pathological Chemistry," 2nd ed., pp. 90-103. McGraw-Hill (Blakiston), New York.

Denton, D. A. (1967). Salt appetite. *In* "Handbook of Physiology" (Am. Physiol. Soc., J. Field, ed.), Sect. 6, Vol. I, pp. 433-459. Williams & Wilkins, Baltimore, Maryland.

Denton, D. A., and Nelson, J. F. (1970). Pituitary-adrenal axis and salt appetite. *Prog. Brain Res.* **2,** 131-140.

Fregly, M. J. (1967). The role of hormones in the regulation of salt intake in rats. *In* "The Chemical Senses and Nutrition" (M. R. Kare and O. Maller, eds.), pp. 115-138. Johns Hopkins Press, Baltimore, Maryland.

Fregly, M. J. (1972). Effect of an oral contraceptive on spontaneous running activity, salt appetite and blood pressure of ovariectomized rats. *J. Pharmacol. Exp. Ther.* **182,** 335–343.

Fregly, M. J. (1973). Effect of an oral contraceptive on NaCl appetite and preference threshold in rats. *Pharmacol., Biochem. Behav.* **1,** 61–65.

Fregly, M. J., and Kim, K. J. (1970). Specificity of the sodium chloride appetite of hydrochlorothiazide-treated rats. *Physiol. Behav.* **5,** 595–599.

Fregly, M. J., and Newsome, D. G. (1974). Oral contraceptive-induced salt appetite in rats. *In* "Oral Contraceptives and High Blood Pressure" (M. J. Fregly and M. S. Fregly, eds.), pp. 141–158. Dolphin Press, Gainesville, Florida.

Fregly, M. J., and Waters, I. W. (1967). Hormonal regulation of the spontaneous sodium chloride appetite of rats. *In* "Olfaction and Taste II" (T. Hayashi, ed.), pp. 439–458. Pergamon, Oxford.

Jalowiec, J. E. (1974). Sodium appetite elicited by furosemide: Effects of differential dietary maintenance. *Behav. Biol.* **10,** 313–327.

Kare, M. R. (1961). Comparative aspects of the sense of taste. *In* "The Physiological and Behavioral Aspects of Taste" (M. R. Kare and B. P. Halpern, eds.), pp. 6–15. Univ. of Chicago Press, Chicago, Illinois.

McCarthy, J. S., Fregly, M. J., and Nechay, B. R. (1967). Effect of diuretics on renal iodide excretion by rats and dogs. *J. Pharmacol. Exp. Ther.* **158,** 294–304.

Richter, C. P. (1942–1943). Total self-regulatory functions in animals and human beings. *Harvey Lect.* **38,** 63–103.

Shulkes, A. A., Covelli, M. D., Denton, D. A., and Nelson, J. F. (1972). Hormonal factors influencing salt appetite in lactation. *Aust. J. Exp. Biol. Med. Sci.* **50,** 819–826.

Wolf, G., and Handal, P. J. (1966). Aldosterone-induced sodium appetite: Dose-response and specificity. *Endocrinology* **78,** 1120–1124.

Chapter 6

Comparative Aspects of Salt Preference and Intake in Birds

B. ROBINZON, M. R. KARE, and G. K. BEAUCHAMP

I. INTRODUCTION

Recently, Dethier (1976) provided a comprehensive comparative review on salt (NaCl) taste. However, the class Aves was not included. Avian species can provide interesting biological and behavioral information on NaCl since they have representatives in the entire dietary spectrum and have unique physiological mechanisms for handling salt. Many of the points to be made concerning birds are directly relevant to a broader comparative outlook.

Carpenter (1956) commented: "In the field of taste, a comparative study is composed of three main variables: the stimulus, the species, and the method of studying the problem—two of which must be held constant in order to make comparisons within the third variable." In approaching the comparative aspects of salt taste, appetite, and avoidance, one becomes confused both by electrophysiological and behavioral methods that have been used and by the fact that they do not permit a simple comparison of results. Behavioral approaches include

ISBN 0-12-397750-9

field observations, and preference and avoidance tests. Some avoidance tests use the motoric reactions of the animal to evaluate certain taste stimuli, while the type and the concentration of the stimuli vary, sometimes beyond any physiological meaning (Gentle, 1978). In preference tests, two methods, which provide very different information, are commonly in use: the two-choice and the one-choice tests. However, even in studies in which the same concentrations of a stimulus and the same preference test methods are used, the duration of the testing period, and the previous experience of the tested animal, as well as its physiological background (which is not always reported) usually vary. All these factors may affect the results. For example, nutritional background or age have been found to affect salt preferences in the human being (Beauchamp, 1979; Beauchamp and Maller, 1977; Desor *et al.*, 1975a,b) and rats (Bernard *et al.*, 1961; Kare and Henkin, 1969). This problem is illustrated in the following study.

II. METHOD

Naive mature male Red-Winged Blackbirds were trapped at Patuxent Wildlife Center, Laurel, Maryland, and transported to the laboratory where they were kept in a group cage at a temperature of 23° ± 1°C and a light cycle of 6 hours light and 18 hours dark for 6 months. Then the birds were individually housed in cages (36 × 41 × 61 cm) under the same environment conditions. Food (Purina Game Bird Flight Conditioning Chow containing 0.5% NaCl) and deionized water were available ad lib. Water was presented from two graduated drinking tubes located at the back of the cage, and food from a cup at the front of the cage. Recording of daily fluid intake started 1 month after introducing the birds to their individual cages. One month later, two-choice preference tests for 0.89% (0.15 *M*) NaCl versus deionized water were performed. Fluid intake was recorded at 1, 2, 4, 24, and 72 hours after exposure. After each recording the position of the drinking tubes was reversed. At the end of the exposure period (72 hours), the birds were given 2 weeks to recover during which only deionized water was available from the two tubes. Subsequently the same preference test procedure was repeated.

III. RESULTS

Figures 1 and 2 present the preference for the saline solution manifested by the birds during the first and the second exposures, respectively. As can be seen, while most of the birds preferred the saline solution during the first exposure, they rejected it during the last 68 hours of the second exposure. This suggests that

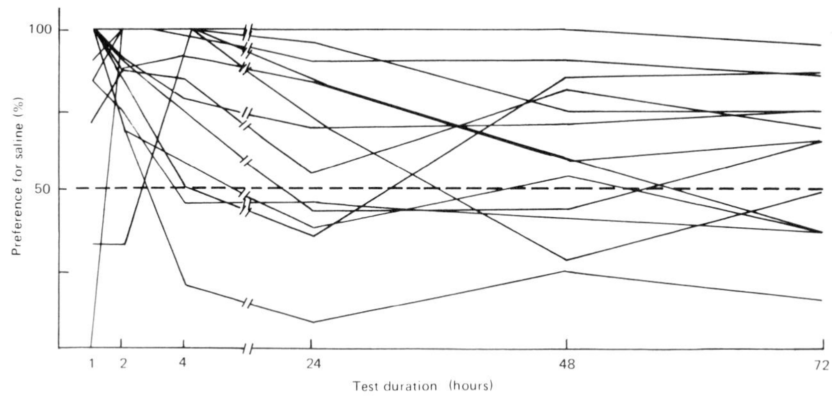

Fig. 1. Individual preference-rejection curves manifested by blackbirds toward 0.9% NaCl solution on their first exposure. The dashed line represents indifference.

the previous experience of the tested animal affects the results. In the second exposure, most of the birds showed a strong preference for the saline solution during the first 2 hours, but at 4 hours and beyond they rejected it (Fig. 2). Thus, the duration of the test (from exposure time until the first recording time) may affect the results and produce conflicting reports varying from acceptance to rejection. Figure 3 presents the total fluid intake before exposures, within exposures, during the recovery period between them, and after termination of exposures. As can be seen, the exposure to saline increased the total fluid intake even during the second period where saline rejection was manifested.

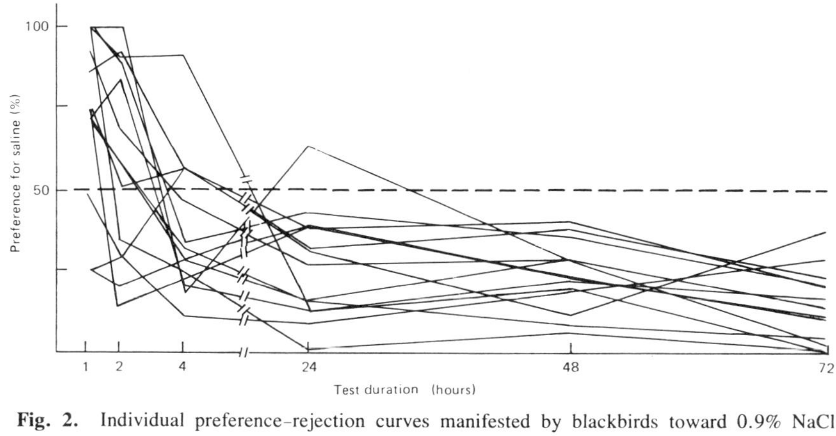

Fig. 2. Individual preference-rejection curves manifested by blackbirds toward 0.9% NaCl solution on their second exposure. The dashed line represents indifference.

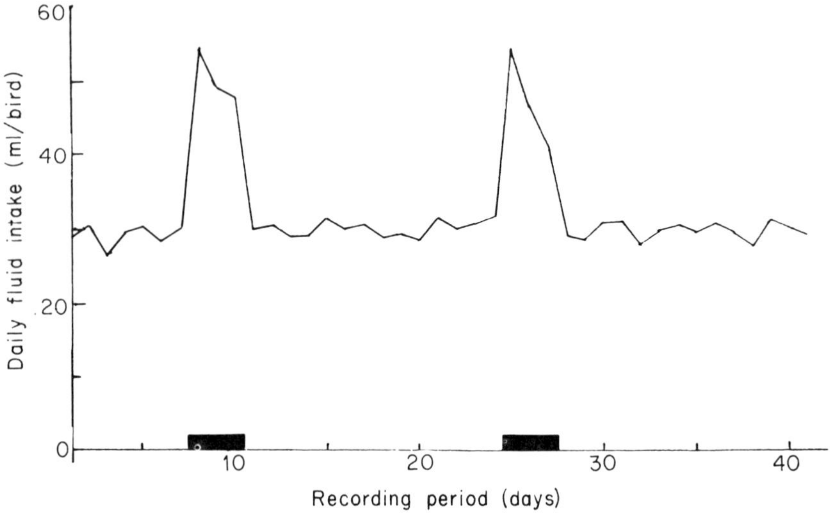

Fig. 3. Average total fluid intake of the blackbirds before, during, between, and after the exposures to 0.9% NaCl solution. The black areas on the time axis represent the exposures to the NaCl solution.

IV. DISCUSSION

Hughes and Wood-Gush (1971) found that in single-choice preference tests, chickens were indifferent to 0.7% saline, while in two-choice tests a strong aversion toward it was manifested. This also suggests that a single bottle preference test for an aversive stimulus will result in more acceptance than a two-choice test. In the same study it was found that under short-term preference tests (a few minutes), Brown Leghorns showed neither preference nor aversion up to 0.6% NaCl, but with long exposure (several days) they exhibited an aversion which intensified from day to day (Hughes and Wood-Gush, 1971). These results are in accordance with those obtained with the blackbirds, and they point out that the testing method, the exposure duration, and the previous experience all may influence the results.

For these reasons, the data from the various publications dealing with NaCl preferences of birds are categorized according to whether they were obtained from one- or two-choice preference tests (Table I) and each category is discussed separately. Values reported for two-choice tests are rejection points, those for one-choice tests are turning points (i.e., the molarity beyond which the fluid consumption starts to decrease and the birds lose weight). As can be seen from the table, most birds that were given two-choice tests rejected saline solutions beginning at concentrations of 0.12–0.25 M. Extremely low levels of rejection,

TABLE I

Bibliographical Comparative Analysis of the Molarity at the Rejection Point, at Two-Choice Situations, and the Molarity of Turning Point (Survival), in One-Choice Experiment, for the Various Birds Which Were Studied

Species	Molarity at rejection point at two-choice exp.	Molarity at turning point one-choice exp.	Reference
Adeline Penguine		⩾0.500	Welty (1967)
Black-Footed Albatross (*Diomedea nigripes*)	⩾0.500	⩾0.500	Frings and Frings (1959)
Laysan Albatross (*Diomedea immitabilis*)	⩾0.500	⩾0.500	Frings and Frings (1959)
Glaucous-Winged Gull (*Larus glaucensceus*)		⩾0.500	Holmes *et al.* (1961)
Laughing Gull (*Larus atricilla*)	0.150	0.250	Harriman (1967)
Herring Gull (*Larus argentatus*)		0.250	Harriman and Kare (1966a)
	0.200		Harriman and Kare (1966b)
Mallard (*Anas platyrhynches*)	0.200		Engelmann (1960)
		⩾0.284	Holmes *et al.* (1968)
		⩾0.470	Donaldson and Holmes (1965)
Snowy Plover (*Charadrius alexandrinus*)		0.250	Purdue and Haines (1977)
Killdeer (*Charadrius vociferus*)		0.100	Purdue and Haines (1977)
Semipalmated Sandpiper (*Calidris pusillus*)		0.250	Purdue and Haines (1977)
Savannah Sparrow (*Passerculus sandwichensis*)			
P.s. beldingi		0.550	Cade and Bartholomew (1959)
	0.250	0.600	Poulson and Bartholomew (1962)
P.s. rostratus		0.550	Cade and Bartholomew (1959)
		0.550	Johnson and Ohmart (1973)

(continued)

TABLE I *(continued)*

Species	Molarity at rejection point at two-choice exp.	Molarity at turning point one-choice exp.	Reference
P.s. brooksi }		0.400	Cade and Bartholomew (1959)
P.s. anthinus }	0.250		
P.s.nevadensis }		0.300	Poulson and Bartholomew (1962)
Sharp-Tailed Sparrow (*Ammospiza caudacuta*)			
A.c. caudacuta	0.100	0.300	Poulson (1969)
		0.500	Trost, in Poulson (1969)
A.c. subvirgata	0.100	0.400	Poulson (1969)
		0.300	Trost, in Poulson (1969)
A.c. nelsoni		0.200	Trost, in Poulson (1969)
Seaside Sparrow (*Ammospiza maritima*)		0.400	Poulson (1969)
Black-Throated Sparrow (*Amphispiza bilineata*)		0.200	Smyth and Bartholomew (1966a)
		0.400	Smyth and Bartholomew (1966b)
Song Sparrow (*Melospiza melodia*)			
M.m. cooperi		0.400	Bartholomew and Cade (1963)
M.m. maxillaris		0.250	Bartholomew and Cade (1963)
M.m. samuelis		0.250	Bartholomew and Cade (1963)
Vesper Sparrow (*Pooecetes gramineusi*)		0.250	Ohmart and Smith (1971)
Brewer's Sparrow (*Spizella breweri*)		0.45–0.55	Ohmart and Smith (1970)
Tree Sparrow (*Spizella arborta*)		0.150	Ohmart and Smith (1970)
Sparrow (*Zonotrichia atricapilla*)		0.250	Bartholomew and Cade (1963)
White-Crowned Sparrow (*Zonotrichia leucophrys gambelii*)	0.087	0.125	MacMillan and Snelling (1966)
		0.200	Okoche *et al.* (1963)
Zebra Finch (*Taeniopygia castanotis*)			

TABLE I (*continued*)

Species	Molarity at rejection point at two-choice exp.	Molarity at turning point one-choice exp.	Reference
Wild type		0.600	Okoche *et al.* (1963)
		0.400	Skadhauge and Bradshaw (1974)
Domesticated			
Nonadapted		0.200	Cade *et al.* (1965)
Adapted		<0.400	Cade *et al.* (1965)
House Finch (*Coprodacus mexicanus*)	0.200	0.400	Bartholomew and Cade (1958)
Black-Rumped Waxbill–Tropical African Finch (*Estrilda troglodytes*)	0.050	0.150	Cade *et al.* (1965)
Red Crossbill	0.100	0.200	Dawson *et al.* (1965)
(*Loxia curvirostra*)	0.050		Willoughby (1971)
Great Tit	0.170		Warren and Vince (1963)
(*Parus major*)	0.170		Vince and Warren (1963)
Stark's Lark (*Spizocorys starki*)		0.200	Willoughby (1968)
Gray-Backed Finch Lark (*Eremopterix verticalis*)		0.300	Willoughby (1968)
Budgerygah		0.300	Cade and Dybas (1962)
(*Melopsittacus undulatus*)		0.300	Greenwald *et al.* (1966)
Starling		0.250	Harriman and Kare (1966a)
(*Sturnus vulgaris vulgaris*)	0.150		Harriman and Kare (1966b)
	0.100		Harriman (1968)
Purple Grackle (*Quiscalus quiscula*)		0.250	Harriman and Kare (1966)
Red-Winged Blackbird (*Agelaius phoeniceus phoeniceus*)			
Marsh type			
Young		0.200	Hesse and Lustick (1972)
Adults		0.200	Hesse and Lustick (1972)
Upland type			
Young		0.200	Hesse and Lustick (1972)
Adults		0.300	Hesse and Lustick (1972)

(*continued*)

TABLE I (*continued*)

Species	Molarity at rejection point at two-choice exp.	Molarity at turning point one-choice exp.	Reference
Cowbird (*Molothrus ater obscurus*)		≤0.300	Lustick (1970)
Mourning Dove (*Zenaidura macroura marginella*)	0.187	0.250	Bartholomew and MacMillan (1960)
		0.1<<0.2	Smyth and Bartholomew (1966b)
White-Winged Dove (*Zenaida asiatica asiatica*)	0.067	0.250	MacMillan and Trost (1966)
Inca Dove (*Scardajella inca*)	0.125	0.187	MacMillan and Trost (1966)
Ground Dove (*Columbia passerina*)		0.150	Willoughby (1966)
Feral Pigeon (*Columba livia*)		0.170	Duncan (1960)
		0.140	Duncan (1962)
	0.100		Englemann (1934)
Bob-White Quail (*Colinus virginianus*)	≤0.340		Brindley (1965), Brindley and Prior (1968)
		0.210	McNabb (1969)
Japanese Quail (*Coturnix coturnix japonica*)	≤0.340		Brindley (1965)
		0.20–0.25	Dunson *et al.* (1976)
	0.150		Harriman (1968)
California Quail (*Lophortyx californicus brunnescens*)	0.188	0.250	Bartholomew and MacMillan (1961)
		0.260	McNabb (1969)
Gambel's Quail (*Lophortyx gambelii*)		0.260	McNabb (1969)
Domestic Fowl (*Gallus domesticus*)	0.250		Engelmann (1934)
	0.175		Pick and Kare (1962)
	0.120		Hughes and Wood-Gush (1971)
Bantham Cock		0.100	Duncan (1962)
Ostrich (*Struthio camelus*)		0.200	Cloudsley-Thompson and El-Rashid (1967)

however, were documented for the Black-Rumped Waxbill (0.05 *M*), Red Crossbill (0.05 *M*), White-Winged Dove (0.067 *M*), and White-Crowned Sparrow (0.087 *M*). On the other hand, the Albatrosses showed no discrimination between fresh water and saline solutions at any concentration that was tested. In these studies the exposure time for the stimuli varied from 2 days (Brindley, 1965; Brindley and Prior, 1968; Harriman, 1957) to 7 days (Bartholomew and MacMillan, 1960, 1961; MacMillan and Trost, 1966), 12 days (Hughes and Wood-Gush, 1971; Dawson *et al.*, 1965), 18 days (Pick and Kare, 1962), or 4–13 days (Bartholomew and Cade, 1958) or were not reported at all (Bartholomew and Cade, 1963).

In none of these reports was the previous experience of the birds documented. As it was pointed out (see Figs. 1 and 2), previous experience drastically affects the discrimination tendency. It was demonstrated with the Red-Winged Blackbird (Fig. 2) and the chicken (Hughes and Wood-Gush, 1971) that in two-choice preference tests for saline solutions, an increase in the exposure time augmented the rejection level, probably due to postingestive cues (Hughes and Wood-Gush, 1971). Thus, without information on previous experiences, a comparative analysis of the data on two-choice discrimination toward saline solutions by birds is extremely problematical.

It is noteworthy that in all the studies reviewed in Table I, *none* of the species showed any preference for any concentration of saline solution that was tested. This phenomenon is confusing. Albatrosses provided with any saline solution less concentrated than seawater continued to lose salt through their salt glands and succumbed (Frings and Frings, 1959). But, even under severe sodium depletion, these birds showed no discrimination between saline solutions and water and increased drinking indiscriminately. In fact, these birds could be saved only by injections of hypertonic saline solutions or by force-feeding with salt (Frings and Frings, 1959). The confusion is even greater for the Red Crossbill. This bird has been observed to eat salt crystals in the nature (Willoughby, 1971) and was easily trapped by using a block of salt as the only bait (Dawson *et al.*, 1965). Yet in two-choice preference tests, this bird showed no preference for saline solutions and rejected them at extremely low concentrations (Dawson *et al.*, 1965; Willoughby, 1971). Thus, it seems that the use of saline solutions in preference tests as a criterion for specific salt appetite in birds may be misleading since the salt appetite of the Red Crossbill (Dawson *et al.*, 1965; Willoughby, 1971) and the physiological need for salt of the Albatross (Frings and Frings, 1959) are not manifested under this procedure.

The one-choice tests for acceptance of saline solutions determine tolerance for salt rather than taste preferences. As can be seen from Table I, the sea birds: the Adeline Penguine, Albatross, and Glaucous-Winged Gull, tolerate seawater salinity, and it may be suggested that these birds are evolutionarily well adapted for their ecological niche. Similar tolerances were found for the salt marsh birds:

Passerculus sandwichensis beldingi and *rostratus, Ammospiza candacuta* and *subvigata,* Seaside Sparrow, and Brewer's Sparrow. The findings that the New World salt marsh birds and the wild Zebra Finch (an Australian desert bird) tolerate seawater while the New World desert birds do not, led Bartholomew and Cade (1963) to suggest that the New World deserts are younger than the Old World ones. Thus, the Old World desert avifaunas are hypothesized to be much better developed. Bartholomew and Cade (1963) continue the argument:

> Coastal salt marshes, in contrast with the New World deserts, are habitats of great antiquity. Long occupancy of salt marshes, in which fresh water is scarce, has favored the evolution of physiological capacities preadaptive for living under desert conditions. Since the desert-adapted renal functions of the Kangaroo rat permit it to drink seawater, it seems likely that the reciprocal is true for Savannah Sparrow: a kidney originally adapted to process a high intake of salt is also adaptive for a minimal intake of water. On the other hand, the ability of a xerophile like the Zebra Finch to maintain water balance while drinking 0.6 *M* NaCl probably is, like the case of the Kangaroo rat, a secondary characteristic of renal functions which evolved in response to low water intake.

In other words, these authors suggest that the lack of tolerance for salty water among the New World desert birds is a result of lack of evolution for xerophilic life, while the Old World desert avifauna is more evolutionarily adapted for lack of water and thus can tolerate higher concentrations of saline.

Data gathered since this hypothesis was proposed, on desert birds from the Namib desert in South-West Africa, do not support this suggestion. The Stark's Lark and the Grey-Backed Finch Lark can maintain their weight without water for at least 30 days, but still do not tolerate salty water any better than Starlings, Grackles, or Red-Winged Blackbirds. Thus, the Zebra Finch appears to be a special case among the investigated desert birds and an extensive study of its natural habitat may give clues to its ability to process salty water. It is strange that in captivity, this bird lost its tolerance for salty water (Cade *et al.,* 1965) in just twenty generations, a tolerance presumably acquired through thousands of years of evolution.

V. SUMMARY

A full comparative evaluation of the responses of birds to NaCl cannot now be made due to a lack of appropriate data. For example, environmental adaptation appears to change the tolerance of the tested bird (Cade *et al.,* 1965). This source of variation is important since in each study (and sometimes even within the same study) a different environmental background and different preadaptation conditions were used for different species (Purdue and Haines, 1977) or even the same species between different tests (Ohmart and Smith, 1970). From the data summarized in Table I the only firm conclusion we wish to draw is that, except for the sea birds, the salt marsh birds and the wild Zebra Finch, none of the birds reviewed can use high saline water to maintain its water economy.

REFERENCES

Bartholomew, G. A., and Cade, T. J. (1958). Effects of sodium chloride on the water consumption of house finches. *Physiol. Zool.* **31,** 304–310.

Bartholomew, G. A., and Cade, T. J. (1963). The water economy of land birds. *Auk* **80,** 504–539.

Bartholomew, G. A., and MacMillan, R. E. (1960). The water requirements of mourning doves and their use of seawater and NaCl solutions. *Physiol. Zool.* **33,** 171–178.

Bartholomew, G. A., and MacMillan, R. E. (1961). Water economy of the California quail and its use of seawater. *Auk* **78,** 505–514.

Beauchamp, G. K. (1980). The development of taste in infancy. *In* "Infant and Child Feeding" (L. J. Filer, Jr. and W. J. Darby, eds.). Academic Press, New York (in press).

Beauchamp, G. K., and Maller, O. (1977). The development of flavor preferences in humans: A review. *In* "The Chemical Senses and Nutrition" (M. R. Kare and O. Maller, eds.), pp. 291–311. Academic Press, New York.

Bernard, R. A., Halpern, B., and Kare, M. R. (1961). Effect of vitamin A deficiency on taste. *Proc. Soc. Exp. Biol. Med.* **108,** 784–786.

Brindley, L. D. (1965). Taste discrimination in Bobwhite and Japanese quail. *Anim. Behav.* **13,** 507–512.

Brindley, L. D., and Prior, S. (1968). Effects of age on taste discrimination in the Bobwhite quail. *Anim. Behav.* **16,** 304–307.

Cade, T. J., and Bartholomew, G. A. (1959). Seawater and salt utilization by Savannah sparrows. *Physiol. Zool.* **32,** 230–238.

Cade, T. J., and Dybas, J. A., Jr. (1962). Water economy of the Budgerygah. *Auk* **79,** 345–364.

Cade, T. J., Tobin, C. A., and Gold, A. (1965). Water economy and metabolism of two estrildine finches. *Physiol. Zool.* **38,** 9–33.

Carpenter, J. A. (1956). Species differences in taste preferences. *J. Comp. Physiol. Psychol.* **49,** 139–151.

Cloudsley-Thompson, J. L., and El-Rashid, M. M. (1967). Water economy of the ostrich. *Nature (London)* **216,** 1040.

Dawson, W. R., Shoemaker, V. H., Tordoff, H. B., and Borut, A. (1965). Observations on the metabolism of sodium chloride in the Red crossbill. *Auk* **82,** 606–623.

Desor, J. A., Green, L. S., and Maller, O. (1975a). Preference for sweet and salty in 9 to 15 year olds and adult humans. *Science* **190,** 686–687.

Desor, J. A., Maller, O., and Andrews, K. (1975b). Ingestive responses of human newborns to salty, sour and bitter stimuli. *J. Comp. Physiol. Psychol.* **89,** 966–970.

Dethier, V. G. (1976). The taste of salt. *Am. Sci.* **65,** 744–751.

Donaldson, E. M., and Holmes, W. N. (1965). Corticosteroidogenesis in the fresh water and saline-maintained duck (*Anas platyrhynchos*). *J. Endocrinol.* **32,** 329–336.

Duncan, C. J. (1960). Preference tests and the sense of taste in the feral pigeon (*Columba livia Van Gmelin*). *Anim. Behav.* **8,** 54–60.

Duncan, C. J. (1962). Salt preferences of birds and mammals. *Physiol. Zool.* **35,** 120–132.

Dunson, W. A., Dunson, M. R., and Ohmant, R. D. (1976). Evidence for the presence of nasal salt glands in the roadrunner and the Coturnix quail. *J. Exp. Zool.* **198,** 209–216.

Engelmann, C. (1934). Versuche uber den Geschmachesinn von Taube, Ente und Huhn. *Z. Vergl. Physiol.* **20,** 626–645.

Engelmann, C. (1960). Weitere Versuche die Futterwahl des Wassergeflugels. Uber die Schmeckempfindlichkeit der Ganse. *Arch. Feflugelzuecht. Kleintiekd.* **9,** 91–102.

Frings, H., and Frings, M. (1959). Observations on salt balance and behavior of Laysen and Black-footed Albatrosses in captivity. *Condor* **61,** 304–314.

Gentle, M. J. (1978). Extra-lingual chemoreception in the chicken. *Chem. Senses Flavor* **3,** 325–329.

Greenwald, L. G., Stone, W. B., and Cade, T. J. (1966). Physiological adjustments of the Badgerygah *Melopsittacus undalatus* to dehydrating conditions. *Comp. Biochem. Physiol.* **22,** 91–100.

Harriman, A. E. (1967). Laughing gull offered saline in preference and survival tests. *Physiol. Zool.* **40,** 273–279.

Harriman, A. E. (1968). Acceptance of cations as chlorides in drinking tests with two species of birds and three species of mammals. *Am. Midl. Nat.* **79,** 396–401.

Harriman, A. E., and Kare, M. R. (1966a). Tolerance for hypertonic saline solutions in herring gull, starlings, and purple grackles. *Physiol. Zool.* **39,** 117–122.

Harriman, A. E., and Kare, M. R. (1966b). Aversion to saline solutions in starlings, purple grackles, and herring gulls. *Physiol. Zool.* **39,** 123–126.

Hesse, W., and Lustick, S. (1972). A comparison of the water requirements of marsh and upland Redwing blackbirds (*Agelaius phoeniceus*). *Physiol. Zool.* **45,** 196–203.

Holmes, W. M., Fletcher, G. L., and Steward, D. J. (1968). The patterns of renal electrolyte excretion in duck (*Anas platyrhynchos*) maintained on fresh water and on hypertonic saline. *J. Exp. Biol.* **48,** 487–508.

Holmes, W. N., Butler, D. G., and Phillips, J. G. (1961). Observations on the effect of maintaining glaucous-winged gulls (*Larus glaucensceus*) on fresh and sea water for long periods. *J. Endocrinol.* **23,** 53–61.

Hughes, B. O., and Wood-Gush, D. M. G. (1971). Investigations into specific appetites for sodium and thiamine in domestic fowls. *Physiol. Behav.* **6,** 331–339.

Johnson, O. W., and Ohmart, R. D. (1973). Some features of water economy and kidney microstructures in the large-billed Savannah sparrow (*Passerculus sandwichensis rostratus*). *Physiol. Zool.* **46,** 276–284.

Kare, M. R., and Henkin, R. I. (1969). The effects of D-penicillamine on taste preference and volume intake of sodium chloride by the rat. *Proc. Soc. Exp. Biol. Med.* **131,** 559–561.

Lustick, S. I. (1970). Energetics and water regulation in the Cowbird (*Molothrus ater obscurus*). *Physiol. Zool.* **43,** 270–287.

MacMillan, R. E., and Snelling, J. C. (1966). Water economy of the White-crowned sparrow and its use of saline water. *Condor* **68,** 388–395.

MacMillan, R. E., and Trost, C. H. (1966). Water economy and salt balance in White-winged and Inca doves. *Auk* **83,** 441–456.

McNabb, F. M. A. (1969). A comparative study of water balance in three species of quail. II. Utilization of saline drinking solution. *Comp. Biochem. Physiol.* **28,** 1059–1074.

Ohmart, R. D., and Smith, E. L. (1970). Use of sodium chloride solutions by the Brewer's sparrow and tree sparrow. *Auk* **87,** 329–341.

Ohmart, R. D., and Smith, E. L. (1971). Water deprivation and use of sodium chloride solutions by Vesper sparrows (*Pooecetes gramineus*). *Condor* **73,** 364–366.

Okoche, A., Farner, D. S., Serventy, D. L., Wolff, F., and Nicholls, C. A. (1963). The hypothalamo-ħypophysial neurosecretory system of the Zebra finch (*Taeniopygia castanotis*). *Z. Zellforsch. Mikrosk. Anat.* **58,** 846–914.

Pick, H. L., and Kare, M. R. (1962). The effect of artificial cues on the measurement of taste preference in the chicken. *J. Comp. Physiol. Psychol.* **55,** 342–345.

Poulson, T. L. (1969). Salt and water balance in Seaside and Sharp-tailed sparrows. *Auk* **86,** 473–489.

Poulson, T. L., and Bartholomew, G. A. (1962). Salt balance in the Savannah sparrow. *Physiol. Zool.* **35,** 109–119.

Purdue, J. R., and Haines, H. (1977). Salt water tolerance and water turnover in the snowy plover. *Auk* **94,** 248–255.

Skadhauge, E., and Bradshaw, S. D. (1974). Saline drinking and cloacal excretion of salt and water in the Zebra finch. *Am. J. Physiol.* **227,** 1263–1267.

Smyth, M., and Bartholomew, G. A. (1966a). The water economy of the black throated sparrow and the Rock Wren. *Condor* **68,** 447–458.

Smyth, M., and Bartholomew, G. A. (1966b). Effects of water deprivation and sodium chloride on the blood and urine of the mourning dove. *Auk* **83,** 597–602.

Welty, J. C. (1967). "The Life of Birds." Saunders, Philadelphia, Pennsylvania.

Willoughby, E. J. (1966). Water requirements of the ground dove. *Condor* **68,** 243–248.

Willoughby, E. J. (1968). Water economy of the Stark's Lark and Grey-backed finch-Lark from the Namib desert of South-West Africa. *Comp. Biochem. Physiol.* **27,** 723–745.

Willoughby, E. J. (1971). Drinking responses of the red crossbill (*Loxia curvirosta*) to solutions of NaCl, $MgCl_2$ and $CaCl_2$. *Auk* **88,** 828–838.

Chapter 7

Sensory Analysis of the Taste of NaCl

LINDA M. BARTOSHUK

I. SOURCE OF SALTINESS: CATIONS

Salts produce complex tastes. Von Skramlik (1922) matched the complex tastes of a variety of salts with mixtures of NaCl, glucose, tartaric acid, and quinine hydrochloride. The ability to analyze the taste of salts into salty, sweet, sour, and bitter components led to the attempt to attribute taste qualities to particular anions, cations, or undissociated molecules.

Höber and Kiesow (1898) and Kahlenberg (1898) both concluded that saltiness is produced by anions, particularly Cl^-. This was also the conclusion of Kionka and Strätz (1922) and Dzendolet and Meiselman (1967). The logic by which they came to this conclusion is demonstrated in a quote from Kahlenberg (1898, p. 20). "It was found that of the persons tested . . . all recognized *n*/25 [0.04 *M*

BIOLOGICAL AND BEHAVIORAL
ASPECTS OF SALT INTAKE

ISBN 0-12-397750-9

NaCl] as a trifle salty. . . . As equivalent solutions of sodium acetate are not salty, possessing hardly any taste, it is clear that the salty taste of the common salt solutions is due to the chlorine ions.''

Kionka and Strätz (1922) added to this conclusion the observation that while the taste quality of salts is determined by anions, the intensity of the taste is determined by the cations. The logic underlying this conclusion rested on thresholds. Salts with a common cation but differing anions produced similar absolute thresholds.

Neural recordings offer a very different point of view about salt taste. First, it is important to note that here the emphasis is on taste responses to the chemical class of salts rather than on the taste quality, saltiness. Beidler (1953, 1954, 1967) identified cations as the active stimuli for neural responses to salts and gave the anion an inhibitory role. The identification of cations as the active part of the salt was based originally on neural responses to a series of salts with sodium in common and a series with chloride in common. Beidler (1954, p. 602) concluded: ``The anion of a salt appears to be of much less consequence than the cation in the stimulation of the 'salt' chemoreceptor. The magnitudes of the responses of many sodium salts are similar. This is in contrast to the magnitudes of the responses to various chloride salts which varied considerably.'' For salts with a common cation, magnitude of neural response tended to decrease as the size of the anion increased (Beidler, 1967). Several mechanisms for this anionic inhibition effect have been proposed (Beidler, 1967; DeSimone and Price, 1976; DeSimone *et al.*, 1979; Mooser, this volume).

This conclusion, that cations are excitatory and anions are inhibitory, contradicts the conclusions from the psychophysical studies discussed above. However, if we reexamine those studies, a logical flaw becomes apparent. The psychophysical studies were all based on the assumption that the taste of a salt is the sum of the tastes of the components. Suppose we reexamine these studies in the light of Beidler's insights concerning the inhibitory role of anions. The same observations take on different meaning. If we assume that saltiness is produced by cations, then in a series of salts with a common cation, the chloride salts are seen to be the saltiest because they are the least inhibitory. The sodium cation produces a pure salty taste. Other cations like K^+ and $NH_4{}^+$ are both bitter and salty.

Could the earlier investigators have proved from psychophysical data alone that anions inhibit the tastes evoked by cations? Consider a comparison of the tastes of potassium chloride (KCl) and potassium bicarbonate ($KHCO_3$). Table I shows the perceived intensities of the various qualities reported for each salt. $KHCO_3$ is less salty (two-tailed, paired t: $p < 0.01$) and less bitter (two-tailed, paired t: $p < 0.001$) than KCl. If we follow the earlier reasoning, KCl tastes bitter-salty because the K^+ is bitter and the Cl^- is salty (note that bitterness must be attributed to K^+ because NaCl is not bitter). $KHCO_3$ is less salty than KCl

TABLE I

Perceived Intensities of Various Qualities for KCl and $KHCO_3$[a]

Salt	Salty	Sweet	Sour	Bitter
KCl	37.1 ± 8.0	0		42.4 ± 6.1
$KHCO_3$	10.3 ± 1.8	3.0 ± 3.0	4.2 ± 2.6	8.1 ± 3.2

[a] Values are mean magnitude estimates ± 1 SEM from 10 subjects.

because HCO^-_3 is a less salty anion. But why would $KHCO_3$ be less bitter than KCl? The earlier reasoning is contradicted by this observation. It should be noted that this observation is interesting for another reason. It demonstrates that Beidler's anionic inhibition works on the bitterness as well as the saltiness evoked by K^+, an observation not previously available.

In addition to the inhibitory role discussed above, some anions must have excitatory roles in taste by virtue of their structure. For example, the sweet taste of Na saccharin is attributed to the saccharin anion. The saccharin anion contains the AH, B, γ structure proposed by Shallenberger and his colleagues (Shallenberger and Acree, 1971; Shallenberger, 1977) to be the basic unit of sweet taste. In general, as molecular weight increases for salts with a common cation, the salts tend to get increasingly bitter (Moncrieff, 1967). There are a variety of structures associated with bitterness.

In summary, saltiness appears to be produced by cations. Sodium (and possibly lithium) does not evoke other qualities. A variety of simple cations (e.g., K^+, NH^+_4) evoke bitterness as well as saltiness. Anions inhibit the effects of cations. Both anions and cations are capable of evoking bitterness and sometimes sweetness when their structures contain groups associated with those qualities.

It is clear, even from this very simplified account, that the contributions of cations and anions to the taste of salts are complicated. The discussion above does not even consider mixture interactions, a phenomenon which almost certainly occurs in salts that have complex tastes. Yet, to a first approximation, particular tastes can be attributed to individual ions but the attributions in the earlier literature are incorrect.

II. SWEETNESS OF SALTS

Dilute NaCl (as well as some other salts) has a sweet taste (Renqvist, 1919; Kionka and Strätz, 1922; Bartoshuk *et al.*, 1964, 1978; Dzendolet and Meiselman, 1967; Bartoshuk, 1974; Cardello and Murphy, 1977). Figure 1 shows the results of an experiment designed to test the suggestion (Dzendolet, 1968; Shal-

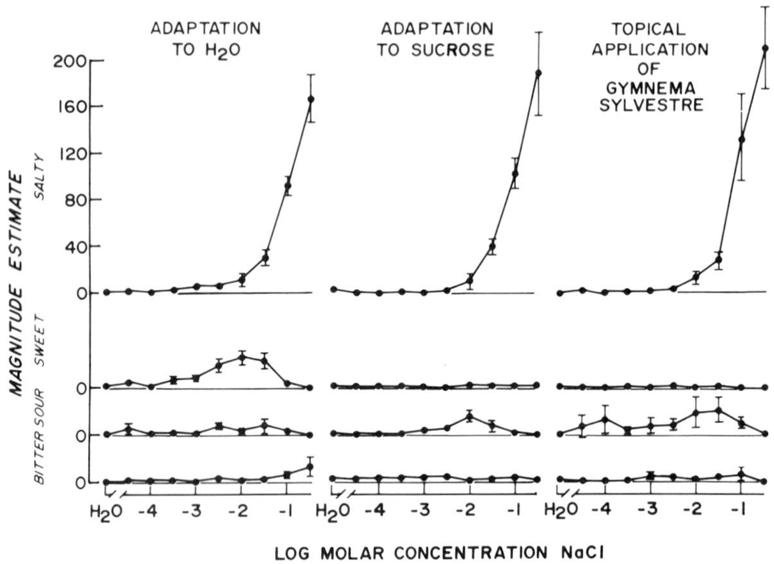

Fig. 1. Magnitude estimates (± 1 SEM) of the perceived intensities of the saltiness, sweetness, sourness, and bitterness of NaCl after adaptation to water and to sucrose and after topical application of *Gymnema sylvestre*. Sucrose at 0.032 *M* was 45.1 ± 6.0 sweet when judged as a stimulus. (From Bartoshuk, Murphy, and Cleveland, 1978).

lenberger and Acree, 1971) that the sweetness of dilute NaCl is produced by water of hydration around the Na^+ ions. If this view is correct, then the sweetness of dilute NaCl is produced by the same structure as that responsible for the sweetness of conventional sweeteners like sucrose, and cross-adaptation with sucrose and topical application of *Gymnema sylvestre* should depress it.

Ten subjects evaluated NaCl (stimuli warmed to body temperature and flowed across the extended tongue) with the method of magnitude estimation (Stevens, 1969). With this method, subjects assign numbers to the perceived intensities of individual taste qualities such that the ratios among the numbers reflect the ratios among the perceived intensities. For example, if the first stimulus was called "10 salty" and the second stimulus was perceived to be twice as intense but half sweet and half salty, then the subject would call it "10 sweet" and "10 salty."

The left part of Figure 1 shows the taste of NaCl after a water rinse. The center and right parts show the effects of adaptation to sucrose and topical application of *Gymnema sylvestre,* respectively. The sweet taste is clearly abolished by both operations.

In summary, the evidence suggests that the saltiness of NaCl is produced by Na^+ ions, and the sweetness of dilute NaCl is produced by water molecules organized around the Na^+ ions such that they produce the structure required for sweet.

III. ADAPTATION

Adaptation to NaCl has two important effects on the taste of NaCl. First, NaCl is salty only at concentrations above the adapting concentration (Hahn, 1934; McBurney and Pfaffmann, 1963). Second, concentrations below the adapting concentration evoke a bitter–sour taste that increases in intensity as the concentration decreases until it reaches a maximum at water (Bartoshuk *et al.*, 1964; McBurney, 1966; Bartoshuk, 1968). These phenomena are shown by the magnitude estimate functions in Fig. 2. The relation between these functions and the relevant thresholds is also shown in Fig. 2. The thresholds were obtained with the up-down method (see Bartoshuk, 1974, for more details). Recognition thresholds, the thresholds for the recognition of a particular quality, are shown above the appropriate quality function. Detection thresholds, the thresholds for the detection of any taste, are shown above the functions for the total taste.

Note that the sweetness of dilute NaCl is abolished by adaptation to 0.01 *M*

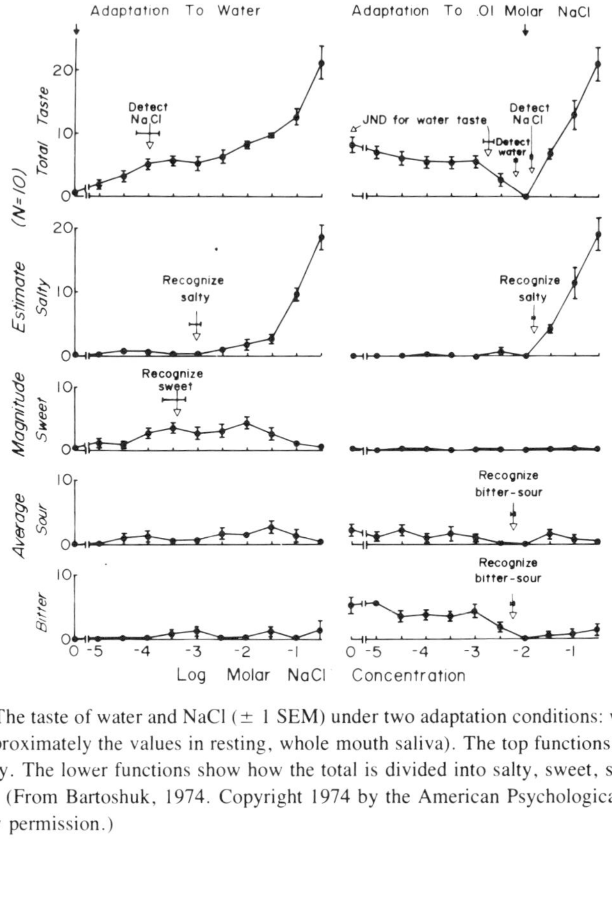

Fig. 2. The taste of water and NaCl (± 1 SEM) under two adaptation conditions: water and 0.01 *M* NaCl (approximately the values in resting, whole mouth saliva). The top functions show the total taste intensity. The lower functions show how the total is divided into salty, sweet, sour, and bitter components. (From Bartoshuk, 1974. Copyright 1974 by the American Psychological Association. Reprinted by permission.)

NaCl. This is consistent with our interpretation of the data in Fig. 1. That is, the sweet stimulus present in dilute NaCl (the water organized around the Na^+ ions) is adapted by the 0.01 *M* NaCl.

The adaptation data show that a salty taste occurs when there is an increment in NaCl concentration and a bitter–sour taste occurs when there is a decrement. The salty taste appears to depend on an increment of Na^+ while the bitter–sour taste may depend on a decrement in Cl^-. Cohen *et al.* (1955) and Bartoshuk (1965) showed that Na acetate following NaCl produced a water response in the cat but choline Cl following NaCl did not. Presumably, Cl^- ions would be removed by Na acetate but not by choline Cl.

A. Adaptation to Saliva

Saliva contains Na^+ and Cl^-. As salivary flow rate increases, the concentration of both ions increases. Resting whole mouth saliva in man contains about 0.01 *M* Na^+ and Cl^- on the average although there is a great deal of intersubject variation. Even with increases in flow rate, human whole mouth saliva cannot reach isotonicity (about 0.15 *M*) because submaxillary and parotid salivas never reach isotonicity (Schneyer *et al.*, 1972).

Figure 3 shows magnitude estimates of NaCl from two subjects adapted to their own saliva (each subject evaluated each concentration once after a water rinse and once while adapted to saliva). Samples of saliva were collected just before each stimulus was tasted. Na^+ was measured with flame photometry and Cl^- was measured with the Schales and Schales (1941) procedure. The salivary Na^+ values were 0.017 ± 0.0006 and 0.016 ± 0.0016 and the Cl^- values were 0.012 ± 0.0004 and 0.016 ± 0.0011. The functions in Fig. 3 look qualitatively similar to those in Fig. 2.

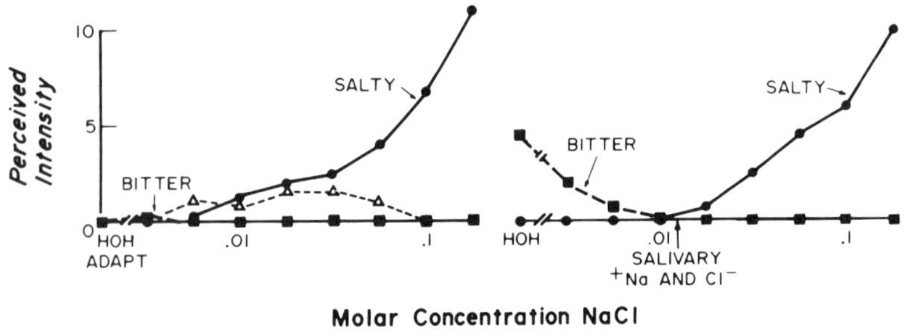

Fig. 3. Taste of NaCl under two adapting concentrations: water and saliva. Stimuli were tasted with the sip and spit method. The sweetness of dilute NaCl is shown by the dotted line. Responses are the means of two subjects, each of whom judged the stimuli once. Salivary Na^+ values were 0.017 ± 0.0006 and 0.016 ± 0.0016 and Cl^- values were 0.012 ± 0.0004 and 0.016 ± 0.0011, respectively.

B. Perceived Saltiness and Changes in Salivary Na^+ and Cl^-

Figure 4 shows the perceived saltiness of NaCl for one subject under three adapting conditions: water, resting saliva (obtained after a 3-min rest), and stimulated saliva (obtained after 1 min of chewing rubber bands). As the concentration of sodium increased, the saltiness responses shifted to the right. Note that just as in Fig. 2, the NaCl concentrations just above the adapting concentration were the most affected. The higher concentrations remain unaffected. That is, adaptation steepens the function by reducing the perceived intensities of the lower concentrations. This phenomenon was first observed in taste by McBurney (1966). It is called recruitment in analogy to a similar phenomenon, recruitment deafness, in audition.

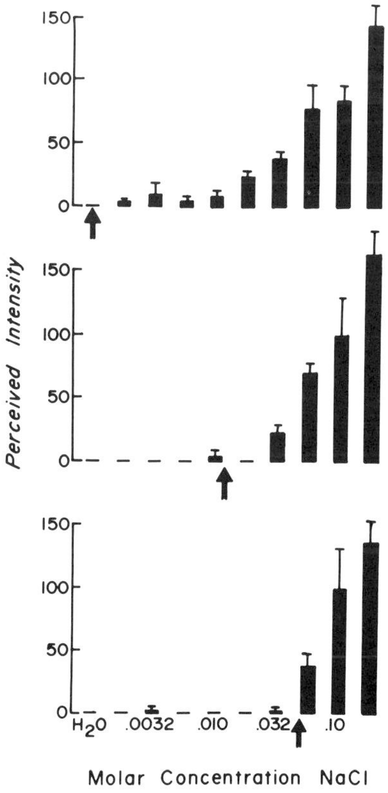

Fig. 4. Perceived intensity (magnitude estimates ± 1 SEM) of the saltiness of NaCl under water adaptation (top function), adaptation to resting saliva (middle function), and adaptation to stimulated saliva (bottom function). Salivary sodium concentrations (0.018 ± 0.002, resting; 0.051 ± 0.003, stimulated) are indicated by the arrows under the middle and bottom functions. Data points are means of five runs ± 1 SEM from a single subject. Stimuli were flowed across the tongue. (From Bartoshuk, 1978).

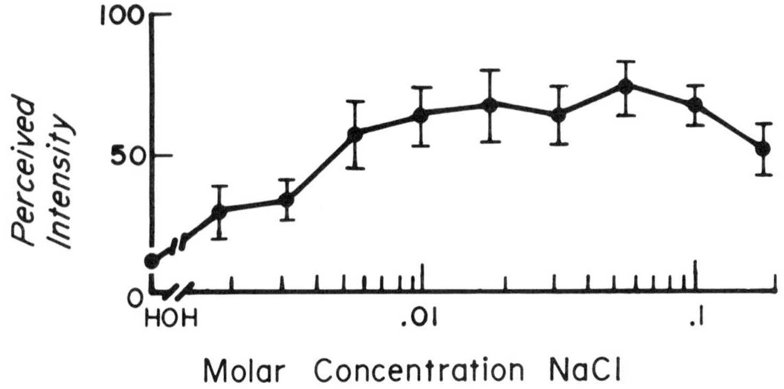

Fig. 5. Magnitude estimates (± 1 SEM) of the perceived intensity of the taste of water after adaptation to various concentrations of NaCl ($N = 6$). (Bartoshuk and Cleveland, International Congress of Physiological Sciences, Paris, 1977.)

C. Taste of Water as a Function of Variation in NaCl Adapting Concentration

Initially, we had hoped to relate individual differences in the perceived intensity of water to individual variation in salivary Na^+ and/or Cl^- levels. Figure 5 shows the perceived intensity of water as a function of the NaCl adapting concentration. This experiment replicates an earlier one (Bartoshuk, 1978) but in this experiment resting and stimulated salivary Na^+ and Cl^- values were measured. The ranges were: resting Cl^-, 0.012–0.020 *M*, Na^+, 0.008–0.019 *M*; stimulated (by 3 min of chewing rubber bands) Cl^-, 0.013–0.039 *M*; Na^+, 0.014–0.051 *M*. Note that the function is quite flat over these ranges of normal salivary electrolyte values. This suggests that Na^+ and Cl^- variation is not likely to be the sole explanation of variation in the perceived intensity of the bitter–sour water taste induced by adaptation to saliva.

D. Taste Thresholds and Adaptation to Saliva

Salivary sodium provides a lower limit for thresholds for the taste of NaCl. Yet there are a variety of studies that give NaCl threshold values below salivary Na^+ values in which subjects appear to be adapted to their own saliva. There are several possible explanations: (1) the saliva may be collected under different conditions than those operating during threshold testing; (2) the theshold testing may provide for shifting adaptation conditions (e.g., permitting a subject to sample back and forth between a water stimulus and a NaCl stimulus) which might remove enough saliva on some trials to permit the tasting of NaCl concentrations below salivary Na^+; (3) when detection thresholds are measured, subjects may detect water instead of NaCl (see Fig. 2). For example, DeWardener and Herx heimer (1957) reported NaCl recognition thresholds that were much lower than measured salivary Na^+ levels. They also failed to find a correlation between salivary Na^+ and NaCl thresholds. However, they stimulated salivation to measure salivary Na^+ which would have raised the values above normal, resting levels and they permitted sampling between water and NaCl stimuli in the threshold test. Similarly, Wotman *et al.* (1967) reported saltiness recognition thresholds that were lower than whole mouth salivary Na^+ levels for their control subjects in a study on hypertension but the saliva was stimulated and subjects sampled both water and NaCl solutions in order to choose the salty stimulus.

Henkin and Powell (1962) reported very low NaCl detection thresholds for children with cystic fibrosis. They used the three-drop technique with no rinse between drops. Salivary Na^+ is elevated in cystic fibrosis (Barbero and Chernick, 1958). The very low detection thresholds may represent water taste thresholds. In support of this, other studies using rinses (Wotman *et al.*, 1964; Hertz *et al.*, 1975) found normal thresholds in children with cystic fibrosis. Another study (Desor and Maller, 1975) permitted subjects to rinse if they chose and found fourteen of sixteen children with cystic fibrosis to have normal detection thresholds. The two children with low thresholds may have detected water or they may have rinsed off saliva.

Studies on Addison's disease have reported abnormally low detection thresholds for NaCl (Henkin *et al.*, 1963) but elevated saltiness recognition thresholds (Henkin, 1975). Since salivary Na^+ is elevated in Addison's disease (Frawley and Thorn, 1951), these results are what would be expected if the subjects were detecting water instead of NaCl but correctly recognizing the saltiness of NaCl.

Studies in which NaCl thresholds are based on actual adaptation to saliva and in which the threshold measure is such that confusions cannot result between NaCl and water taste (McBurney and Pfaffmann, 1963; Morino and Langford, 1978) show the expected relation between salivary Na^+ and NaCl thresholds.

It should be noted that the clinical studies that appeared to violate the laws of taste adaptation were done before these laws were understood.

IV. CROSS-ADAPTATION AMONG SALTS

Cross-adaptation among salts was studied systematically for the first time by Hahn *et al.* (1940). They reported that adaptation to any one of twenty-four salts did not elevate the thresholds for the others (i.e., there was no cross-adaptation). McBurney and his students (McBurney and Lucas, 1966; Smith and McBurney, 1969) studying the saltiness of suprathreshold concentrations of salts came to a very different conclusion. They found that NaCl completely cross-adapted the saltiness of all salts tested.

Figures 6 and 7 show the results of an experiment run by B. Bierer as part of a Senior Thesis Project at Yale University. The experiment was designed to show how Hahn's reliance on detection thresholds could have led him to erroneous conclusions. Hahn used a Geschmacksluppe to deliver taste stimuli. The device was actually a small, inverted cup (1.5 cm in diameter) with tubes to introduce and drain away solutions. We flowed stimuli through tubing with an opening similar in size to that used by Hahn. When a limited area of the tongue is stimulated, stimuli taste less intense than when the whole tongue is stimulated, but the rate at which taste intensity grows with concentration remains the same (Smith, 1971). Thus the left part of Fig. 6 looks similar to the left parts of Figs. 1 and 2. However, the water taste was reduced relatively more (i.e., the center part of Fig. 6 does not show the typical bitter–sour taste of the NaCl concentrations below the adapting concentration.)

The right parts of Figs. 6 and 7 show cross-adaptation between NaCl and KCl. Figure 7 shows that adaptation to NaCl abolishes the saltiness of KCl below 0.1 *M*. However, the bitterness of KCl is not abolished and, if anything, is increased. The detection threshold for KCl would be changed little, if any, by NaCl adaptation.

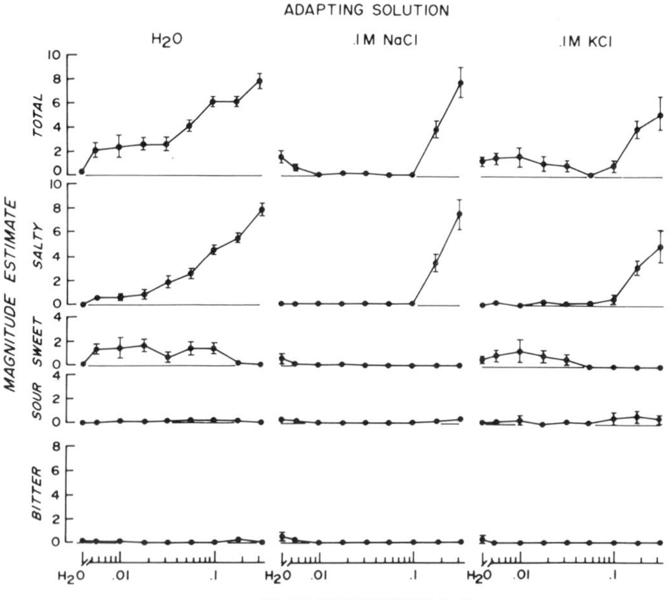

Fig. 6. Magnitude estimates (± 1 SEM) of the taste of NaCl under three adapting solutions: water, 0.1 *M* NaCl, and 0.1 *M* KCl ($N = 8$). Solutions were warmed to body temperature and flowed (4 ml/sec) across the tongue through a "Hahn Geschmacksluppe." (Data collected by B. Bierer as part of her senior thesis at Yale University.)

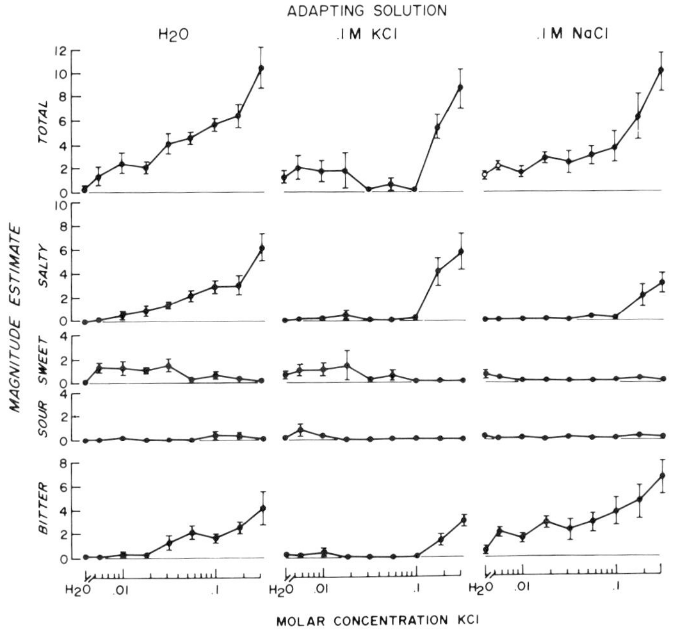

Fig. 7. Magnitude estimates (± 1 SEM) of the taste of KCl under three adapting solutions: water, 0.1 *M* KCl, and 0.1 *M* NaCl ($N = 8$). Solutions were warmed to body temperature and flowed (4 ml/sec) across the tongue through a "Hahn Geschmacksluppe." (Data collected by B. Bierer as part of her senior thesis at Yale University.)

The reverse case is less clear. Figure 6 shows that adaptation to KCl abolishes the saltiness of NaCl below 0.1 *M* NaCl. In addition, adaptation to KCl produces a sweet water taste. Although we cannot draw any conclusions for certain because we do not know the exact way in which Hahn's thresholds were determined, Hahn's subjects may have somehow confused the water taste with NaCl taste.

V. CROSS-ADAPTATION AMONG NaCl, CITRIC ACID, SUCROSE, CAFFEINE, AND UREA

"Successive contrast" between substances with different taste qualities was reported in early work (Kiesow, 1894; Henning, 1927). This phenomenon, believed to be analogous to colored afterimages in vision, referred to an intensification of the taste of a solution after the tasting of a solution of a different quality.

A later study with controls for water tastes (McBurney and Bartoshuk, 1973) suggested that the apparent enhancement was actually the addition of a water taste to the normal solute taste. This study was designed as follows. First, solutions of five substances were matched for perceived intensity. These were: 0.1 *M* NaCl, 0.82 *M* urea, 0.004 *M* citric acid, 0.1 *M* caffeine, and 0.18 *M* sucrose. These concentrations, the concentrations 1/2 and 1 log step weaker, and water were evaluated after adaptation to each of the five matched solutions and water. The effects of adaptation to each of these substances on the taste of NaCl are shown in Fig. 8. The total intensity functions (top of Fig. 8) show clear effects of adaptation (compare the water-adapted NaCl function on the left to the other functions in the top row). However, an examination of the individual qualities shows that apparent enhancement effects are water tastes. For example, water tastes salty after adaptation to urea (see the leftmost point in the third function from the left in the bottom row). Thus the increases in the saltiness of the two weakest concentrations of NaCl are actually due to the addition of a salty water taste and not enhancement of the salty taste of NaCl. Kiesow's contrast appears to have been a water taste artifact. That is, cross-enhancement among different qualities does not appear to be a major taste phenomenon.

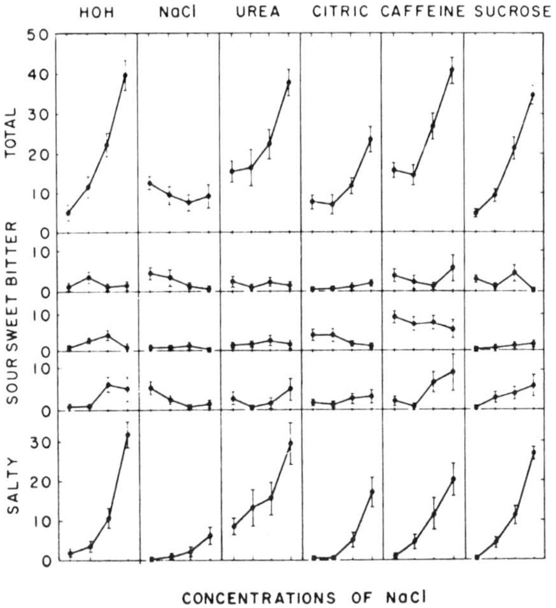

Fig. 8. Effects of adaptation to water and to five compounds on the taste of water and NaCl. The top row shows the effects on the total taste intensity. The other rows show the effect on bitterness, sweetness, sourness, and saltiness, respectively. Each column shows the effects of one adapting condition. Within each cell, the four points show the effects of a particular adapting solution on the total intensity, or the intensity of one quality, on water and NaCl. The leftmost point in each cell represents water, followed by the three concentrations of NaCl, in order. Data are means (± 1 SEM) of ten subjects. (From McBurney and Bartoshuk, 1973.)

What about cross-adaptation among qualities? In the experiment described above, adaptation to any one of the five substances did not abolish the tastes of any of the other four; however, the tastes of some substances were reduced in intensity. In particular, the saltiness of NaCl was significantly reduced by adaptation to citric acid and caffeine. The meaning of these reductions is complicated by mixture interactions. That is, both citric acid and caffeine produce sweet water tastes. Thus NaCl following either citric acid or caffeine will be a mixture of sweet and salty. The reduction in saltiness could be a consequence of the presence of sweetness.

VI. MIXTURES CONTAINING NaCl

When substances with different taste qualities are mixed, the perceived intensities are usually reduced. The amount of the reduction appears to depend on several variables including the shapes of the psychophysical functions (Bartoshuk, 1975; Bartoshuk and Cleveland, 1977). For example, if the perceived intensity of the taste of a substance grows with concentration in a simple linear fashion, then doubling concentration will double the perceived intensity. However, if perceived intensity grows more slowly than concentration (this kind of psychophysical function is said to show compression), then doubling concentration will not double perceived intensity. In our first experiment on substances with different tastes, the degree to which the taste of a substance showed compression was closely related to the degree to which the taste of that substance was suppressed in mixtures (Bartoshuk, 1975). In order to test this relation more fully, we changed the degree of compression by varying temperature and tasting method. The degree of compression continued to be a good predictor of mixture suppression for some pairs of substances, particularly sucrose and QHCl, but failed to predict mixture suppression in others, particularly NaCl and QHCl. In these mixtures, the bitterness of quinine was usually substantially reduced (often to 50% or less of its unmixed taste) while the saltiness of NaCl was much less reduced. In one mixture experiment (done in combination with the data reported in Bartoshuk, 1975), the tongue was adapted to one of the components in the

TABLE II

Effect of NaCl on Bitterness of Quinine

Stimulus	Adaptation condition	Bitterness of stimulus
QHCl	H_2O	23.31 ± 2.21
NaCl + QHCl	H_2O	12.80 ± 3.59
NaCl + QHCl	NaCl	8.92 ± 3.08

mixture before the mixture was tasted. In general, this released the suppression. But there was one exception: adaptation to NaCl did not return the bitterness of a mixture of NaCl and quinine to the normal bitterness of quinine (Table II). This suggests the possibility of a peripheral effect of NaCl on the mechanism underlying the taste of QHCl.

VII. SUMMARY

Early analyses of the sources of taste in salts, assumed that the taste of a salt is the sum of the tastes of its components. Beidler (1953, 1954, 1967) suggested that cations are excitatory and anions inhibitory in taste. This logic, applied to human evaluation of the tastes of salts, produces an internally consistent assignment of tastes to ions. Saltiness can be attributed to sodium and lithium. Cations like potassium taste both salty and bitter. The simple anion chloride is the least inhibitory and has no taste of its own. More complex anions both inhibit the responses produced by the cations and can take on their own tastes (primarily bitter). Water organized around cations appears to account for the sweet tastes reported for some dilute salts.

When mixtures are constructed from substances with different taste qualities, most salts evoke more than one quality. Complex interactions which we are just beginning to understand change the perceived intensities of the components. These kinds of interactions may also occur in salts with complex tastes.

REFERENCES

Barbero, G. J., and Chernick, W. (1958). Function of the salivary gland in cystic fibrosis of the pancreas. *Pediatrics* **22,** 945–952.

Bartoshuk, L. M. (1965). Effects of adaptation on responses to water in cat and rat. Doctoral dissertation. Brown University, Providence, Rhode Island. No. 16–13,630 (University Microfilms, Ann Arbor, Michigan, 1965).

Bartoshuk, L. M. (1968). Water taste in man. *Percept. & Psychophys.* **3,** 69–72.

Bartoshuk, L. M. (1974). NaCl thresholds in man: Thresholds for water taste or NaCl taste? *J. Comp. Physiol. Psychol.* **87,** 310–325.

Bartoshuk, L. M. (1975). Taste mixtures: Is mixture suppression related to compression? *Physiol. Behav.* **14,** 643–649.

Bartoshuk, L. M. (1977). Water taste in mammals. *In* "Drinking Behavior" (J. A. W. Weijnen and J. Mendelson, eds.), pp. 000–000. Plenum, New York.

Bartoshuk, L. M. (1978). Psychophysics of taste. *Am. J. Clin. Nutr.* **31,** 1068–1077.

Bartoshuk, L. M. and Cleveland, C. T. (1977). "Taste of water: Effects of saliva." Paper presented at the International Congress of Physiological Sciences, Paris, 1977.

Bartoshuk, L. M., and Cleveland, C. T. (1977). Mixtures of substances with similar tastes: A test of a new model of taste mixture interactions. *Sens. Proc.* **1,** 177–186.

Bartoshuk, L. M., McBurney, D. H., and Pfaffmann, C. (1964). Taste of sodium chloride solutions after adaptation to sodium chloride: Implications for the "water taste." *Science* **143,** 967–968.

Bartoshuk, L. M., Murphy, C., and Cleveland, C. T. (1978). Sweet taste of dilute NaCl: Psychophysical evidence for a sweet stimulus. *Physiol. Behav.* **21,** 609-613.

Beidler, L. M. (1953). Properties of chemoreceptors of tongue of rat. *J. Neurophysiol.* **16,** 595-607.

Beidler, L. M. (1954). A theory of taste stimulation. *J. Gen. Physiol.* **38,** 133-159.

Beidler, L. M. (1967). Anion influences on taste receptor response. *In* "Olfaction and Taste II" (T. Hayashi, ed.), pp. 509-534. Pergamon, Oxford.

Cardello, A. V., and Murphy, C. (1977). Magnitude estimates of gustatory quality changes as a function of solution concentration of simple salts. *Chem. Senses Flavor* **2,** 327-339.

Cohen, M. J., Hagiwara, S., and Zotterman, Y. (1955). The response spectrum of taste fibres in the cat: A single fibre analysis. *Acta Physiol. Scand.* **33,** 316-332.

DeSimone, J. A., and Price, S. (1976). A model for the stimulation of taste receptor cells by salt. *Biophys. J.* **16,** 869-880.

DeSimone, J. A., Heck, G. L., and DeSimone, S. K. (1979). A surface chemical model of salt, acid, and "water taste." *In* "Advances in Chemistry. Monograph of the American Chemical Society" (M. Blank, ed.) (in press).

DeSor, J. A., and Maller, O. (1975). Taste correlates of disease states: Cystic fibroses. *J. Pediatr.* **87,** 93-96.

DeWardener, H. E., and Herxheimer, A. (1957). The effect of a high water intake on salt consumption, taste thresholds and salivary secretion in man. *J. Physiol. (London)* **139,** 53-63.

Dzendolet, E. (1968). A structure common to sweet-evoking compounds. *Percept. & Psychophys.* **3,** 65-68.

Dzendolet, E., and Meiselman, H. L. (1967). Cation and anion contributions to gustatory quality of simple salts. *Percept. & Psychophys.* **2,** 601-604.

Frawley, T. F., and Thorn, G. W. (1951). The relation of the salivary sodium-potassium ratio to adrenal cortical activity. *Proc. Clin ACTH Conf., 2nd, 1950* Vol. 1, 115-122.

Hahn, H. (1934). Die adaptation des Geschmackssinnes. *Z. Sinnesphysiol.* **65,** 8-145.

Hahn, H., Kuckulies, G., and Bissar, A. (1940). Eine systematische Untersuchung der Geschmacksschwellen. II. *Z. Sinnesphysiol.* **68,** 185-260.

Henkin, R. I. (1975). The role of adrenal corticosteroids in sensory processes. *In* "Handbook of Physiology" (S. R. Geiger, ed.), Sect. 7, Vol. VI, pp. 209-230. Am. Physiol. Soc., Washington, D. C.

Henkin, R. I., and Powell, G. F. (1962). Increased sensitivity of taste and smell in cystic fibrosis. *Science* **138,** 1107-1108.

Henkin, R. I., Gill, J. R., and Bartter, F. C. (1963). Studies on taste thresholds in normal man and in patients with adrenal cortical insufficiency: The role of adrenal cortical steroids and of serum sodium concentration. *J. Clin. Invest.* **42,** 727-735.

Henning, H. (1927). Psychologische studien am Geschmackssinn. *In* "Handbuch der biologischen Arbeitsmethoden" (E. Aberhalden, ed.), pp. 627-740. Urban & Schwarzenberg, Berlin.

Hertz, J., Cain, W. S., Bartoshuk, L. M., and Dolan, T. F. (1975). Olfactory and taste sensitivity in children with cystic fibrosis. *Physiol. Behav.* **14,** 89-94.

Höber, R., and Kiesow, F. (1898). Ueber den Geschmack von Salzen und Laugen. *Z. Phys. Chem.* **27,** 601-616.

Kahlenberg, L. (1898). The action of solutions on the sense of taste. *Bull. Univ. Wis.* **2,** 3-31.

Kiesow, F. (1894). Beiträge zur physiologischen Psychologie des Geschmackssinnes. *Philos. Stud.* **10,** 523-561.

Kionka, H., and Strätz, F. (1922). Setzt der Geschmack eines Salzes sich Zusammen aus dem Geschmack der einzelnen Ionen odor schmeckt man jedes Salz als Gesamtmolekül. *Arch. Exp. Pathol. Pharmakol.* **95,** 241-257.

McBurney, D. H. (1966). Magnitude estimation of the taste of sodium chloride after adaptation to sodium chloride. *J. Exp. Psychol.* **72,** 869-873.

McBurney, D. H., and Bartoshuk, L. M. (1973). Interactions between stimuli with different taste qualities. *Physiol. Behav.* **10,** 1101-1106.
McBurney, D. H., and Lucas, J. A. (1966). Gustatory cross adaptation between salts. *Psychon. Sci.* **4,** 301-302.
McBurney, D. H., and Pfaffmann, C. (1963). Gustatory adaptation to saliva and sodium chloride. *J. Exp. Psychol.* **65,** 523-529.
Moncrieff, R. W. (1967). "The Chemical Senses." Leonard Hill, London.
Morino, T., and Langford, H. G. (1978). Salivary sodium correlates with salt recognition threshold. *Physiol. Behav.* **21,** 45-48.
Renqvist, Y. (1919). Über den Geschmack. *Skand. Arch. Physiol.* **38,** 97-201.
Schales, O., and Schales, S. S. (1941). A simple and accurate method for the determination of chloride in biological fluids. *J. Biol. Chem.* **140,** 879-884.
Schneyer, L. H., Young, J. A., and Schneyer, C. A. (1972). Salivary secretion of electrolytes. *Physiol. Rev.* **52,** 720-777.
Shallenberger, R. S. (1977). Chemical clues to the perception of sweetness. *In* "Sensory Properties of Foods" (G. G. Birch, J. G. Brennan, and K. J. Parker, eds.), pp. 91-100. Appl. Sci. Publ. Ltd., London.
Shallenberger, R. S., and Acree, T. E. (1971). Chemical structure of compounds and their sweet and bitter taste. *In* "Handbook of Sensory Physiology" (L. M. Beidler, ed.), Vol. 4, Part 2, pp. 221-277. Springer-Verlag, Berlin and New York.
Smith, D. V. (1971). Taste intensity as a function of area and concentration: Differentiation between compounds. *J. Exp. Psychol.* **87,** 163-171.
Smith, D. V., and McBurney, D. H. (1969). Gustatory cross-adaptation: Does a single mechanism code the salty taste? *J. Exp. Psychol.* **80,** 101-105.
Stevens, S. S. (1969). Sensory scales of taste intensity. *Percept. & Psychophys.* **6,** 302-308.
von Skramlik, E. (1922). Mischungsgleichungen im Gebiete des Geschmackssinnes. *Z. Psychol. Physiol. Sinnesorg.* **53,** 36-78.
Wotman, S., Mandel, I. D., Khotim, S., Thompson, R. H., Kutscher, A. H., Zegarelli, E. V., and Denning, C. R. (1964). Salt taste thresholds and cystic fibrosis. *Am. J. Dis. Child.* **108,** 372-374.
Wotman, S., Mandel, I. D., Thompson, R. H., and Laragh, J. H. (1967). Salivary electrolytes and salt taste thresholds in hypertension. *J. Chron. Dis.* **20,** 833-840.

Chapter 8

Contribution of the Anion to the Taste Quality of Sodium Salts

SUSAN S. SCHIFFMAN

I. INTRODUCTION

According to the traditional theory of taste, the realm of taste sensations is spanned by four so-called primaries: salty, sweet, sour, and bitter. All other tastes are assumed to be mixtures of these four "primaries." Henning (1916) proposed a gustatory model commonly used today to represent the traditional conception of the taste realm based on four "primary" tastes. His model is a tetrahedron with salty, sweet, sour, and bitter stimuli located at the four corners. Intermediate sensations consisting of mixtures of two primaries are situated on the edges of the tetrahedron, and sensations consisting of three primaries are located on the surfaces. Henning specified that the tetrahedron must be hollow because he believed that gustatory stimuli with sensations produced by four primaries did not exist.

The traditional viewpoint implies that the tastes of sodium salts can also be conceptualized by the tetrahedral model because their taste sensations should fall

BIOLOGICAL AND BEHAVIORAL
ASPECTS OF SALT INTAKE

ISBN 0-12-397750-9

within the salty, sweet, sour, bitter range. Von Skramlik (1922) concluded that the taste sensations of a series of salts which he tested could be matched by mixtures of four standards: salty (NaCl), sweet (glucose), sour (tartaric acid), and bitter (quinine). Sensations comprised of mixtures of four primaries could be represented by the tetrahedral model, falling within the body of the tetrahedron, even though Henning had specified that it was hollow. Other experimenters have not concurred with Von Skramlik's conclusion. Kionka and Strätz (1922) concluded that salts had a very wide range of taste sensations, far greater than the traditional four.

The difficulties encountered in describing salts so that they fall within the traditional taste realm indicate that Henning's tetrahedron is troublesome as a complete gustatory model. Although it is a convenient means of conceptualizing gustatory data, it is closed-ended so that many stimuli, including salts which cannot be described phenomenologically in terms of the four "primaries," cannot be ordered by the model.

A recently developed methodology called "multidimensional scaling" can systematically order taste stimuli without requiring that their sensations be describable in terms of four primaries. Multidimensional scaling procedures are open-ended so that all stimuli can be placed in a space utilizing experimental measures of similarity among the stimuli. These procedures do not require the *a priori* assumption that the taste realm is spanned by a tetrahedron based on "primaries."

Multidimensional scaling procedures require measures of similarity among all pairs of stimuli as input. They arrange stimuli whose sensations are judged to be similar near one another in a resultant space or map. Stimuli whose sensations are judged to be dissimilar are located distant from one another. Several studies in which multidimensional scaling has been applied to gustatory data reveal that the traditional primaries represented by Henning's tetrahedron do not span the range of taste. Yoshida (1963) found that potassium alum and monosodium glutamate fell outside the tetrahedral structure. Schiffman and Erickson (1971) found that Na_2CO_3 and NaOH also fell outside. Schiffman and Dackis (1975) and Schiffman *et al.* (1975) found amino acids, acetylated amino acids, and other nutrients which were not contained within the closed system represented by a tetrahedral structure.

The purpose of this chapter is to demonstrate that the taste sensations of sodium salts do not fall within the salty, sweet, sour, bitter domain. The study reported here is described in more detail by Schiffman *et al.* (1980).

II. METHODS

Thirteen sodium salts, as well as several traditional stimuli—sour (citric acid), sweet (sucrose), and bitter (quinine HCl)—were paired with one another two at a time at two concentrations in two separate experiments. The concentrations used in the two experiments are shown in Table I. In the first experiment, all the sodium salts were paired at 0.2 *M* Na^+. In the second experiment, they were presented at equal overall intensity equated to 0.15 *M* NaCl as determined by pretesting. The sodium salts in the two experiments which had a pH above 7 were also neutralized with their corresponding acids. Sodium acetate, sodium ascorbate, sodium bicarbonate (and carbonate), sodium citrate, and sodium phosphate were presented at natural pH and were also neutralized with acetic acid, ascorbic acid, CO_2, citric acid, and phosphoric acid, respectively. The stimuli were prepared in deionized water and presented in plastic cups at 72°F. Twelve subjects, ranging in age from 19 to 26, took part in each of the experiments.

Ten milliliters of each stimulus were tasted in pairs. The subjects were asked to make judgments of the similarity in overall quality for the two stimuli in a pair by making ratings along a 5-inch line as shown below.

Same ——————————— (5-inch) ——————————— Different

If two stimuli were perceived to taste similar to one another, an X was placed toward the left. If the stimuli were perceived to taste different, an X was placed

TABLE I

The Concentrations of Stimuli Used in the Two Experiments

	Concentrations used	
	Experiment 1	Experiment 2
Monosodium glutamate (MSG)	0.2 *M* Na^+	0.30 *M*
Na acetate	0.2 *M* Na^+	0.47 *M*
Na acetate (neutralized)	0.2 *M* Na^+	0.47 *M*
Na ascorbate	0.2 *M* Na^+	0,50 *M*
Na bicarbonate	0.2 *M* Na^+	0.45 *M*
Na bicarbonate (neutralized)	0.2 *M* Na^+	(—)
Na bromide	0.2 *M* Na^+	0.15 *M*
NaCl	0.2 *M* Na^+	0.15 *M*
Na citrate	0.2 *M* Na^+	0.22 *M*
Na citrate (neutralized)	0.2 *M* Na^+	(0.22 *M*)
Na carbonate	0.2 *M* Na^+	(0.075 *M*)
Na carbonate (neutralized)	0.2 *M* Na^+	(—)
Na phosphate—dibasic	0.2 *M* Na^+	(0.36 *M*)
Na phosphate—dibasic (neutralized)	0.2 *M* Na^+	(0.36 *M*)
Na phosphate (monobasic)	0.2 *M* Na^+	(0.15 *M*)
Na tartrate	0.2 *M* Na^+	(0.34 *M*)
Na succinate	0.2 *M* Na^+	(0.075 *M*)
Na sulfate	0.2 *M* Na^+	(0.25 *M*)
Citric acid	0.2 *M* Na^+	0.006 *M*
Quinine HCl	0.2 *M* Na^+	0.0006 *M*
Sucrose	0.2 *M* Na^+	0.65 *M*

toward the right. These ratings were transcribed from "0" to "100" (a mark at "same" was transcribed as "0" and a mark at "different" was transcribed as "100"). The ratings were used as input for ALSCAL, a multidimensional scaling procedure designed by Takane *et al.* (1977). Judgments were also made on a series of adjective scales used previously in taste experiments (Schiffman and Erickson, 1971; Schiffman *et al.*, 1975, 1978; Schiffman and Dackis, 1975; Schiffman and Engelhard, 1976; Schiffman, 1977). These ratings were also made on 5-inch lines with opposites of the adjectives at each end of the line.

III. RESULTS

ALSCAL was applied to the twelve similarity matrices (for each of the twelve subjects) for both experiments. The spatial arrangements derived were similar in that the sodium salts fell outside the traditional salty, sweet, sour, bitter domain for both experiments. The arrangement for experiment 2 (salts equated in overall intensity to 0.15 *M* NaCl) is shown in Fig. 1. This multidimensional space represents the communalities in the similarity data among the twelve individual subjects participating in the experiment. A three-dimensional space was considered appropriate because no new relationships among the stimuli were found in spaces of higher dimensionality. The spatial arrangement for the salts at equal intensity is preferable for illustration here because some of the salts at 0.2 *M* Na^+ were quite weak in intensity.

Figure 1 clearly illustrates that the traditional standards—NaCl, citric acid, sucrose, and quinine HCl—do not span the taste realm. Monosodium glutamate (MSG) and sodium succinate are located above the standards while the rest of the sodium salts fall toward the right. Neutralization tends to pull the salts toward the traditional range but not within it.

ALSCAL also provides weights for individual subjects which indicate how each person idiosyncratically emphasizes the three dimensions of the space in Fig. 1. The weight spaces are shown in Figs. 2A and B. Each letter represents a subject. If a subject (such as G) weights dimension I more than dimension II, his/her solution is similar to that in Fig. 1 but stretched out eliptically along dimension I. The weight spaces as well as individual solutions found by ALSCAL indicate that only minor individual differences were found in the relative arrangement of stimuli apart from idiosyncratic stretching along the axes.

Much more variation among individuals was found when adjective ratings rather than similarity judgments were employed. Figure 3 shows the individual variation on adjective scales for the stimuli in experiment 2 (salts equated in overall intensity to 0.15 *M* NaCl). The dots indicate the distribution of the individual subject's ratings. The adjective given at the top of each section of the figure indicates the adjective relevant to the subjects located toward the left of the

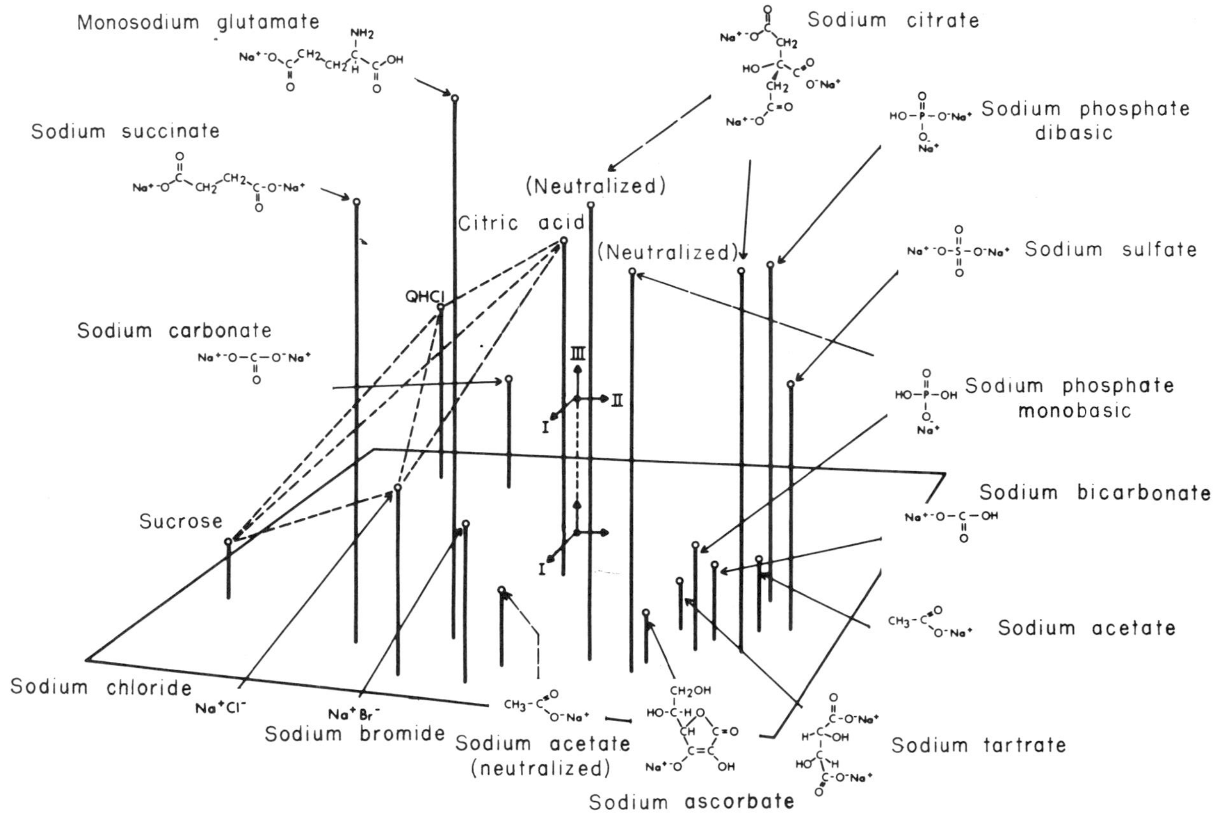

Fig. 1. Multidimensional arrangement of sodium salts and traditional standards achieved by ALSCAL. The sodium salts are not contained within the closed system defined by the four so-called primary tastes represented by: NaCl (salty), citric acid (sour), quinine HCl (bitter), and sucrose (sweet).

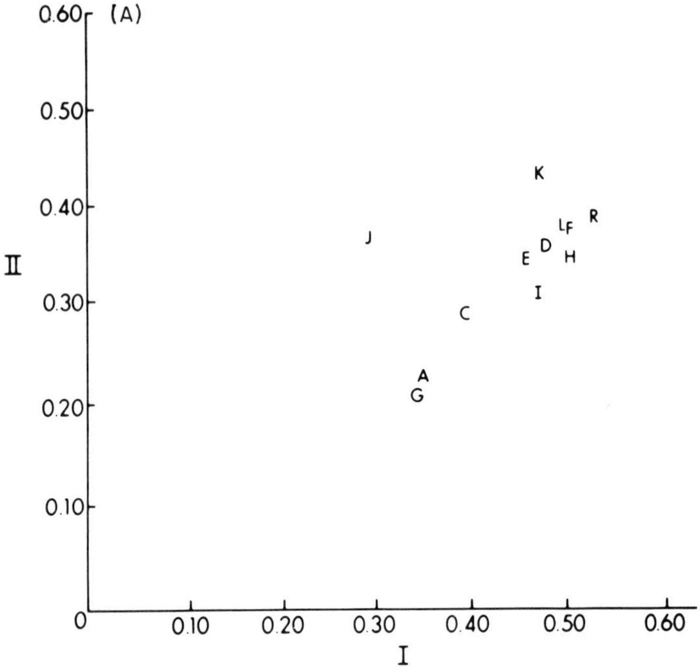

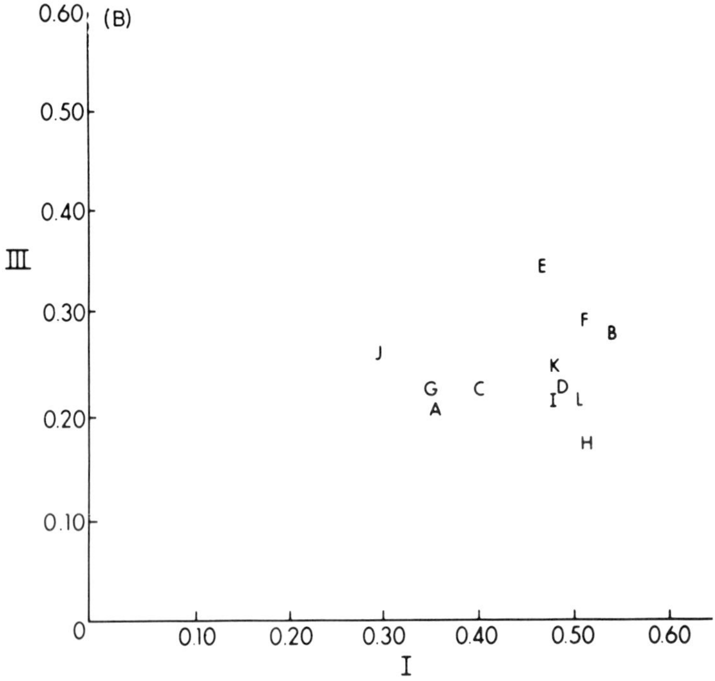

Fig. 2A and B. Weight spaces which indicate the emphasis individual subjects place on the individual dimensions of the three-dimensional space in Fig. 1. Each letter represents a subject.

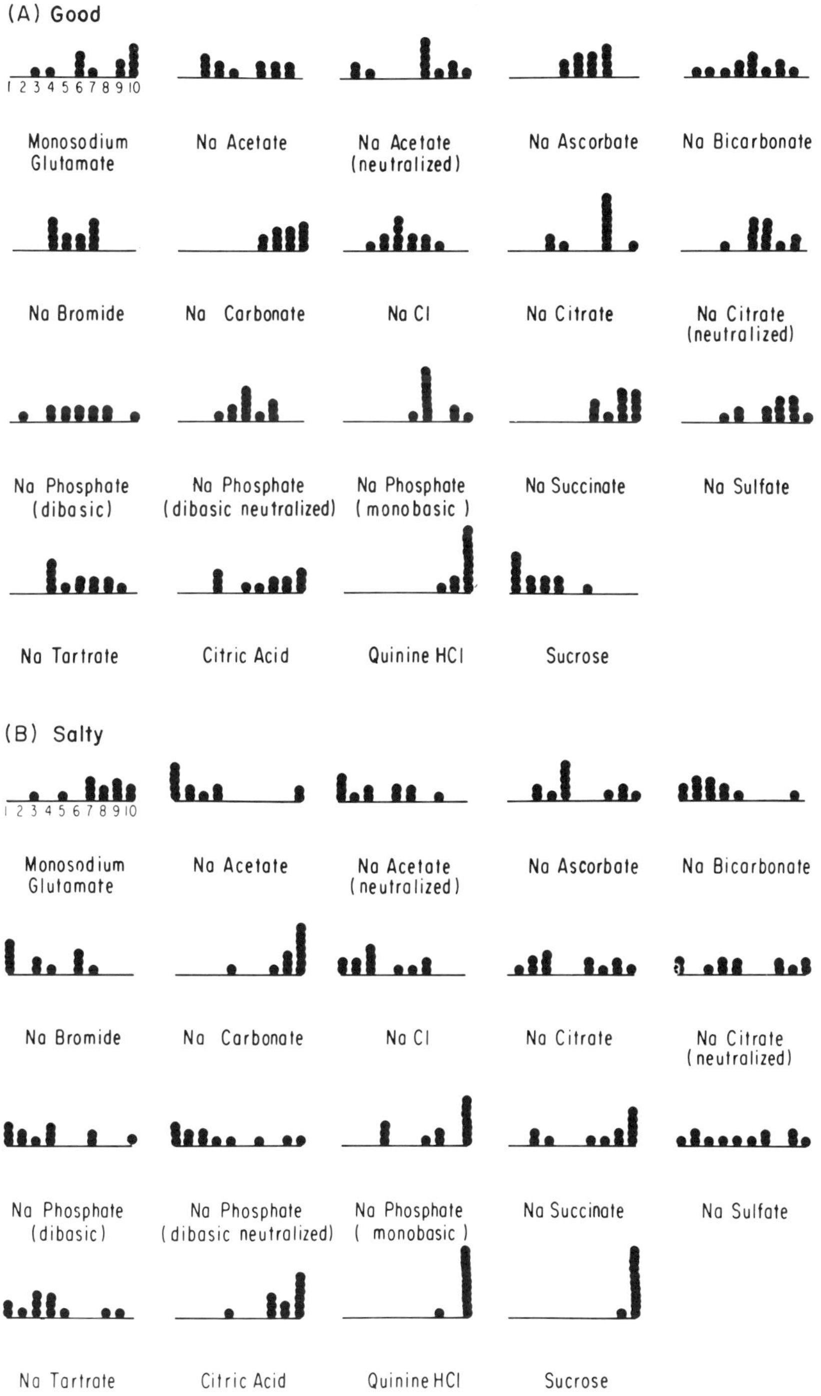

Fig. 3 (See text for explanation.) *(continued)*

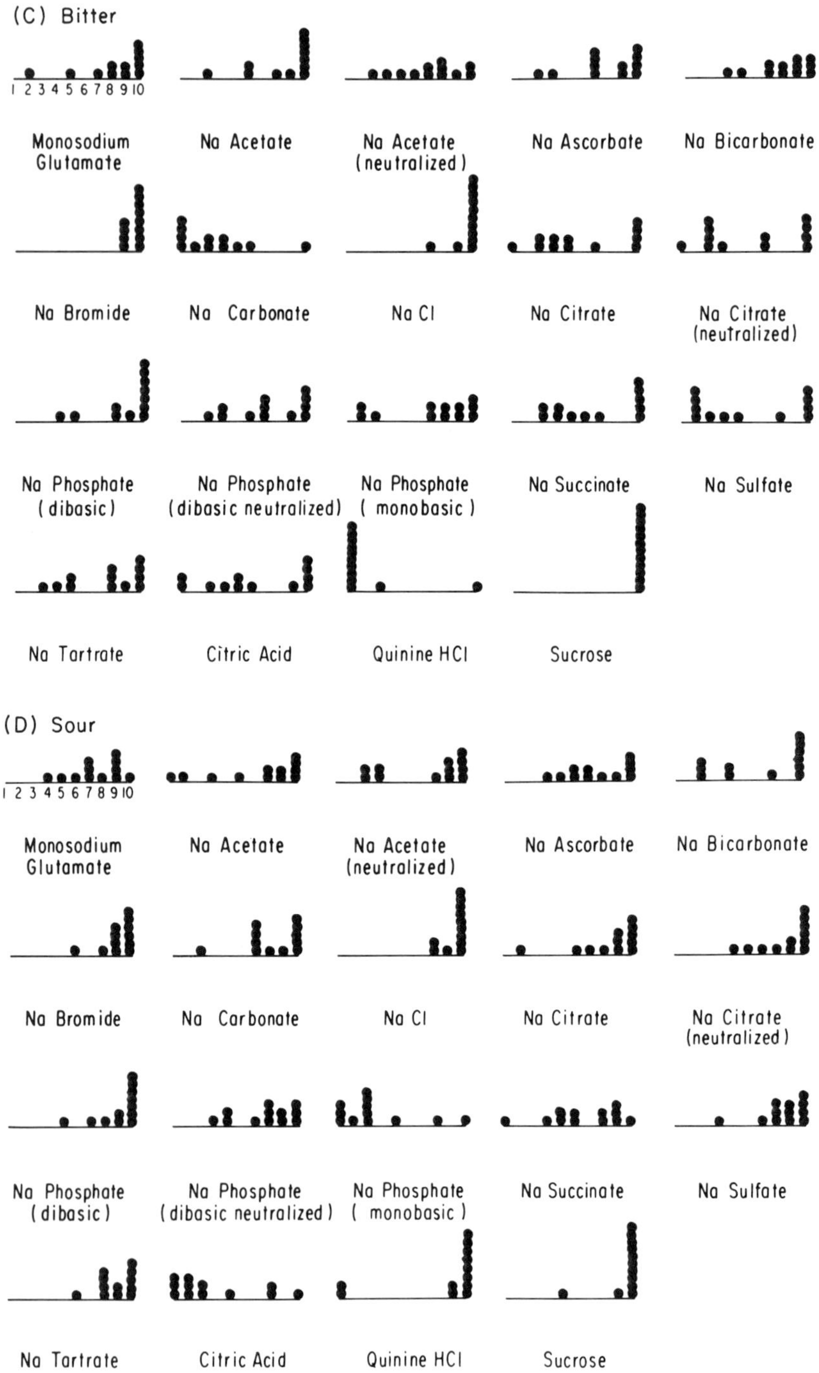
(C) Bitter
1 2 3 4 5 6 7 8 9 10
Monosodium Glutamate
Na Acetate
Na Acetate (neutralized)
Na Ascorbate
Na Bicarbonate
Na Bromide
Na Carbonate
Na Cl
Na Citrate
Na Citrate (neutralized)
Na Phosphate (dibasic)
Na Phosphate (dibasic neutralized)
Na Phosphate (monobasic)
Na Succinate
Na Sulfate
Na Tartrate
Citric Acid
Quinine HCl
Sucrose
(D) Sour
1 2 3 4 5 6 7 8 9 10
Monosodium Glutamate
Na Acetate
Na Acetate (neutralized)
Na Ascorbate
Na Bicarbonate
Na Bromide
Na Carbonate
Na Cl
Na Citrate
Na Citrate (neutralized)
Na Phosphate (dibasic)
Na Phosphate (dibasic neutralized)
Na Phosphate (monobasic)
Na Succinate
Na Sulfate
Na Tartrate
Citric Acid
Quinine HCl
Sucrose

Fig. 3

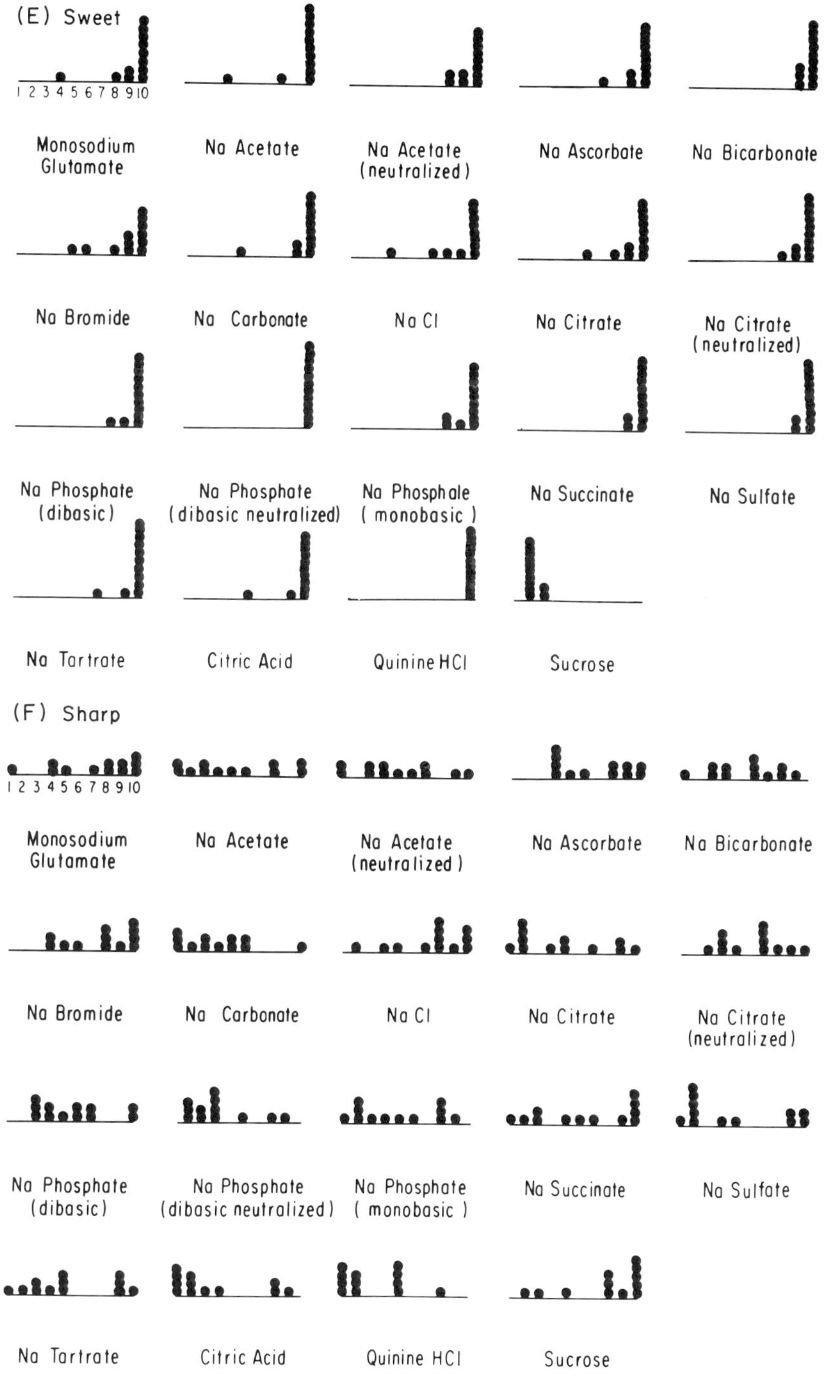

Fig. 3 *(continued)*

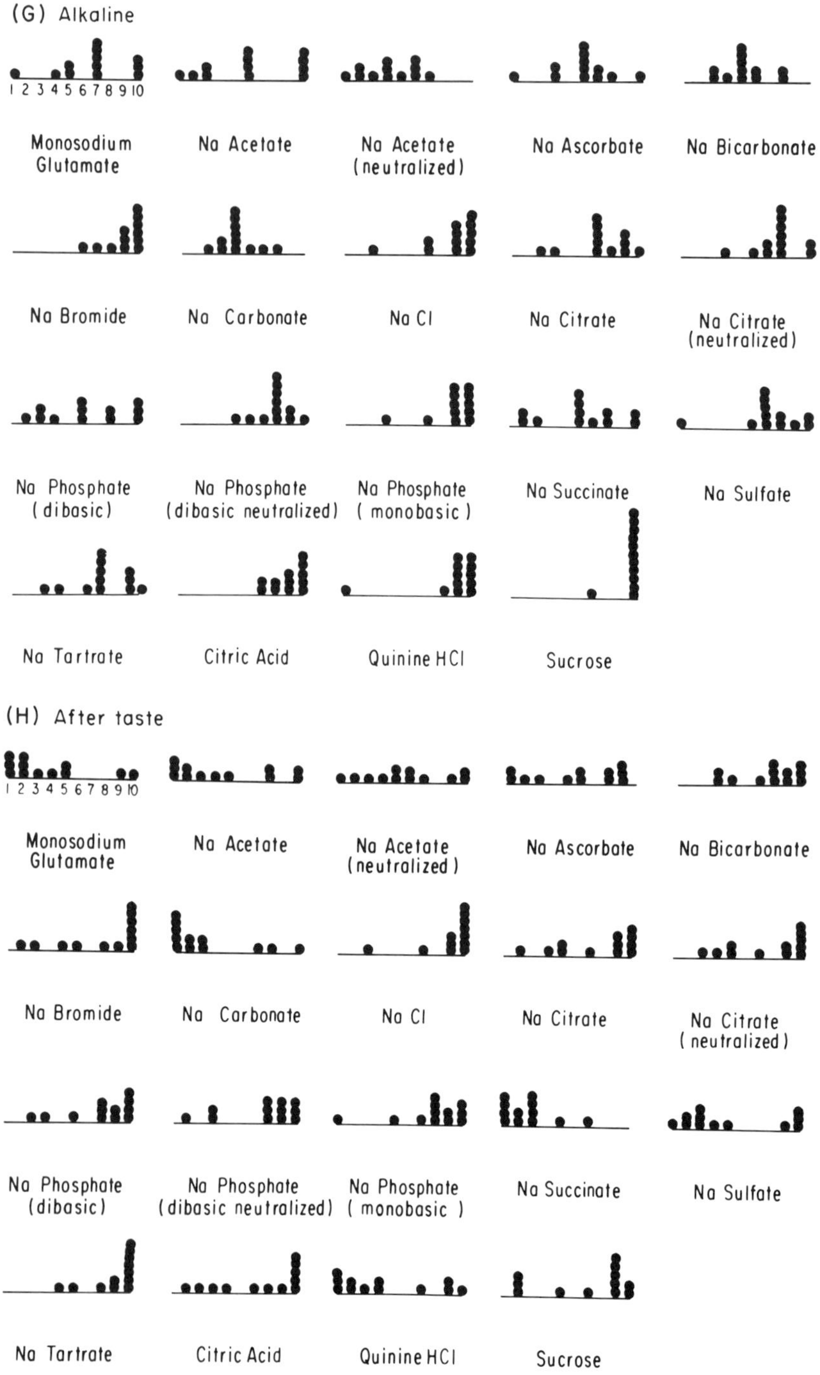
(G) Alkaline
1 2 3 4 5 6 7 8 9 10
Monosodium Glutamate
Na Acetate
Na Acetate (neutralized)
Na Ascorbate
Na Bicarbonate
Na Bromide
Na Carbonate
Na Cl
Na Citrate
Na Citrate (neutralized)
Na Phosphate (dibasic)
Na Phosphate (dibasic neutralized)
Na Phosphate (monobasic)
Na Succinate
Na Sulfate
Na Tartrate
Citric Acid
Quinine HCl
Sucrose
(H) After taste
1 2 3 4 5 6 7 8 9 10
Monosodium Glutamate
Na Acetate
Na Acetate (neutralized)
Na Ascorbate
Na Bicarbonate
Na Bromide
Na Carbonate
Na Cl
Na Citrate
Na Citrate (neutralized)
Na Phosphate (dibasic)
Na Phosphate (dibasic neutralized)
Na Phosphate (monobasic)
Na Succinate
Na Sulfate
Na Tartrate
Citric Acid
Quinine HCl
Sucrose

Fig. 3

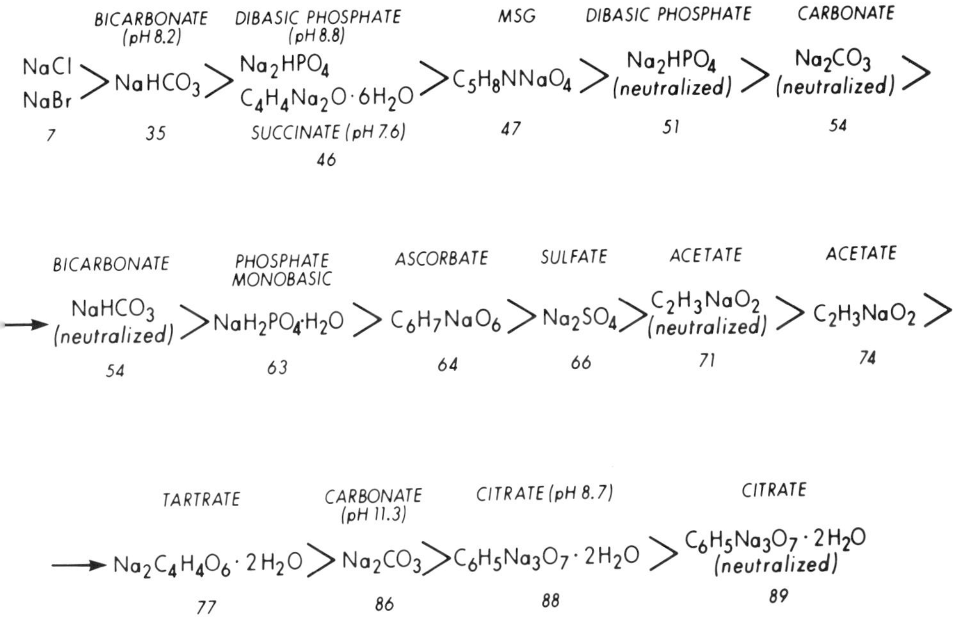

Fig. 4. The rank order for saltiness for 0.2 *M* Na^+ salts from most salty to least salty.

line. For example, dots located toward the left indicate individual subject ratings of "good." Dots toward the right indicate ratings of "bad."

Adjective ratings were also found for the stimuli in experiment 1 (0.2 *M* Na^+ salts). The rank order for saltiness ratings from most salty to least salty is given in Fig. 4.

IV. DISCUSSION

The spatial arrangement in Fig. 1 indicates that the anion greatly contributes to the overall taste sensation of sodium salts. This is confirmed by the diverse positioning of sodium salts with different anions within the taste "map" derived by the application of ALSCAL to the similarity judgments. The arrangement, however, does not reveal an unequivocal relationship between the chemical

---

Fig. 3. Individual variation on adjective scales for the sodium salts equated in overall intensity to 0.15 *M* NaCl. Ratings on three traditional standards are shown as well. The dots indicate distribution of individual subject's ratings. Dots located toward the left represent high ratings on the adjective at the top of a section, e.g., "good." Dots toward the right indicate ratings on the opposite adjective, e.g., "bad." (A) Good; (B) salty; (C) bitter; (D) sour; (E) sweet; (F) sharp; (G) alkaline; (H) aftertaste.

structure of the anion and the taste of the sodium salts. Sodium salts with moderately large anions, such as sodium tartrate, fall proximate to salts with smaller anions, such as sodium phosphate monobasic, on the basis of similarity in taste quality.

The range of the taste sensations of sodium salts is not contained within the closed system defined by the four so-called primary tastes: salty, sweet, sour, and bitter. This suggests that Henning's tetrahedron is incomplete as a taste model because it cannot order the stimuli used in this study. On the other hand, ordering the sodium salts by a multidimensional scaling technique presented no difficulty because this methodology is open-ended and thus allows ordering of all the stimuli.

In addition to the fact that the anion contributes its own taste to sodium salts, the anion can also reduce the salty taste sensation of sodium salts as seen in Fig. 4. Application of multidimensional scaling to similarity judgments among tastes of sodium salts yields greater agreement among subjects than adjective ratings as seen in Figs. 2 and 3. This may be due to the manner in which language-based labels are learned for tastes. Although there may be agreement among individuals on the degree of similarity or difference between tastes, the manner in which language-based labels such as "bitter" or "sour" are learned or extracted from perceptions may vary among individuals.

V. SUMMARY

Application of multidimensional scaling to similarity judgments among a series of sodium salts reveals that the anion contributes significantly to the overall taste quality. The anion can also reduce the salty taste sensation of sodium salts. The taste range of the sodium salts extends beyond the traditional range defined by the four so-called primaries: salty, sweet, sour, and bitter.

ACKNOWLEDGMENT

This research was supported by a grant to the author, NIA AG 00443.

REFERENCES

Henning, H. (1916). Die Qualitatenreihe des Geschmacks. *Z. Psychol.* **74,** 203-219.

Kionka, H., and Strätz, F. (1922). Setzt der Geschmack eines Salzes sich zusammen aus dem Geschmack der einzelnen Ionen oder schmeckt man jedes Salz als Gesamtmolekül? *Arch Exp. Pathol. Pharmakol.* **95,** 241-257.

Schiffman, S. S. (1977). Food recognition by the elderly. *J. Gerontol.* **32,** 586-592.

Schiffman, S. S., and Dackis, C. (1975). Taste of nutrients: Amino acids, vitamins, and fatty acids. *Percept. & Psychophys.* **17,** 140–146.

Schiffman, S. S., and Engelhard, H. H. (1976). Taste of dipeptides. *Physiol. Behav.* **17,** 523–535.

Schiffman, S. S., and Erickson, R. P. (1971). A psychophysical model for gustatory quality. *Physiol. Behav.* **7,** 617–633.

Schiffman, S. S., Moroch, K., and Dunbar, J. (1975). Taste of acetylated amino acids. *Chem. Senses Flavor* **1,** 387–401.

Schiffman, S. S., Musante, G., and Conger, J. (1978). Application of multidimensional scaling to ratings of foods for obese and normal weight individuals. *Physiol. Behav.* **21,** 417–422.

Schiffman, S. S., McElroy, A. E., and Erickson, R. P. (1980). The range of taste quality of sodium salts. *Physiol. Behav.* (in press).

Takane, Y., Young, F. W., and de Leeuw, J. (1977). Nonmetric individual differences in multidimensional scaling: An alternating least squares method with optimal scaling features. *Psychometrika* **42,** 7–67.

von Skramlik, E. (1922). Mischungsgleichungen im Gebiete des Geschmackssinnes. *Z. Psychol. Physiol. Sinnesorg.* **53,** 36–78.

Yoshida, M. (1963). Similarity among different kinds of taste near threshold concentration. *Jpn. J. Psychol.* **34,** 25–35.

Chapter 9

Salivary Chloride Levels, Taste Thresholds for Salt, and Food Ingestion

HOWARD H. CHAUNCEY, SHARON WALLACE, and JOHN E. ALMAN

I. INTRODUCTION

Previous studies have indicated that human NaCl detection threshlds increase with age. Cooper *et al.* (1959) studied 100 subjects in the age range 15–89 years, and noted that there was a significantly higher NaCl threshold for persons 60- to 74-years than for individuals in the age range of 45- to 59-years. Hinchcliffe (1962) subsequently observed that the NaCl threshold appeared to increase exponentially with age.

More recently Fikentscher and co-workers (1977) tested 140 male and female subjects, 20 in each of 7 age decades from 10 to 80 years, and observed an age-related significant decrease in salt sensitivity for both men and women. Furthermore, it was found that the women exhibited a lesser sensitivity deficit

ISBN 0-12-397750-9

than men. A pilot study conducted by Kare and Wallace (1976), which utilized the "whole mouth" threshold test procedure devised by Desor and Maller (1975), indicated that a group of men ranging in age from 80 to 85 years had significantly higher NaCl thresholds than a group of men in the age range 37–45 years. In contrast, Hermel and co-workers (1970), using a "drop stimulus" technique, stated that there was no change in sensitivity to NaCl among 4 age groups with a range of 4 to 60 years.

In general, the taste literature suggests that the NaCl threshold increases with age. The degree of change in NaCl sensitivity does not appear to be consistent, but varies according to the test procedure employed. Changes noted with NaCl sensitivity do not correlate with changes observed with the other taste modalities, and these age-associated threshold changes may not be related to supra-threshold preference (Meiselman, 1972). However, in the pilot study by Kare and Wallace (1976), which included preference for suprathreshold tastant solutions, older subjects tended to prefer higher concentrations of NaCl.

Although there are a few frequently cited reports of a shift in taste preference with aging (Shultz and Pilgrim, 1953; Schiffman, 1977), these studies were conducted with foods and contained both olfactory and gustatory stimuli. Unfortunately, no data regarding the possible effect of denture status were presented. Information is available indicating the full upper dentures can affect the olfactory component in flavor, but do not alter taste thresholds (Giddon *et al.*, 1954; Kapur *et al.*, 1967; Chauncey *et al.*, 1967; Shannon *et al.*, 1969; Feller and Shannon, 1970).

Most taste studies suffer from a failure to define subject health and/or denture status. In many disease states (Henkin *et al.*, 1963; Schelling *et al.*, 1965; Carson and Gormican, 1976a,b; Conger, 1974), and with a number of medications (Rollin, 1978), altered general taste receptivity, saliva flow rate and/or composition occur (Minaire *et al.*, 1975; Abelson *et al.*, 1976; Brown *et al.*, 1976). Although saliva composition has been shown to be an important factor in gustatory perception (McBurney and Pfaffman, 1963), there is a paucity of information relative to the interaction of saliva composition and dietary habits.

Salt use has been implicated in the etiology of hypertension, which is considered to be a serious national health problem. The restriction of NaCl intake has been proposed as a national dietary goal (U.S. Select Committee on Nutrition and Human Needs, 1977). Therefore, the authors believed that it might be of value to define further the relationship between salivary sodium and chloride levels, taste threshold for NaCl and patterns of salt ingestion in healthy aging individuals.

II. METHODS

Two hundred participants from the V.A. "Longitudinal and Cross-Sectional Study of Oral Health in Healthy Veterans" were requested to participate in the present study. The ''Longitudinal Dental Study,'' initiated in 1969 as a companion study to the ''Veterans Administration Normative Aging Study,'' contains 1200 subjects. It includes salivary analysis, preference for thirteen foods (taste, texture, ease of chewing, and ingestion frequency) and masticatory performance tests. The age distribution of the participants is quite similar to the general veteran population, and when the study was initiated they ranged in age from 25 to 75 years. They were selected for the ''Normative Aging Study'' because they met specific health criteria, represented a broad range of socioeconomic strata, and exhibited geographic stability. Oral health was not a consideration in the selection of the original participants.

A. Salt Intake Scoring

One hundred and fifty-three participants in the ''Longitudinal Dental Study'' volunteered to participate and returned a completed comprehensive food intake questionnaire designed to elicit use frequency of high salt food items and perceived table salt use (Wallace, 1979). A comprehensive salt intake score for each participant was developed from the responses obtained to the various questions. The first contribution to the intake score was the ordinal equivalent of the answer to the 3 questions presented in Table I.

Table II shows the format used to elicit a food intake pattern for both working and leisure days. The number of times that code 5, or salty snacks, was entered on the form contributed to the intake score. Intake frequency of salty snacks ranged from 0 to 2 per day.

The third table shows the source of another major contribution to the intake

TABLE I

Questionnaire Items for Eliciting Amount and Frequency of Salt Use

Score contribution	Question
	How often do you add salt to your food at the table?
1	Never
2	Occasionally
3	Most of the time
4	Always
	Do you usually salt your food before you taste it?
0	No
4	Yes
	How would you describe your use of salt?
1	Do not use
2	Light
3	Moderate
4	Heavy

TABLE II

Questionnaire Items Eliciting Food Intake Pattern

Use the codes below to report your meal pattern for working days. Write the times you usually eat. Write the number code for the kind of meal you typically eat at that time . . . PLEASE READ ALL THE CHOICES BEFORE YOU BEGIN.

CODES FOR KIND OF MEAL

1 = Light Breakfast (three items or less—example: coffee, juice, toast)
2 = Full Breakfast (four items or more—example: coffee, juice, cereal, milk)
3 = Fruit or Vegetable Snack (examples: apple, carrot sticks)
4 = Sweet Snack (examples: donut, brownie, cookies, cake, ice cream, candy)
5 = Salty Snacks (examples: saltines, chips, pretzels, popcorn)
6 = Light Lunch or Supper Meal
7 = Heavy Luncheon or Dinner Meal
8 = Mini Meal (examples: bowl of soup, cheese and fruit, half sandwich)
9 = Beverage Alone

FOR WORKING DAYS CODE NUMBER:

Time I arise on working days: ________AM/PM

Time I first eat or drink something: ________ AM/PM What I usually have at that time: ________

Time I next eat or drink: ____________AM/PM What I usually have at that time: ________

TABLE III

Questionnaire Items Eliciting Use Frequency of High Salt Foods

Write the one LETTER CODE that best describes how often you use each item, in the box provided.

Items used, *daily*	Used less than daily, but used, *every week*	Used *less often*
A = 4 or more times/day	E = 6 times/week	K = 2–3 times/month
B = 3 times/day	F = 5 times/week	L = rarely or never
C = 2 times/day	G = 4 times/week	
D = 1 time/day	H = 3 times/week	
	I = 2 times/week	
	J = 1 time/week	

☐ SALTED SNACKS (chips, nuts, crackers)
☐ CHEESE (not cottage)
☐ CANNED SOUP
☐ PICKLES, OLIVES, RELISH
☐ CATSUP, MUSTARD
☐ LUNCHMEAT OR FRANKS (salami, bologna, liverwurst, etc.)
☐ HAM, BACON, SAUSAGE

TABLE IV

Form for Recording Food Intake Diary

FOOD DIARY FOR: ______________ ______________
NAME DATE

Time I got up: ______________

Time I ate and/or drank	Items I ate and/or drank	How prepared	Approximate amount

score. Ordinal equivalents for the letter code answer to the questions shown in Table III were added into the score. Letter codes A–C were valued at 3, D–G were assigned a value of 2, H–J were given a value of 1, and K–L were considered to be 0. Subjects were also asked how often they would like to use these items; responses to this question also contributed to the total score.

Table IV shows the format used to record a 24-hour intake diary. The number of high salt items entered in this diary also contributed to the total salt intake score. Score contributions from this source ranged from 0 to 6. A high salt item was defined as a serving of a food or beverage that would be excluded from a sodium restricted diet.

B. Threshold Determination

The range of observed composite scores was 2–33, with mean of 17.43 and standard deviation 6.52, for the 153 respondents. The range of scores was divided into triads. Representatives from each triad were tested for taste threshold. Twenty-four from the bottom triad, 15 from the middle triad and 26 from the top triad were tested. The total number of persons tested was 65. More subjects from the top and bottom triads were used to maximize the opportunity to observe differences.

Each subject was presented with 20 paper cups. Ten contained 10 ml of distilled deionized water, while 10 contained 10 ml of a NaCl solution, at room temperature. Each subject was asked to swish the liquid in his mouth and report whether the solution was "plain," or "salt." Samples of water and salt solution were presented prior to the first test cup to task-orient the subjects. During the testing, subjects were advised whether they were correct or incorrect after each cup trial. Order of presentation for water and salt trials in each concentration series was random. The base or starting salt solution was the 0.015 *M* sodium chloride concentration. When the subject responded correctly on 16 or more of the 20 trials at one concentration, a lower concentration was used for the next 20-cup trial; if less than 16 correct responses were obtained, the next higher concentration was used. The concentration series is presented in Table V. Test-

TABLE V

Concentrations of Test Solutions and Assigned Threshold Value

Concentrations of NaCl solutions used to determine threshold (*M*)	Assigned threshold value (*M*)
0.0001	
	0.0005
0.001	
	0.0030
0.005	
	0.0075
0.010	
	0.0125
0.015 (starting concentration)	0.0175
0.020	
	0.030
0.040	
	0.060
0.080	

ing continued until a break, i.e., 16 or more correct responses in an ascending series, or 15 or fewer correct responses in a descending series, was obtained. Threshold was defined as the concentration midway between the 2 test concentrations where the break occurred.

C. Salivary Analysis

Stimulated parotid and whole saliva collections were made at random in the morning or afternoon, at least 1.5 hours postprandial. Ten milliliters of rubber band-stimulated whole saliva were collected. Subsequently, a vacuum-maintained metal collection device (Shannon and Chauncey, 1967) was positioned over the orifice of Stenson's duct. The gustatory stimulus employed was a sour lemon flavored lozenge.* Each subject was given a one minute "acquaintance" interval of stimulation to clear the collection apparatus and to allow the gland to accommodate to stimulation. After the "acquaintance" interval, the plastic collection tubule was transferred to a graduated tube and 10.0 ml of parotid fluid were collected. The lozenge was changed every 5 min to maintain a con-

*Regal Crown Imported Lemon Sours, Murray Allen Imports, New York City, NY.

stant level of stimulation. Both whole and parotid saliva flow rates (ml/min) were calculated by recording the time necessary to collect a standard 10.0 ml volume.

Immediately after collection, the saliva pH value and bicarbonate level were measured. Bicarbonate was determined by the automated method for the estimation of carbon dioxide detailed by Skeggs (1960a,b), while the pH was measured with a Corning Model 12 Research pH meter. The saliva sample was then stored at 4°C until the remaining variables could be measured, usually within 24 hours. Sodium and potassium were measured by flame photometry (I L Digital Flame Photometer). Calcium and inorganic phosphorus were determined by the automated method of Kessler and Wolfman (1964); the latter procedure involved a modification of the method described by Fiske and Subbarow (1925). Chloride analysis was conducted by the procedure described by Cotlove *et al.* (1958).

III. RESULTS

Pearson correlation coefficients among age, salt taste threshold, salt intake scores, and whole saliva chloride levels are shown in Table VI. Correlation coefficients were low, particularly those between threshold and both salt intake and whole saliva chloride. The highest correlation obtained was 0.35; this was between age and taste threshold. The only negative coefficients were between age and salt intake, and between age and whole saliva chloride.

The data were further examined using contingency table analysis. Table VII illustrates the results obtained in the tabulation of threshold versus age. Age was split at 55 years since this was the median age for the 153 questionnaire respondents. The breakpoint for salt taste threshold was based on whether an ascending or descending concentration series was used in the testing procedure, which, in turn, was based on subject response to the starting test concentration of NaCl. The 0.015 *M* NaCl used as the starting concentration is considered to be the average threshold for normal adults (Pfaffmann *et al.*, 1971). The chi square for

TABLE VI

Pearson Correlation Coefficients of Age, Threshold, Salt Use Score, and Salivary Chloride Level

	Threshold	Salt intake score	Whole saliva Cl^{+b}
Age	0.35[a]	−0.23	−0.25
Threshold		0.17[a]	0.13[a]
Salt intake score			0.26

[a] Statistic based on 65 cases.
[b] Statistic based on 141 cases.

TABLE VII

Tabulation of Subjects by Age and NaCl Threshold[a]

Age (years)	Threshold for NaCl: 0.0125 M or less	0.0175 M or more	Total
<55	26	12	38
55+	14	13	27
Total	40	25	65

[a] $\chi^2 = 1.20$, 1 d.f., $p > 0.05$.

Table VII shows no significant relationship between age and threshold in the 65 subjects tested. It may be that the age range of this subset of subjects is too narrow to demonstrate an age effect on threshold. For example, the 27 subjects 55 years and older split about equally between the 2 threshold categories. However, of the 10 subjects who were 60 years or older, 2 exhibited thresholds of 0.0125 M or less, while 8 had thresholds of 0.0175 M or greater.

Table VIII shows cross tabulation of the salt intake score versus age for all 153 respondents. The intake score was divided into approximately equal triads. The age breakpoints were chosen to highlight differences between the top and bottom 20% of the age distribution. Chi square analysis shows a significant relationship between these 2 variables with the effect dominated by a high intake for the youngest group and low intake for the oldest group. The contingency coefficient for this table is moderately low, 0.30.

In the 2 × 2 contingency table of age versus whole saliva chloride level (Table IX) the age breakpoint was based on the median age for the 153 respondents (55 years). Whole saliva chloride levels were divided using the median value of the

TABLE VIII

Tabulation of Subjects by Age and Salt Intake Score[a]

Age (years)	Composite salt intake score by triad: 2–13	14–19	20–23	Total
33–44	5	5	17	27
45–64	32	30	36	98
65–83	10	14	4	28
Total	47	49	57	153

[a] $\chi^2 = 14.84$, 4 d.f., $p < 0.01$.

TABLE IX

Tabulation of Subjects by Age and Whole Saliva Chloride (mEq/liter)[a]

Age (years)	Whole saliva chloride 7.5–19.6	19.7–48.6	Total
<55	39	34	73
55+	32	36	68
Total	71	70	141

[a] $\chi^2 = 0.34$, 1 d.f., $p > 0.05$.

141 respondents measured in the second analysis cycle of the "Dental Study." The results indicated no trend between whole saliva chloride and age. A Pearson correlation utilizing 1,050 participants in Cycle 2 of the "Longitudinal Dental Study" confirmed this.

In Table X, the composite salt intake score was divided using the triad values obtained for the 153 questionnaire respondents, as seen in Table VIII. The 3 categories for the taste threshold values were based on a division of the observed thresholds into approximately equal numbers of participants. A significant chi square was obtained for the salt intake score versus taste threshold. The contingency coefficient for this table is 0.46. The significant effect is primarily derived from the individuals with low thresholds, who tended to use less salt.

Analysis of salt taste thresholds versus whole saliva chloride levels (Table XI) yields a significant chi square, with a contingency coefficient of 0.36. This relationship appears to be primarily due to a concentration of persons in the low taste threshold and low whole saliva chloride group and the high threshold, high chloride group.

TABLE X

Tabulation of Subjects by Salt Intake Score and Threshold[a]

Threshold for NaCl (*M*)	Composite salt intake score by triad 2–13	14–19	20–33	Total
0.00055–0.0075	13	6	2	21
0.0125 –0.0175	4	3	16	23
0.030 –0.060	7	6	8	21
Total	24	15	26	65

[a] $\chi^2 = 17.47$, 4 d.f., $p < 0.002$.

TABLE XI

Tabulation of Subjects by Threshold and Whole Saliva Chloride (mEq/liter)[a]

Threshold for NaCl (M)	Whole saliva chloride		
	7.5–19.6	19.7–48.6	Total
0.00055–0.0075	16	5	21
0.0125 –0.0175	13	10	23
0.030 –0.060	6	15	21
Total	35	30	65

[a] $\chi^2 = 9.68$, 2 d.f., $p < 0.01$.

TABLE XII

Tabulation of Subjects by Salt Intake Score and Whole Saliva Chloride (mEq/liter)[a]

Composite salt intake score	Whole saliva chloride		
	7.5–19.6	19.7–48.6	Total
2–13	19	23	42
14–19	22	22	44
20–33	32	23	55
Total	73	68	141

[a] $\chi^2 = 1.68$, 2 d.f., $p > 0.05$.

The contingency table for whole saliva chloride levels and salt intake scores (Table XII) showed a nonsignificant chi square.

IV. DISCUSSION

The results suggest relationships among certain of the variables examined; specifically, a relationship between salt intake and age, salt intake and threshold, and between threshold and salivary chloride. Age versus threshold should be examined further because of the clustering of subjects in the age range 45–55 years.

It has been noted that pleasantness and intensity ratings of tastant solutions follow different functional curves, and thus are not predictive of one another (Dillon, 1976). The data here suggest that perhaps, in young subjects, salt intake may be guided, in part, by the chloride environment in the oral cavity. Older subjects tested frequently mentioned a voluntary restriction of salt intake as a preventive health care practice. Preference testing and threshold determination of older subjects with high salivary chlorides might confirm this.

Dietary surveys confirm the need for concern that older individuals may not select foods that provide adequate amounts of all nutrients (O'Hanlon and Kohrs, 1978; Hartsook, 1974). Altered taste perception has been implicated in this problem (Langan and Yearick, 1976). It is often taken as established fact that diminished taste acuity contributes to oral complaints and low nutrient intake in the elderly (Soremark and Nilsson, 1972). The data here demonstrated that the NaCl taste acuity and intake patterns of young adults may be more deleterious than that of older adults.

Alterations in salivary composition and taste acuity have been reported for several disease states. Recognition threshold for salt has been reported to be increased in cancer (Carson and Gormican, 1976b). In patients with Addison's disease, the threshold has been reported to be decreased (Henkin *et al.*, 1963). Medications can alter taste (Carson and Gormican, 1976a) or salivary composition (Wotman *et al.*, 1971), as can administration of various hormones (Denton *et al.*, 1976).

Schechter *et al.* (1974) found the preference for salt was increased in hypertension. It may be that young adults who display exquisite sensitivity and have a low salt intake are protected from developing hypertension.

If salivary composition and/or taste thresholds are to be used as markers for disease, studies of normal subjects are essential. Behavioral correlates of changes in salivary composition and of changes in taste perception must be identified. The present study is a step in this direction. Further studies of the interaction between diet, taste thresholds, preferences, and salivary variables are warranted.

V. SUMMARY

This investigation was conducted to determine if relationships existed among age, salivary chloride level, taste threshold for NaCl, and salt intake. Low intake, low threshold, and low salivary chloride appeared to be related. However, further study is necessary to define the interaction of intake pattern, threshold and age.

ACKNOWLEDGMENTS

This research was supported by the Medical Research Service of the Veterans Administration. The authors would like to acknowledge the assistance of Carol Conway, Dorothea L. Malone, and Helen G. Oskin.

REFERENCES

Abelson, D. S., Mandel, I. D., and Karmiol, M. (1976). Salivary studies in alcoholic cirrhosis. *Oral Surg., Oral Med. Oral Pathol.* **41,** 188–192.

Brown, L. R., Dreizen, S., Rider, L. J., and Johnston, D. A. (1976). The effect of radiation induced xerostomia on saliva and serum lysozyme and immunoglobulin levels. *Oral Surg., Oral Med. Oral Pathol.* **41,** 83–92.

Carson, J. S., and Gormican, A. (1976a). Disease-medication relationships in altered taste sensitivity. *J. Am. Diet. Assoc.* **68,** 550–553.

Carson, J. S., and Gormican, A. (1976b). Taste acuity and food attitudes of selected patients with cancer. *J. Am. Diet. Assoc.* **70,** 361–365.

Chauncey, H. H., Shannon, I. L., and Feller, R. P. (1967). Effect of oral and nasal chemoreception on parotid secretion. *In* "Secretory Mechanism of Salivary Glands" (L. H. Schneyer and C. A. Schneyer, eds.), pp. 351–364. Academic Press, New York.

Conger, A. D. (1974). Loss and recovery of taste acuity in patients irradiated to the oral cavity. *Radiat. Res.* **53,** 338–347.

Cooper, R. M., Bilash, J. P., and Zubek, J. P. (1959). The effect of age on taste sensitivity. *J. Gerontol.* **14,** 56–58.

Cotlove, E., Trantham, H. V., and Bowman, R. C. (1958). An instrument for and method for automatic rapid, accurate, and sensitive trituration of chloride in biologic samples. *J. Lab. Clin. Med.* **51,** 461–468.

Denton, D. S., Abraham, S. F., Blaine, E. H., McKinley, M. J., Nelson, R. S., Weisinger, R. S., and Whipp, G. T. (1976). Taste and hormones. *Clin. Exp. Pharmacol. Physiol.* **3,** 375–381.

Desor, J. A., and Maller, O. (1975). Taste correlates of disease: Cystic fibrosis. *J. Pediatr.* **87,** 93–97.

Dillon, K. M. (1976). Some historical, physiological and psychological correlates of NaCl consumption. Doctoral Dissertation, University of Massachusetts, Boston.

Feller, R. P., and Shannon, I. L. (1970). Taste, tactile stimulation, and parotid flow in the human. *J. Oral Med.* **25,** 37–88.

Fikentscher, R., Roseburg, B., Spinar, H., and Bruchmuller, W. (1977). Loss of taste in the elderly: Sex differences. *Clin. Otolaryngol.* **2,** 183–189.

Fiske, C. H., and Subbarow, Y. (1925). The colorimetric determination of phosphorus. *J. Biol. Chem.* **66,** 375–400.

Giddon, D. B., Dreisbach, M. E., Pfaffman, C., and Manly, R. S. (1954). Relative abilities of natural and artificial dentition patients for judging sweetness of solid foods. *J. Prosthet. Dent.* **4,** 263–268.

Hartsook, E. I. (1974). Food selection, dietary adequacy and related dental problems of patients with dental prostheses. *J. Prosthet. Dent.* **32,** 32–40.

Henkin, R. I., Gill, J. R., and Batter, F. C. (1963). Studies on taste thresholds in normal man and in patients with adrenal cortical insufficiency: The role of adrenal cortical steroids and of serum sodium concentration. *J. Clin. Invest.* **42,** 727–735.

Hermel, J., Schonwetter, S., and Samueloff, S. (1970). Taste sensation and age in man. *J. Oral Res.* **25,** 39–41.

Hinchcliffe, R. (1962). Aging and sensory thresholds. *J. Gerontol.* **17,** 45–50.

Kapur, K. K., Collister, T., and Fischer, E. E. (1967). Masticatory and gustatory reflex secretion rates and taste thresholds of denture wearers. *J. Prosthet. Dent.* **18,** 406–410.

Kare, M., and Wallace, S. (1976). Taste thresholds in aging (personal communication).

Kessler, G., and Wolfman, M. (1964). An automated procedure for the simultaneous determination of calcium and phosphorus. *Clin. Chem.* **11,** 624–627.

Langan, M. J., and Yearick, E. S. (1976). The effects of improved oral hygiene on taste perception and nutrition of the elderly. *J. Gerontol.* **31,** 413–418.

McBurney, D. H., and Pfaffman, C. (1963). Gustatory adaptation to saliva and sodium chloride. *J. Exp. Psychol.* **65,** 523–529.

Meiselman, H. R. (1972). Human taste perception. *Crit. Rev. Food Technol.* **89,** 119.

Minaire, U., Descos, L., and Lambert, R. (1975). Chronic pancreatitis, alcoholic liver cirrhosis and salivary secretion. *Digestion* **12,** 57–60.

O'Hanlon, P., and Kohrs, M. B. (1978). Dietary studies of older Americans. *Am. J. Clin. Nutr.* **31,** 1257–1269.

Pfaffmann, C. Bartoshuk, L. M., and McBurney, D. H. (1971). Taste psycho-physics. *In* "Handbook of Sensory Physiology" (L. Biedler, ed.), Vol. 10, Part 2, pp. 75–101. Springer-Verlag, Berlin and New York.

Rollin, H. (1978). Drug related gustatory disorders. *Ann. Otol., Rhinol., & Laryngol.* **87,** 37–42.

Schechter, P. J., Horwitz, D., and Henkin, R. I. (1974). Salt preference in patients with untreated and treated essential hypertension. *Am. J. Clin. Med.* **267,** 320–326.

Schelling, J. L., Tetrault, L., Lasagna, L., and Davis, M. (1965). Abnormal taste threshold in diabetes. *Lancet* **1,** 508–512.

Schiffman, S. (1977). Food recognition by the elderly. *J. Gerontol.* **32,** 586–592.

Shannon, I. L., and Chauncey, H. H. (1967). A parotid fluid collection device with improved stability characteristics. *J. Oral Ther. Pharmacol.* **4,** 93–97.

Shannon, I. L., Terry, J. M., and Chauncey, H. H. (1969). Effect of a maxillary mouthguard on the parotid flow rate response to flavored solutions. *Proc. Soc. Exp. Biol. Med.* **130,** 1052–1054.

Shultz, H. G., and Pilgrim, F. J. (1953). Psychophysiology in food acceptance research. *J. Am. Dent. Assoc.* **29,** 1126–1134.

Skeggs, L. T., Jr. (1960a). The determination of carbon dioxide in blood serum. *Ann. N.Y. Acad. Sci.* **87,** 650–657.

Skeggs, L. T., Jr. (1960b). An automatic method for the determination of carbon dioxide in blood plasma. *Am. J. Clin. Pathol.* **33,** 181–185.

Soremark, R., and Nilsson, B. (1972). Dental status and nutrition in old age. *In* "Nutrition in Old Age" (L. A. Carlson, ed.), pp. 147–164. Almqvist & Wiksell, Stockholm.

U.S. Select Committee on Nutrition and Human Needs (1977). "Dietary Goals for the United States," 2nd ed. US Govt. Printing Office, Washington, D.C.

Wallace, S. (1979). Taste threshold and food habits. Doctoral Dissertation, Harvard University, Cambridge, Massachusetts.

Wotman, S., Bigger, J. T., Mandel, I. D., and Bartelstone, H. F. (1971). Salivary electrolytes in the detection of digitalis toxicity. *N. Engl. J. Med.* **285,** 871–878.

Chapter 10

Measuring Taste Sensitivity and the Effects of Adrenalectomy in Rats

G. ROLFE MORRISON

I. INTRODUCTION

I first would like to present the data that a former student of mine, Douglas Barnes, and I collected some time ago concerning the question of whether adrenalectomy affects the rat's taste sensitivity to sodium. Following this, some of the problems involved in the measurement of sensory capacity in animals, and the reservations that these problems cause in the interpretation of our data and those of others are discussed.

Richter (1939) suggested the possibility that the change in the rat's NaCl preference function found following adrenalectomy might be attributed in part to an altered sensitivity to NaCl. However, a number of experiments, particularly those of Pfaffmann and Bare (1950), Carr (1952), and Harriman and McLeod (1953) had failed to find any differences in the NaCl thresholds between normal and adrenalectomized rats, and others demonstrated that the NaCl detection thresholds for normal animals were at or below the preference thresholds for

BIOLOGICAL AND BEHAVIORAL
ASPECTS OF SALT INTAKE

ISBN 0-12-397750-9

adrenalectomized animals (Koh and Teitelbaum, 1961; Morrison and Norrison, 1966; Shaber *et al.*, 1971). The general consensus at this time was that the effect of adrenalectomy was on preference only, not on sensitivity; that is, on how the animal evaluates the taste, not on how well he can taste.

Our initial reason for believing the question might be worth reexamining was that these prior experiments were concerned with measuring absolute thresholds, which is not the only possible measure of sensitivity. Possibly there are changes that do not affect the threshold but which would show up in the response to suprathreshold stimuli. After we had completed the experiments and started contemplating what we and others had done, I argued further that: (1) these experiments had not in fact measured thresholds, and (2) in any event threshold is a poor index of sensitivity. These two points were dealt with in detail in a previous paper (Morrison, 1974) and I will refer back to them in the last section of this chapter.

Somewhat unfortunately, from my point of view, I subsequently continued the line of reasoning that had raised these two points, and this in turn, along with some additional experiments, led to some reservations about the interpretation of our data. I will describe our experiments and then come back to this point.

At the time of these experiments I had developed a procedure for scaling sensitivity (or what seemed to be sensitivity) to suprathreshold taste stimuli which worked reliably and well in a number of experiments with normal rats (Morrison and Norrison, 1966; Morrison, 1967, 1969, 1972). We used this method to compare normal and adrenalectomized animals.

II. METHOD

The first experiment was part of Barnes' (1969) B.Sc. (Hons.) thesis and the procedure has been described there in detail. Briefly the method is as follows: Animals were first trained in a discrete trial procedure in a two-lever Skinner box. On each trial a drinking spout projected into the box and remained until the animal had licked at it for 2 seconds; then it was removed. To complete the trial, the rat had to then press one of the two levers. On a given trial the spout contained either distilled water or a high concentration of NaCl, and these two varied randomly from trial to trial. A response on the left hand lever was correct if the bottle contained water and on the right if NaCl. The first lever press response, whether correct or incorrect, terminated the trial and brought a new spout into the box for the next trial.

If the animal made the correct response on a trial, it was reinforced with a food pellet; if it made the incorrect one, it received nothing. The rats were always tested under 23-hour food deprivation.

After the animal mastered the task, test trials were begun in which the concentration of NaCl was systematically decreased from session to session, a single concentration being used in each test session. Test sessions consisted of 50 trials, 25 in which the stimulus was water, 25 with NaCl.

In this first experiment, 12 animals were trained as above to discriminate between distilled water and a 3.2% solution of NaCl. They were then tested successively with 1, 0.1, 0.01, and 0.001% solutions. After this test series, the animals were retrained on the 3.2% solution and then divided into 2 groups. Five of the animals were successfully bilaterally adrenalectomized and formed the ADX group. Five others were subjected to a sham operation. The remaining 2 were discarded, one failing to show evidence of a successful adrenalectomy, the other failing to recover from the operation.

After a recovery period, the 2 groups were run through the test series again. Throughout the postoperative period, all animals had access to a 2% NaCl solution as well as water in their home cages.

III. RESULTS

The results of this part of the experiment are shown in Figs. 1 and 2 where percentage correct responses are plotted as a function of concentration pre- and postoperatively.

As Fig. 1 shows, there are no pre or post differences for the sham animals. In Fig. 2 however, it can be seen that there are substantial and significant differences in the ADX group. The postoperative curve is much flatter for these animals, with poorer performance at the higher concentrations.

It is not at all certain at this point, however, that the observed change in performance can be attributed to a change in NaCl sensitivity. Our immediate reaction to these results was that the most likely explanation was that an adrenal-

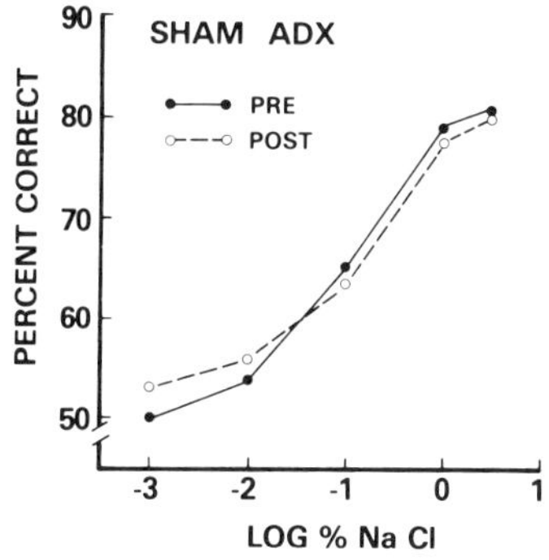

Fig. 1. Percentage correct responses pre- and postoperatively in the sham adrenalectomized rats as a function of NaCl concentration.

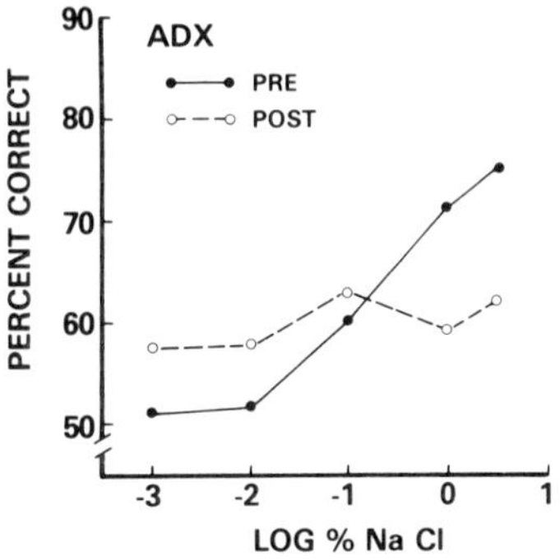

Fig. 2. Percentage correct responses pre- and postoperatively in the adrenalectomized rats as a function of NaCl concentration.

ectomized rat is not capable of performing as well as a normal one in any complex task, and the nature of the discriminative stimuli is irrelevant.

We decided however that, before writing off these results, we should test the possibility that the nature of the stimuli is relevant. We did this by retaining the animals in the same task, except that they were now required to discriminate between distilled water and a 20% sucrose solution. They were then tested with a series of decreasing sucrose concentrations.

Over the retraining sessions there was no difference in the rate at which the 2 groups acquired the new discrimination or in their final level of performance. The results of the sucrose test series are shown in Fig. 3.

It is apparent from this figure that there is no difference between the groups on

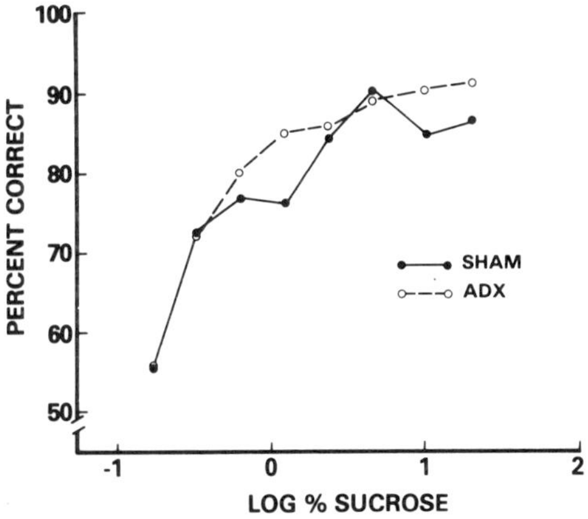

Fig. 3. Percentage correct responses postoperatively in the sham and adrenalectomized rats as a function of sucrose concentration.

these sucrose discriminations. In fact, the ADX animals are slightly superior to the controls. The differences observed in the first experiment do not seem to be due to an inability of the ADX animals to perform a complex task.

What about the possibility that the differences between the NaCl and sucrose tests could be due to different stages of recovery? To consider this we retrained the animals on the original NaCl discrimination and ran through the test series a final time.

Over the retraining trials with 3.2% NaCl, the ADX group was consistently poorer than the sham group. The results of this final test series are shown in Fig. 4.

Once again the ADX group showed significantly poorer performance than the controls at the higher concentrations. At this stage we decided to see whether we could replicate the results with a new set of animals while controlling for any effects of stages of recovery.

Eight new animals were trained in a similar manner except that they were taught the NaCl-water and sucrose-water discriminations simultaneously. In each training session the taste stimulus on a given trial could be either water, 3.2% NaCl, or 10% sucrose. The animals were trained to respond on the left hand lever if it were water and the right hand lever for either sucrose or NaCl. Following training they were again tested with a range of NaCl and sucrose concentrations. NaCl and sucrose test days were alternated so that on one day a test concentration of sucrose was present, the next NaCl, etc. After this all animals were adrenalectomized and the test series repeated.

Adrenalectomy was successful in 6 of the 8 animals and the results of the pre and post tests for these 6 are shown in Figs. 5 and 6.

These results show the same pattern as in the previous experiment. Figure 5

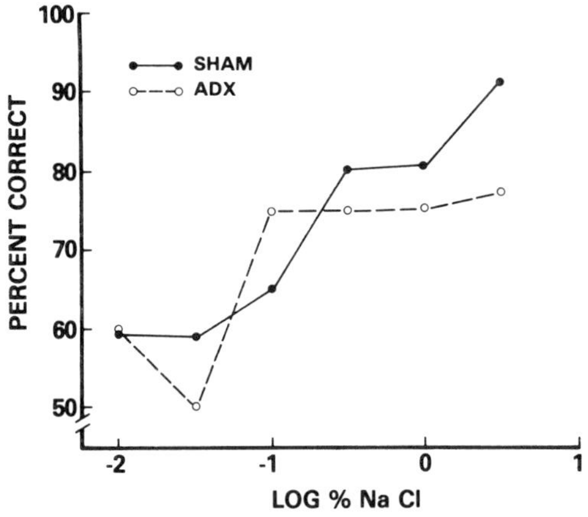

Fig. 4. Percentage correct responses on the second postoperative test as a function of NaCl concentration.

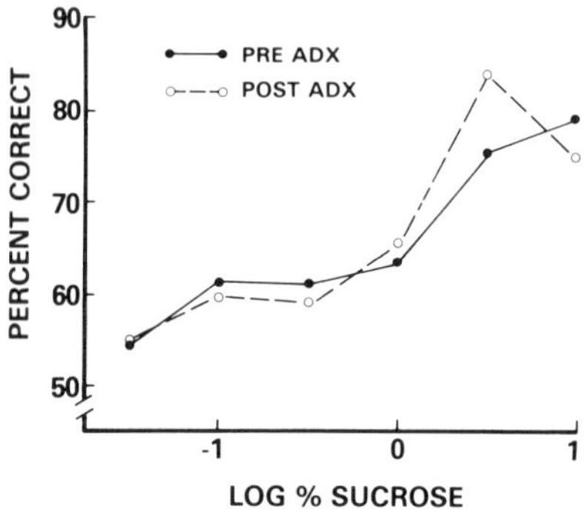

Fig. 5. Percentage correct responses pre- and postadrenalectomy as a function of sucrose concentration.

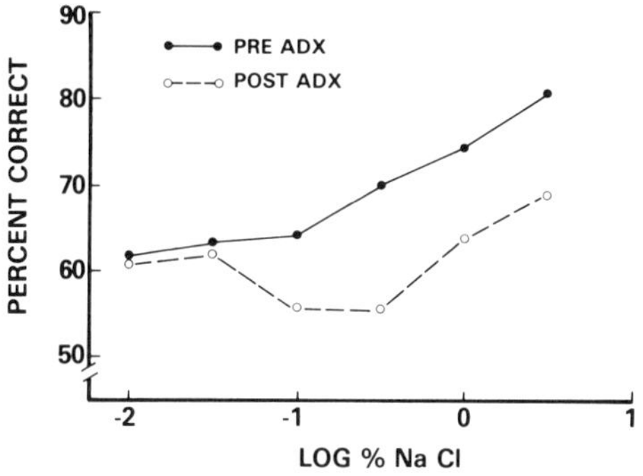

Fig. 6. Percentage correct responses pre- and postadrenalectomy as a function of NaCl concentration.

shows that there are no pre–post differences for the sucrose discriminations, while Fig. 6 shows the significantly poorer postadrenalectomy performance at higher NaCl concentrations.

These experiments demonstrate that adrenalectomy affects the discrimination of NaCl at high concentrations although there is no evidence for a change in threshold. We cannot be certain, of course, that this change is specific to NaCl or sodium, but it does not occur with sucrose. As I indicated earlier, however, there are some reservations about whether these observed differences truly represent differences in sensitivity.

IV. DISCUSSION

In a previous paper (Morrison, 1974) I raised some questions about interpretations of experiments which looked at absolute thresholds. I would suggest that if one wishes to ask whether 2 animals differ in sensitivity, the starting point for this should be to consider the type of psychophysical model which might be appropriate to describe the behavior and to derive the methodology from the model. A failure to do so may lead to an erroneous interpretation of the results. Too often it appears that the starting point has been the utilization of a method which seems reasonable on practical grounds without considering the theoretical implications. This is often compounded by the fact that the data analysis is then influenced implicitly if not explicitly by a particular model even though the procedures have not been derived from that model.

Let me illustrate this point in the following way. If one were to approach the problem completely uninfluenced by any theoretical considerations, the most logical way to proceed would be to take one or more stimulus intensities and determine if the behavior of the 2 groups differs at these intensities, which is in fact what we did. This is not, however, what has been done in the other experiments to which I have referred. Instead of proceeding in this way, they utilize what must seem to the completely psychophysically naive observer a much more tortuous approach which is to specify a particular criterion for behavior and ask if the stimulus intensity at which this criterion is met differs for the groups. Why would one proceed in this way?

At the time the earliest of these experiments was done, there was an almost universally accepted psychophysical model, the "high threshold" model which defined the absolute threshold as a meaningful construct. Quite obviously this model was the basis for this approach. The developments in psychophysics since the mid 1950's have, however, made it increasingly clear that for both humans and animals this model and construct can no longer be considered tenable. To measure absolute threshold as it is specified by this model is at best to be measuring the stimulus intensity at which the animal's response meets some arbitrary criterion. The subject's response, however, is dependent on at least two things, sensitivity and bias. If we wish to look at the former, the data must be corrected for the latter. But the appropriate correction for response bias depends on the form of the psychophysical model.

It is quite easy to picture results that, when corrected for bias using the dictates of the high threshold model, will show rat A to be more sensitive than rat B. But the reverse would be true if the data were analyzed in accordance with, for example, the signal detection model.

To interpret results as reflecting differences or lack thereof in sensitivity, at least one of three things must be true with respect to response bias. The psychophysical model and the correction factor derived from it must be an adequate representation of how the animals are behaving; bias must be reasonably constant from rat to rat and be uninfluenced by the independent variable; or the response differences are of such a form and extent that no reasonable correction for bias will eliminate them. In the case of the threshold experiments, it can be argued that the first condition does not hold. The second one is very doubtful—variations in response bias tend to be substantial in discriminations of this type and may well be affected by the experimental treatments. The form of data analysis precludes the examination of the third. There is a good possibility that, had these experiments been analyzed differently, differences might well have been observed between the groups.

As presented, our data are not tied to any particular model and the curves shown in the various figures are not pure measures of sensitivity. However, it does seem to meet the third of the three criteria. These data can be subjected to a variety of bias corrections as suggested by different models without changing either the pattern or the significance of the results. The hesitancy I have in the interpretation of our results is not in terms of the response bias problem.

I became interested in the psychophysical modeling question in part because of this type of consideration and in part due to some observations from this and similar experiments; and at least one result from some model building experiments turned out to have a direct bearing on the present data.

In a typical human psychophysical experiment almost all of the response variation can be attributed to a combination of sensitivity and response bias. A 2-parameter model typically will account for something on the order of 95% of the variance. This of course explains the emphasis on controlling or accounting for the effects of bias. It appears strongly, however, that rats differ from humans, at least in their psychophysical characteristics. There is at least one additional factor of equivalent importance in the rat's behavior which requires the model to have at least three parameters to achieve the same level of predictability. This third factor is something that might be called the attention (or inattention) parameter. Little attention has been paid to this parameter. Church *et al.* (1976), for example, mention it as a factor but do not attempt to deal with it systematically.

What I mean by attention is that, in a discrimination situation, it usually appears that the animal is using only part of the available sensory information even when thoroughly familiar with the task. Two aspects of our data and those of others initially suggested this.

First, although I could obtain very nice looking and close fitting functions relating performance to stimulus intensity in taste, vision and audition, these are never as steep as I think they should be. The slope constants of these psychometric functions are always considerably lower than those for human subjects in equivalent situations. Second, regardless of either the extent of training or the intensity of the stimuli, animals never seem to maintain perfect performance. They will maintain 95–97% correct response for session after session for weeks or months without rising above this. Both these effects show up in the present data. Starting from these observations we have done several experiments to consider how an attention parameter might be incorporated into a psychophysical model, and more importantly for present purposes, what are some of the variables that affect the level of attention.

One result that has some bearing on these data is that attention seems to vary inversely with discriminability. The harder a discrimination, the more the rat will attend to it. This would account for the lack of steepness in the psychometric functions. It also suggests that the lower the stimulus intensity or concentration, the more closely the results reflect sensitivity. Unfortunately, it also seems to be true that the effects of response bias are in the opposite direction.

A second, more significant result came from an auditory discrimination experiment done with John Kane (Morrison and Kane, 1969). In this experiment the animals were trained to discriminate between noise and noise plus tone in basically the same procedure as used in the taste experiments. Correct responses were reinforced by a 0.1 ml drop of 0.5 *M* glucose. The animals were given 100 trial daily sessions for several months and their behavior was very stable. At this point they were divided into 2 groups. The concentration of the glucose reinforcement was halved to 0.25 *M* for one group; it was doubled to 1.0 *M* for the other. Both groups were then tested for 10 additional days with constant stimulus conditions. The results of these 10 sessions are shown in Fig. 7.

By the tenth session the difference in performance between the 2 groups is of the same order of magnitude as the differences between our normal and ADX rats. This difference cannot reasonably be attributed to sensitivity, response bias, or degree of training but must reflect something along the lines of our attention factor.

Note that this is not equivalent to the situation where changing the reinforcer might well be expected to change response rate or the probability that a response occurs. All animals must respond on all trials. A correct response is still reinforced in both groups, incorrect responses are not. It seems that the 1.0 *M* group is willing to put more effort into the decision or pay more attention to the stimuli.

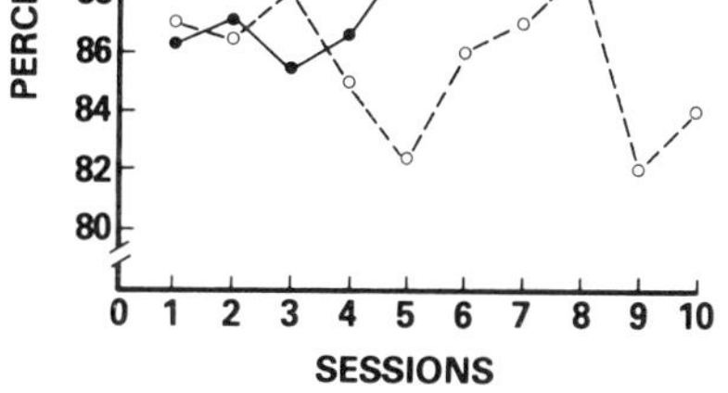

Fig. 7. Percentage correct responses as a function of trials for the two reinforcement conditions.

Given these data, we are forced to consider the possibility that in the present experiment, adrenalectomizing an animal may be functionally equivalent to changing the reinforcing value of the stimuli. In this case the effect would not depend so much on what we, as experimenters, have designated as the reinforcing stimulus, i.e., the foot pellet (and in fact the sucrose results suggest this is unimportant), but on the reinforcing aspects of the discriminative stimuli, the NaCl solutions. In an equivalent human experiment, it may well be possible for a subject to keep separate the discriminative and hedonic aspects of a stimulus and continue to respond to the former as the latter is changed. But this may well not be true for the rat.

It could even be argued that if differential attention is influencing the differences between the groups, the most likely effect would be in the opposite direction to the observed ones. Until we know more about the rat's psychophysical behavior, the variables that affect it, and how these interact, caution must be observed in interpreting results.

Our data are certainly consistent with the idea that adrenalectomy affects NaCl sensitivity by reducing the effectiveness of high concentrations. This possibility is now strongly reinforced by Contreras' results (1977) on the changes in responsiveness in salt-sensitive fibers as a result of NaCl deprivation. At least they suggest the problem is worthy of further consideration.

V. SUMMARY

I would like to emphasize that measuring sensory capacity in animals is not as simple as it sometimes appears. There are a variety of pitfalls which are not always immediately obvious. Some of the difficulties are in the method, but others are in the model. Models of human discrimination, upon which methods tend to be based, may turn out to be quite inadequate when applied to the nonhuman. Applied problems in rat measurement will require a theoretical rat psychophysics.

REFERENCES

Barnes, D. S. (1969). Altered discriminability for suprathreshold salt stimuli in the rat following bilateral adrenalectomy. B.Sc. (Hons.) Thesis, McMaster University.

Carr, W. J. (1952). The effect of adrenalectomy upon the NaCl taste threshold in the rat. *J. Comp. Physiol. Psychol.* **45,** 377-380.

Church, R., Getty, D. J., and Lerner, N. D. (1976). Duration discrimination by rats. *J. Exp. Psychol.: Anim. Behav. Process.* **2,** 303-312.

Contreras, R. J. (1977). Changes in gustatory nerve discharges with sodium deficiency: A single unit analysis. *Brain Res.* **121,** 373-378.

Harriman, A. E., and McLeod, R. B. (1953). Discriminative thresholds of salt for normal and adrenalectomized rats. *Am. J. Psychol.* **66,** 465-476.

Koh, S. D., and Teitelbaum, P. (1961). Absolute behavioral taste thresholds in the rat. *J. Comp. Physiol. Psychol.* **54,** 223-229.

Morrison, G. R. (1967). Behavioural response patterns to salt stimuli in the rat. *Can. J. Psychol.* **21,** 141-152.

Morrison, G. R. (1969). Relative discriminability of sugars for the rat. *J. Comp. Physiol. Psychol.* **68,** 45-49.

Morrison, G. R. (1972). Detectability and preference for sodium chloride and sodium carbonate. *Physiol. Behav.* **8,** 25-28.

Morrison, G. R. (1974). Taste thresholds, taste sensitivity and the effects of adrenalectomy in rats. *Chem. Senses Flavor* **1,** 77-88.

Morrison, G. R., and Kane, J. (1969). Auditory detection response bias and attention in the rat. Presented at the Canadian Psychological Association Meeting, Winnipeg.

Morrison, G. R., and Norrison, W. (1966). Taste detection in the rat. *Can. J. Psychol.* **20,** 208-217.

Pfaffmann, C., and Bare, J. K. (1950). Gustatory nerve discharges in normal and adrenalectomized rats. *J. Comp. Physiol. Psychol.* **43,** 320-324.

Richter, C. P. (1939). Salt taste thresholds of normal and adrenalectomized rats. *Endocrinology* **24,** 367-371.

Shaber, G. S., Brent, R. L., and Rumsey, J. A. (1971). Conditioned suppression taste thresholds in the rat. *J. Comp. Physiol. Psychol.* **73,** 193-201.

Part III
Factors Affecting Salt Preference

Chapter 11

Salt Intake and Equilibration

E. F. ADOLPH

A parallelism exists between salt intake and salt excretion. As is widely recognized, an excess of salt in the body is excreted. The larger the excess or load (L), the faster the output (uU) in urine (Fig. 1A), or, $uU \propto L$.

In a steady state of load, Cl^- or Na^+ output also bears a linear relation to increment of plasma Cl^- or Na^+ concentration (P) above a threshold (P_t). Data were provided for dog (Wolf, 1943; Adolph, 1957) (Fig. 1B), and for rat (Adolph *et al.*, 1954)—or, $uU \propto (P - P_t)$. Although $uU/(P - P_t) = C_d$, C_d is not the traditional renal clearance; it is analogous to clearance once a threshold of excretion (P_t) is estimated.

The load L is related to the increment of plasma concentration by the factor termed b, i.e., the volume of distribution within which the excess solute is contained. Therefore, $L = (P - P_t)b$.

Thus, $C_d = uUb/L$ is the slope of the regression line in Fig. 1C. Figure 1C represents data equivalent to those of Fig. 1A, though actually derived from measurements of plasma concentrations.

The analogy of intake to output is shown when a deficit of Na^+ in the body leads to drinking of a salt solution. Denton *et al.* (1969) measured $NaHCO_3$ ingested by a sheep at the end of 24 or 48 hours during which saliva rich in $NaHCO_3$ was drained away through a parotid fistula. Within 15 minutes the

ISBN 0-12-397750-9

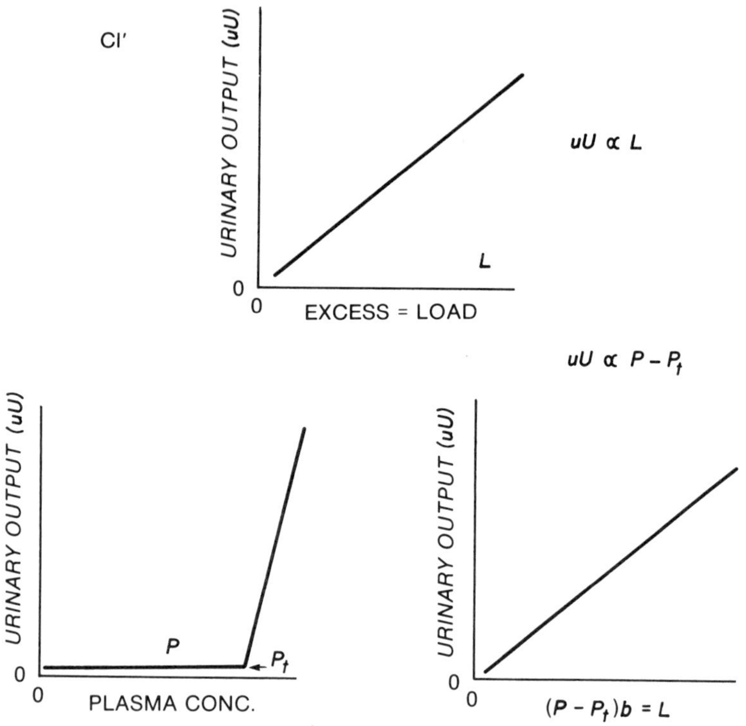

Fig. 1. Relations of chloride output to excess chloride in the body of dogs infused by vein with NaCl solutions. Data of Wolf (1943) as plotted by Adolph (1957). u = urine flow; U = Cl^- concentration in urine; L = Cl^- retained in body; P = Cl^- concentration in plasma; P_t = apparent threshold for excretion of Cl^- from plasma; b = volume of Cl^- distribution in body.

sheep made up the body's deficit of Na^+ by drinking $NaHCO_3$ solution containing that amount of Na^+ (Fig. 2A).

For convenience Denton's correlation graph was shifted from second quadrant (Fig. 2A) to first quadrant (Fig. 2B). Then the data on Cl^- or Na^+ excess (Fig. 1A) and the data on Na^+ deficit (Fig. 2B) were combined. On the ordinates (Fig. 2C) are the rates of exchange (intake, output), and on the abscissae are the loads (negative, positive). Intake and output have the same units.

The combined result (Fig. 2C) is the familiar equilibration diagram. This diagram was created to coordinate the measurements of water exchanges after various body water contents had been established. The diagram helped physiologists to regard what intake organs do as the mirror image of what output organs do. Here it does the same for Na^+.

One corollary of the diagram is that the clearance-like C_d for output has a counterpart for intake, which can be called "replenishment," S. Thus, a shop

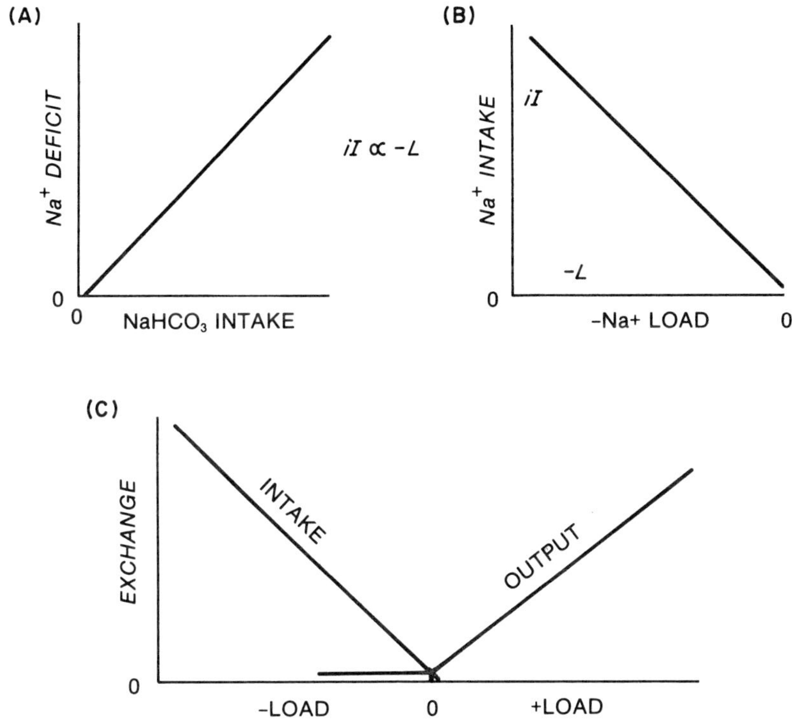

Fig. 2. (A and B) Relations of sodium intake to deficit of sodium in the body of sheep deprived of saliva by means of a fistula. Data of Denton *et al.* (1969). i = solution drunk; I = Na^+ concentration in drink; $-L$ = Na^+ deficit in body. (**C**). Combination of Figs. 1A and 2B to form an equilibration diagram, as explained in text.

that has a clearance of goods, and a turnover at which imports equal the average of goods sold, has a periodic "replenishment" that restores the equality between imports and sales of each article of commerce. $C_d = uU/(P - P_t)$ for output is positive; $S = iI/(P - P_t)$ for intake is negative.

For example, in the sheep "Cecil" of Denton *et al.*, P and P_t were 136 and 145 mEq of Na^+ per liter of plasma, respectively, after and before depletion. The 15-minute ingesta contained 1100 mEq of $NaHCO_3$, and furnished enough Na^+ to replenish the Na^+ of plasmalike fluid at

$$S = \frac{1100 \text{ mEq/15 min} \cdot 30 \text{ kg}}{(136\text{–}145) \text{ mEq/liter}} = -0.27 \text{ liters/min} \cdot \text{per kg of body}$$

Of course, the salt ingested was metered by the alimentary tract long before an appreciable amount had been absorbed into the blood.

I believe our thinking about intakes can profit by the realization that intakes relate to body contents in a manner analogous to outputs. The relation plainly says, *load* or $(P - P_t)b$, which is the independent variable, arouses *intake iI*.

REFERENCES

Adolph, E. F. (1957). Regulation in fluid exchange. *In* "Metabolic Aspects of Transport Across Cell Membranes" (Q. R. Murphy, ed.), pp. 3–22. University of Wisconsin, Madison.

Adolph, E. F., Barker, J. P., and Hoy, P. A. (1954). Multiple factors in thirst. *Am. J. Physiol.* **178,** 538–562.

Denton, D. A., Orchard, E., and Weller, S. (1969). The relation between voluntary sodium intake and body sodium balance in normal and adrenalectomized sheep. *Commun. Behav. Biol.* **3,** 213–221.

Wolf, A. V. (1943). The relative retention of infused chloride, urea and water. *Am. J. Physiol.* **138,** 191–204.

Chapter 12

Factors Affecting Salivary Sodium Concentration, NaCl Intake, and Preference Threshold and Their Interrelationships

TERRY N. THRASHER and MELVIN J. FREGLY

I. INTRODUCTION

Adrenalectomy (Richter, 1936, 1939), administration of deoxycorticosterone (DOC) (Herxheimer and Woodbury, 1960), or chronic treatment with oral con-

ISBN 0-12-397750-9

traceptives (Fregly, 1973) lower the preference threshold and induce a spontaneous appetite for NaCl solution in the rat. Sodium depletion (Falk, 1961) and hypovolemia (Stricker and Wolf, 1966; Fitzsimons, 1969) also stimulate increased intake of NaCl solution. A common feature of all the above conditions, with the exception of adrenalectomy, is an increased blood level of aldosterone.

Aldosterone is the principal sodium-retaining hormone of the body. It has also been proposed to play a role in regulating the appetite for NaCl solution (Fregly, 1967). One possible way aldosterone could influence salt intake in the rat is via effects on the concentration of sodium or the sodium-to-potassium ratio in saliva. It is well established that mineralocorticoids can influence salivary concentrations of sodium and potassium in man (Frawley and Thorn, 1951), dog (Yoshimura *et al.*, 1963), and sheep (Blair-West *et al.*, 1963). Studies on humans have demonstrated that the recognition threshold for NaCl (McBurney and Pfaffmann, 1963) and the taste intensity of a given concentration of NaCl solution (McBurney, 1963) are dependent on the concentration of sodium to which the taste receptors are adapted. Furthermore, rats made desalivate by duct ligation, which could lower the sodium concentration of the oral cavity, are reported to develop an enhanced preference for NaCl solution (Vance, 1965).

Evidence has accumulated that salt appetite in the rat is innate (Epstein and Stellar, 1955; Nachman, 1962) and that the appetite may be related to altered responses to the taste of salt (Finger and Mook, 1971). Therefore, it seems reasonable to investigate the influence of sodium concentration in saliva on preference for NaCl solution.

The aim of the studies reported here was to determine whether manipulating the level of sodium in the oral cavity could influence NaCl preference in the rat. This was accomplished both by surgical removal of the salivary glands and by perfusion of the oral cavity with solutions containing differing concentrations of sodium. In addition, measurements were made of the effects of adrenalectomy, administration of DOC, and chronic treatment with oral contraceptives on salivary sodium levels.

II. EFFECTS OF PARTIAL OR TOTAL SALIVARIECTOMY ON SODIUM CHLORIDE PREFERENCE

A. Methods

1. Experiment 1

The effects of secretions of the salivary gland on both the intake of 0.15 *M* NaCl solution and the preference threshold for NaCl solution were studied in rats subjected to partial or total salivariectomy. Twenty-four male rats (Sprague-Dawley) were housed individually, provided ground Purina Laboratory Chow and offered a choice between water and 0.15 *M* NaCl solution ad lib. Food and fluid intakes were recorded daily at which time the position of each drinking bottle was rotated. Following 10 days of control measurements, the rats were randomly assigned to four treatment groups of 6 each. Parotid and submaxillary-major sublingual glands (the desalivate group) were removed from one group; the submaxillary-major sublingual glands were removed from a second group (the submandibular group); the parotid glands were removed from a third group; and the control group underwent a sham operation. Daily measurements of the intakes of food, water, and 0.15 *M* NaCl solution were continued for 10 additional days.

In conjunction with these studies, a procedure was developed for sampling the oral secretions of the rats. The rats were lightly anesthetized with ether, and 1.0 ml of distilled water was injected into the mouth, above and below the tongue. The effluent was collected immediately and averaged consistently better than 90% of injected volume. These samples were then analyzed for sodium and potassium concentrations by flame photometry. All collections were made in the morning and were repeated at intervals throughout the postoperative experimental period.

2. *Experiment 2*

The effects of either partial or total salivariectomy on the preference threshold for NaCl solution was determined on the rats used in Experiment 1. However, the usual procedure for determining preference threshold was modified for the following reason. The desalivate rats drank very large volumes of fluid due to the necessity of moistening food in order to facilitate swallowing. Therefore, the rats were adapted to a schedule in which premoistened food (ground food mixed with water in a 2:1 proportion) was available for 4 hours in the absence of drinking fluid. A two-bottle choice between water and saline solution was available during the remaining 20 hours in the absence of food. This schedule reduced total fluid intake in the desalivate group to a level which was similar to the control group.

Initially each rat was offered a choice between two bottles containing distilled water to ensure lack of bottle or position preference. Next, the rats were offered NaCl solution in one bottle, over an ascending concentration range of 1 to 350 m*M*/liter, and distilled water in the other. The bottles were rotated daily and the concentration of NaCl changed on alternate days. The criterion chosen for determining the preference threshold was similar to the one described by Richter (1939). The preference threshold for NaCl was defined to be that concentration of NaCl at which the absolute volume intake of NaCl solution significantly ($p <$ 0.05) exceeded the volume of water drunk. A second criterion, the cross-over concentration, was also used as a check of the former method. The cross-over concentration is the lowest concentration of NaCl solution ingested by each rat, in excess of water, and beyond which the intake of NaCl solution continued to increase. Thus, this method determines the individual threshold for each rat from which a mean threshold concentration may be calculated for all rats.

3. *Experiment 3*

In order to test whether the enhanced preference for NaCl solution produced by desalivation was specific or extended to other ions, the rats were offered a choice between 0.15 *M* KCl solution and water for 2 days. The rats used in Experiments 1 and 2 were also used here. Next, the rats were again offered a choice between 0.15 *M* NaCl solution and water. Preference was defined as a significantly greater volume intake of the electrolyte solution compared to water.

4. *Experiment 4*

Salivary glands have been reported to contain significant amounts of renin (Schneyer *et al.*, 1972), which is known to be involved in the regulation of aldosterone secretion. Therefore, it is possible that salivariectomized rats could have increased urinary sodium loss which might account for the altered salt preference. To test this possibility, the same groups of rats used in previous experiments were administered an intraperitoneal load of 0.15 *M* NaCl solution equivalent to 3% of body weight while lightly anesthetized with ether. Urine was collected for 5 hours and the concentration of sodium and potassium determined by flame photometry.

B. Results

1. *Experiment 1*

The acute effects of total or partial salivariectomy on the intake of 0.15 *M* NaCl solution are shown in Fig. 1. During the control period there were no significant differences in either body weight or intake of food, water, or 0.15 *M* NaCl solution among the groups. The control group (Fig. 1A) showed no change in intake of water or saline solution during the 8 days of observation. A small decline in food intake, observed only during the first 2 days, was probably due to the combined effects of surgical stress and anesthesia. In contrast, total desalivation (Fig. 1D) was associated with a significantly greater intake of 0.15 *M* NaCl solution compared to water intake. Food intake and body weight declined rapidly during the immediate postoperative period. The large increase in saline intake observed during the last 4 days of the experiment was apparently associated with the act of learning to use fluid to aid swallowing. During this phase of the experiment, food intake returned to control levels and the decline in body weight was lessened.

The effect of removal of the submaxillary gland was similar to, but less dramatic than that of total desalivation (Fig. 1C). Food intake was depressed during the first 2 postoperative days but returned to preoperative levels during the

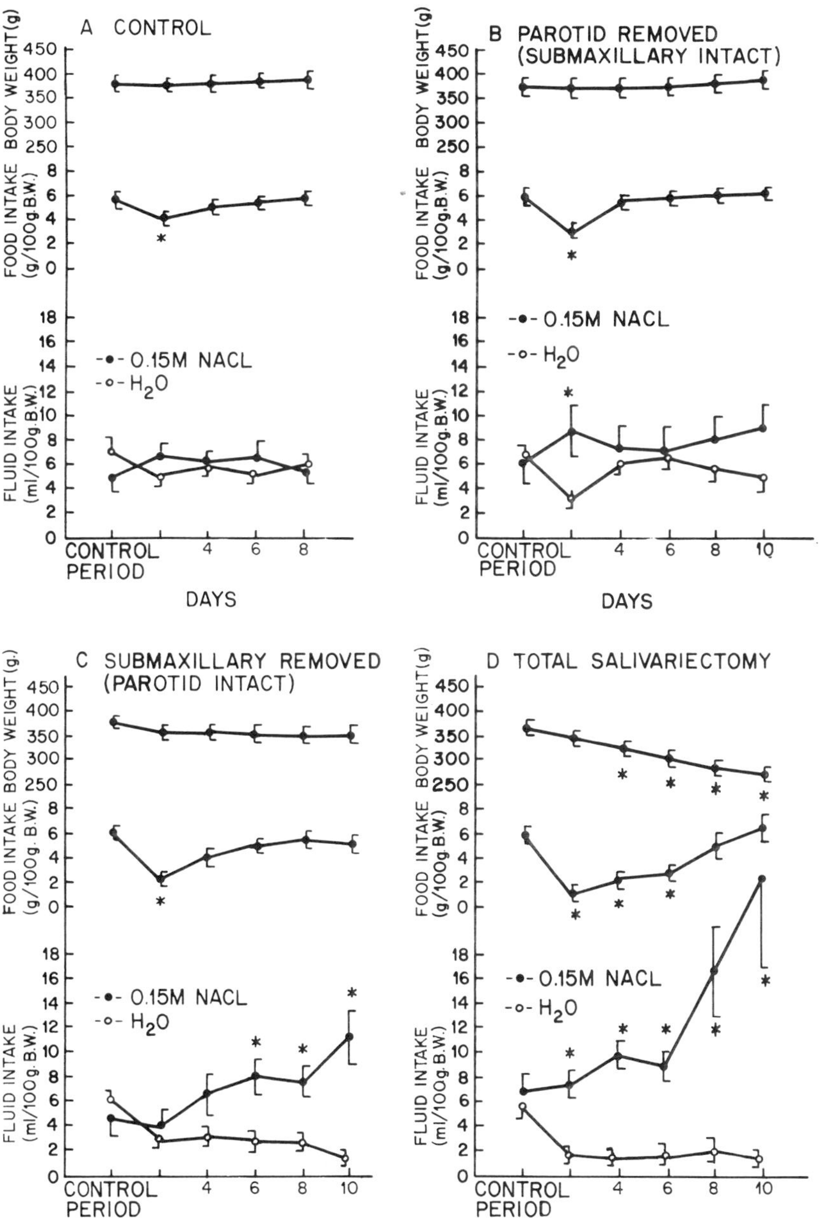

Fig. 1. Effect of sham salivariectomy (A), parotid gland removal (B), submaxillary gland removal (C), or total salivariectomy (D), on body weight and on intake of food, water, and 0.15 *M* NaCl solution. One standard error is set off at the means. Asterisks on body weight or food intake indicate a significant ($p < 0.01$) difference from preoperative control level. Asterisks on intake of NaCl solution indicate a significant difference from corresponding water intake.

TABLE I

Effect of Total or Partial Salivariectomy on the Relative Concentration of Sodium, Potassium, and the Na/K Ratio in Male Rats

Group	N	[Na] mEq/liter[a]	[K] mEq/liter[a]	Na/K
Control	6	0.43 ± 0.05	0.85 ± 0.07	0.51 ± 0.04
Parotids removed	6	0.31 ± 0.08	0.76 ± 0.08	0.39 ± 0.07
Submaxillary-major sublingual removed	6	0.15 ± 0.02[c]	0.20 ± 0.01[c]	0.81 ± 0.12[b]
Desalivate	6	0.11 ± 0.01[c]	0.20 ± 0.01[c]	0.58 ± 0.03

[a] Mean ± one standard error of the concentration in sample of oral rinse.
[b] Significantly different from control ($p < 0.05$).
[c] Significantly different from control ($p < 0.01$).

remainder of the experiment. An increase in saline intake compared to water intake was observed postoperatively and became significant by the sixth day. Water intake declined and remained depressed throughout the 10 days of observation. Body weight was unchanged during the experiment.

Removal of the parotid glands also produced a transient decline in food intake as noted in the other groups (Fig. 1B). However, saline intake exceeded water intake only during the first 2 postoperative days. Body weight was also well maintained in this group.

The concentrations of sodium and potassium in oral samples obtained from the groups are shown in Table I. Five separate collections were made from each rat. Comparison of the sodium and potassium concentrations obtained indicated good repeatability and individual values proved remarkably consistent. Therefore, the concentrations for each rat were averaged and the values shown represent the mean and standard error of each rat's mean concentration of sodium and potassium in the salivary samples. In addition, Table I shows the sodium-to-potassium ratio calculated from the concentration of these ions in each sample. The concentrations of sodium and potassium in samples collected from the desalivate rats were significantly ($p < 0.01$) lower than those of the control group. The concentrations of these two ions were also significantly ($p < 0.01$) reduced in the group without submaxillary glands. No significant differences were detected between the parotidectomized and the control groups. Comparison of the sodium-to-potassium ratios indicated that only the submaxillary group differed from control.

2. *Experiment 2*

The initial choice in the preference threshold experiment was between two bottles containing distilled water. All groups drank equal volumes from both bottles when both contained water (Fig. 2). Furthermore, there were no significant differences in total fluid intake among the groups. When offered a choice

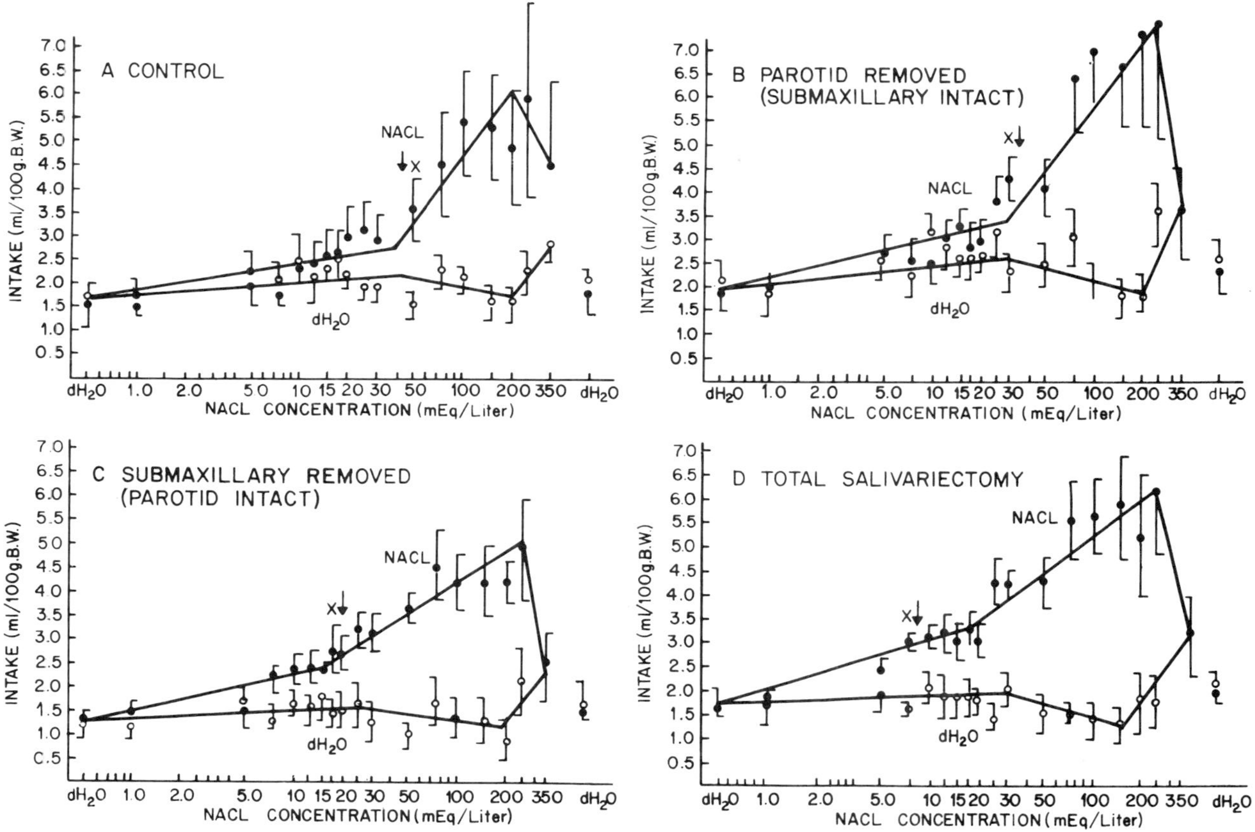

Fig. 2. Determination of preference threshold concentration for NaCl solution in control rats (A), or rats without parotid glands (B), submaxillary glands (C), or both parotid and submaxillary glands (D). One standard error is set off at the means. Arrow indicates threshold determined by the method of Richter, and X indicates threshold determined by the cross-over concentration.

between water and NaCl solution in ascending concentrations, the rats without salivary glands showed a preference for NaCl solution at a concentration of 7.5 m*M*/liter (Fig. 2D). Therefore, the preference threshold for this group lies between 5 and 7.5 m*M* NaCl/liter. In comparison, the control group did not show a preference for NaCl solution until the concentration reached 50 m*M*/liter, which indicates a threshold between 30 and 50 m*M* NaCl/liter. Partial desalivation, following removal of the submaxillary glands, also reduced the preference threshold when compared to control. This group showed a preference at 17.5 m*M*/liter, indicating a threshold between 15 and 17.5 m*M* NaCl/liter (Fig. 2C). The parotidectomized group chose 30 m*M* NaCl/liter and thus had a threshold between 25 and 30 m*M*/liter, which was slightly below the control group (Fig. 2B).

Comparison of the preference thresholds determined by the method of Richter (indicated by the arrows in Fig. 2) with those obtained by the cross-over concentration (indicated by x's) shows very good agreement. Therefore, total or partial desalivation does affect the preference threshold concentration for NaCl solution.

Spontaneous intake of NaCl solution peaked at 250 m*M*/liter in all groups and declined sharply at higher concentrations. Finally, when both bottles contained water, the rats drank equal volumes from each bottle. Measurements of food intake during the experiment indicated no significant differences among the groups. Therefore, dietary sodium deficiency could not have been a factor in these results.

3. *Experiment 3*

The results of preference tests between water and either 0.15 *M* NaCl or 0.15 *M* KCl solution, are shown in Table II. All groups showed a significant preference for the NaCl solution over water. However, none of the groups displayed a similar preference for the KCl solution. Therefore, these data indicate that the preference for NaCl solution after total or partial salivariectomy is not generalized to solutions containing potassium salts.

TABLE II

Effect of Partial or Total Salivariectomy on Intake of NaCl and KCl Compared to Water

		Intake (ml/100 g body wt)[a]			
Group	N	Water	0.15 *M* NaCl	Water	0.15 *M* KCl
Control	6	1.6 ± 0.4	5.3 ± 1.1[b]	2.5 ± 0.4	2.7 ± 0.5
Parotids removed	6	1.7 ± 0.4	6.7 ± 1.3[b]	3.6 ± 0.8	2.4 ± 0.5
Submaxillary-major sublingual removed	6	1.4 ± 0.4	4.3 ± 0.7[b]	1.8 ± 0.6	2.8 ± 0.5
Desalivate	6	1.3 ± 0.4	5.9 ± 1.1[b]	2.7 ± 0.6	2.6 ± 0.3

[a] Mean ± 1 S.E.
[b] Significantly different from corresponding water intake ($p < 0.01$).

TABLE III

Effect of Partial or Total Salivariectomy on Renal Response to an Acute Load of 0.15 *M* NaCl Solution[a]

Group	N	Urine volume (ml)	Urinary output (mEq/kg body wt)[b]		
			Na	K	Na/K
Control	7	9.2 ± 1.7	2.3 ± 0.5	0.8 ± 0.1	2.6 ± 0.4
Parotids removed	6	9.0 ± 1.5	2.1 ± 0.5	1.0 ± 0.1	2.2 ± 0.6
Submaxillary-major sublingual removed	4	9.7 ± 1.3	2.3 ± 0.5	1.2 ± 0.2	2.0 ± 0.4
Desalivate	7	9.8 ± 0.9	2.2 ± 0.2	1.1 ± 0.1	2.0 ± 0.2

[a] Load administered ip equivalent to 3% of body weight.
[b] Mean ± 1 S.E.

4. *Experiment 4*

The renal response to an acute intraperitoneal load of 0.15 *M* NaCl solution is shown in Table III. No significant differences were evident with respect to either urine volume, urinary sodium or potassium output, or the sodium-to-potassium ratio of the urine. Thus, these data suggest that salivariectomized rats do not have increased urinary loss of sodium.

C. Discussion

Desalivation is known to produce a large increase in fluid intake (Epstein *et al.*, 1964; Vance, 1965). The excess drinking is associated with eating dry food and is used as an aid to facilitate swallowing. The results shown in Fig. 1 demonstrate that acute removal of the salivary glands has a dramatic effect on the intake of NaCl solution. The fact that total fluid intake increases in the desalivate rat could account for the increased volume intake of NaCl solution. However, in these experiments the rat had a choice between water and NaCl solution and chose to drink from the salt bottle almost exclusively. Water intake declined from preoperative levels and remained depressed throughout the 10 days of observation. Therefore, the enhanced preference for NaCl solution cannot be due to increased fluid intake alone.

The group without submaxillary glands (Fig. 1C) also demonstrated an enhanced preference for NaCl solution and a decline in water intake. However, the total fluid intake by this group was not significantly different from preoperative levels. Thus, as with the desalivate group, the altered preference behavior appears unrelated to changes in total fluid intake. The group without parotid glands (Fig. 1B) differed from these two groups in that a slight increase in saline intake occurred initially but was unchanged over the final 8 days of observation.

The enhanced preference for NaCl solution seen in both the desalivate and submandibular groups could be explained in three ways: (1) The decreased food intake produced a state of dietary sodium deficiency and the preference was secondary to sodium depletion; (2) removal of salivary glands eliminated a source of renin and, therefore, increased urinary loss of sodium produced a sodium deficit; or (3) the reduction in concentration of sodium in fluids bathing the taste receptors altered the taste response to NaCl solution. The possibility of dietary sodium deficiency does not appear to be the primary cause since food intake of the desalivate group, while depressed for the first 6 postoperative days, was, nevertheless, sufficient to provide the minimal requirement of 4 mg/day (Spector, 1956). Furthermore, in the submandibular group, food intake was depressed for only the first 2 days postoperatively, as in all groups, yet these rats showed an enhanced preference for NaCl throughout the study (Fig. 1C).

The possibility that increased renal sodium excretion was responsible for the NaCl appetite was tested. No differences in the rate of renal sodium excretion were observed among the groups in response to an intraperitoneal load of 0.15 *M* NaCl solution. This study suggests that the desalivate and submandibular groups were not losing excessive amounts of sodium in urine.

The results support the notion that the level of sodium in saliva may play a role in determining the preference for NaCl solution. Measurements of the sodium concentration in oral samples taken from the rats (Table I) suggest an inverse relationship between sodium concentration and preference for 0.15 *M* NaCl solution. For example, the desalivate group had the lowest oral sodium concentration and the greatest increase in NaCl intake. The oral sodium concentration in the group without submaxillary glands was significantly below control levels but above that of the desalivate group. This group increased its intake of NaCl solution but not as dramatically as the desalivate group. The oral sodium concentration of the parotid group was not different from the control group and intake of NaCl solution did not differ between the two groups. These results suggest that preference for NaCl solution may be affected by the level of sodium in the fluid bathing the tongue.

The enhanced NaCl preference observed in desalivate rats could reflect a nonspecific response to decreased saliva and might, therefore, be extended to other electrolyte solutions. A test of this possibility indicated that KCl solution was not preferred over water but NaCl solution was (Table II). Therefore, the enhanced preference for NaCl is not a nonspecific response to loss of salivary secretions.

Many conditions which cause an increased sodium appetite have also been shown to lower the preference threshold concentration for NaCl solution, e.g., treatment with mineralocorticoids, oral contraceptives, and adrenalectomy. Therefore, the effect of partial or total salivariectomy on the preference threshold for NaCl solution was examined. The results (Fig. 2) clearly indicate that removal of the salivary glands lowers the preference threshold concentration.

The possibility of a relationship between the salivary concentrations of sodium, potassium, or the Na/K ratio, and the preference threshold for NaCl solution was tested by regression analysis. The line equating X (salivary sodium concentration) and Y (preference threshold) was computed using the salivary sodium concentration and preference threshold of each rat. The resulting equation was $Y = 95.7\ X + 0.88$. The correlation coefficient was $r = 0.93$, which was significant ($p < 0.01$, $n = 24$), and suggests that the two variables are related. A plot of each group's mean preference threshold against the mean salivary sodium concentration is shown in Fig. 3. The correlation coefficient (r) of the regression of preference threshold on salivary potassium concentration and on the Na/K ratio was 0.62 and −0.22, respectively. Since the correspondence between sodium and threshold was considerably higher than that with either potassium or the Na/K ratio, it suggests that the sodium level is the principal determinant of the preference threshold concentration in the rat.

The relationship between preference threshold and sodium concentration in the rat (Fig. 3) is very similar to that described for NaCl recognition threshold in humans by McBurney and Pfaffmann (1963). They observed that the concentration at which a solution was recognized as containing NaCl just exceeded the concentration of NaCl solution to which the taste receptors had been adapted. Furthermore, when the threshold concentration, obtained with the tongue adapted to the subject's saliva, was plotted against the sodium concentration in that same subject's saliva, the point fell on the line relating adapting concentration to threshold. Although it is impossible to equate human recognition threshold to rat preference threshold for NaCl solution, the similarity between the

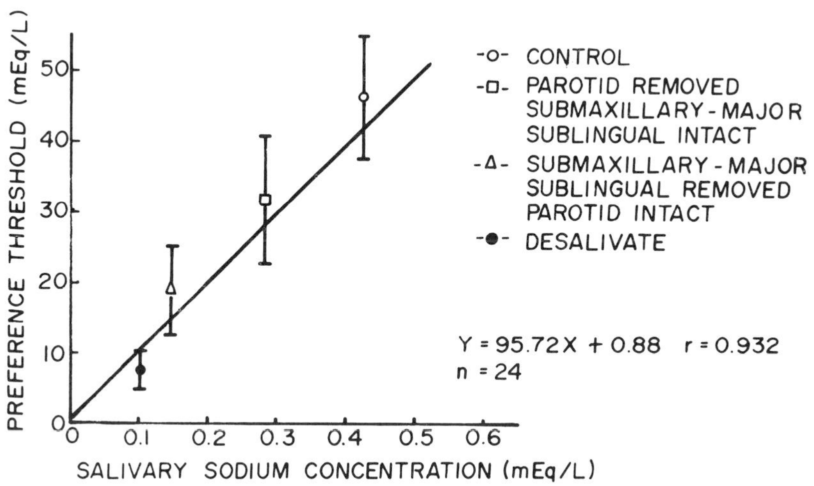

Fig. 3. Relationship between salivary sodium concentration (mEq/liter) and preference threshold in partially or totally desalivate rats. Points and standard error bars are the mean preference thresholds of the groups determined by the cross-over concentration method.

results with respect to the influence of salivary sodium concentration is striking.

Electrophysiologic studies have also suggested a relation between adaptation concentration and taste receptor response to NaCl solution (Pfaffmann, 1961). Measurements of integrated electrical activity of the chorda tympani nerve have shown that the steady-state level of activity depends on the concentration of the solution to which the taste receptors are adapted. For example, adaptation to water produced the lowest level of activity. Applying a stimulating solution containing sodium in higher concentration than the adapting solution produced an increment in activity. Conversely, applying a solution with a lower than adapted sodium concentration decreased nerve activity. Thus, recognition and preference thresholds for sodium may be reached only when the test solution contains a higher concentration of this ion compared to the adapting fluid.

Returning to the results of Experiment 1, the large increase in volume intake seen in the desalivate rats is certainly related to prandial drinking. Thus, substituting a wet-mash diet (Experiment 2) for the dry food returned volume intake to normal. However, the fact remains that when drinking prandially, the desalivate rat preferred NaCl solution almost totally to water (Fig. 1D). These results are at variance with those reported in the literature. Vance (1965) noted that preference for NaCl solution peaked 4 days after ligating the salivary ducts and then declined, reaching the level of water intake after about 50 days. Kissileff (1967) also reported that desalivate rats failed to show a preference for saline solution. He suggested that the loss of preference was due to masking the taste of salt during prandial drinking because preference returned if food was removed. Whether the enhanced preference for NaCl would have disappeared in Experiment 1 is unknown because it was terminated after 10 days. However, it is possible that the differences are due to the method of producing desalivation. Both Vance and Kissileff reduced salivary flow by ligating the salivary ducts as opposed to surgical desalivation used in the present study. The answer to this question is unresolved and awaits further study.

The results of these studies suggest that the concentration of sodium to which the taste receptors are adapted may influence the rat's preference for NaCl solution. A more direct test of this proposition would be to determine preference for NaCl after sequential alterations in salivary electrolyte concentration. An experimental approach to this question is described next.

III. EFFECT OF SEQUENTIAL ALTERATIONS IN SALIVARY ELECTROLYTE CONCENTRATION ON PREFERENCE FOR NaCl

A. Methods

A method was developed to allow continuous perfusion of the oral cavity in the unanesthetized, unrestrained rat via a chronically implanted catheter in the submaxillary duct. The submaxillary major-sublingual and parotid glands were removed after placement of the catheter in the duct. The experimental protocol consisted of perfusing the oral cavity with various solutions containing sodium and potassium chloride while measuring intake of water and 0.15 *M* NaCl solution. The perfusion rate was set at 2.06 μl/min, which totaled 3 ml/day, or less than 5% of the average daily fluid intake. Five different perfusion solutions were used and were made up to contain sodium in the following concentrations: less than 10^{-6} *M* NaCl and 25, 50, 75, and 100 m*M* NaCl. Each solution also contained 50 m*M* KCl/liter.

Perfusion was begun immediately after surgery but a 3-day recovery period was allowed before measurements were begun. The rat was perfused with each solution in ascending order for 20 hours, during which time water and saline were restricted but food (moistened with water in a 2:1 proportion) was available. The food was removed in the morning and the rat was offered a choice between water and 0.15 *M* NaCl solution during a 4-hour test period. After the drinking test, the perfusion solution was changed and the sequence repeated. Drinking, in response to each perfusion solution, was replicated three times in each of three rats.

B. Results and Discussion

Perfusing the oral cavity with a solution containing less than 1 m*M* sodium/liter produced a large intake of NaCl solution and a small water intake (Fig. 4). Preference for NaCl solution, expressed as intake of saline/total fluid was 85% (Fig. 4). Graded increases in the sodium concentration of the perfusion solution was accompanied by graded decreases in the intake of NaCl solution and concomitant increases in water intake. The preference ratio of NaCl to total fluid intake also declined as sodium concentration in the perfused solution increased. Intake of water and NaCl solution was about equal when the perfusion solution contained 75 and 100 m*M* sodium/liter.

The results of this experiment provide direct evidence for a relationship between the levels of sodium to which the taste receptors are exposed and preference for NaCl solution. When the concentration of sodium in the perfusion solution was low, intake of NaCl solution represented about 85% of total fluid intake. An increase in the concentration of sodium in the solution perfusing the tongue was accompanied by a decrease in the preference for NaCl solution. The results of this experiment are also compatible with the suggestion of an inverse relationship between the level of salivary sodium and preference for NaCl proposed previously. Thus, each group of rats in the previous experiment (Fig. 1) had a different level of salivary sodium, and each group had a different preference for NaCl solution. This experiment shows that exposing the rat to various levels of sodium systematically alters the preference for NaCl solution in the same inverse fashion.

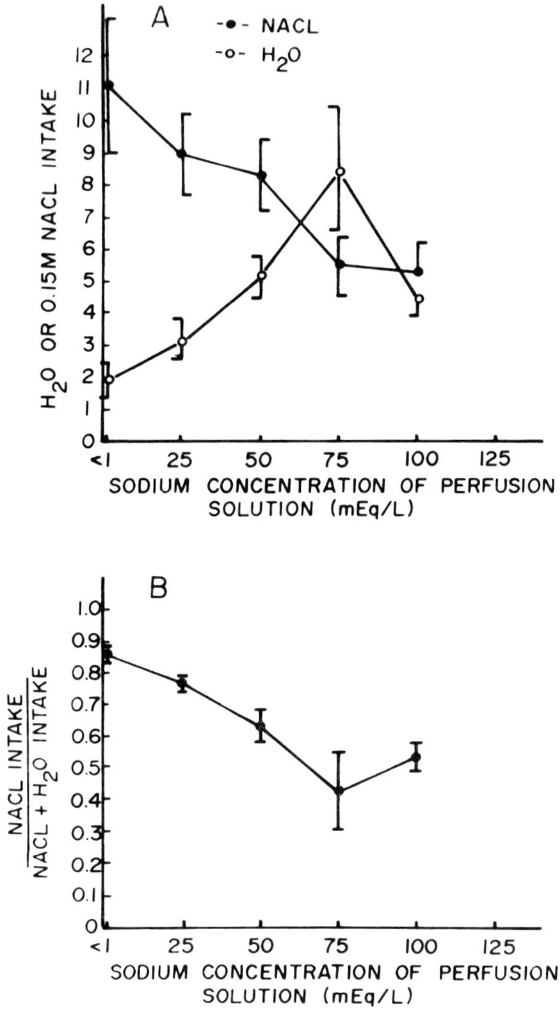

Fig. 4. Effect of chronic infusion of the oral cavity with various concentrations of sodium on intake of 0.15 *M* NaCl solution (A) and the ratio of NaCl intake to total fluid intake (B). One standard error is set off at the means.

If our interpretation of these results is correct, one could predict that procedures which lower the preference threshold for NaCl and stimulate a salt appetite might also lower the sodium concentration of saliva. This prediction was tested in adrenalectomized rats and in rats administered either deoxycorticosterone (DOC) or oral contraceptives.

IV. EFFECT OF ADRENALECTOMY AND DOC OR ORAL CONTRACEPTIVES ON SALIVARY SODIUM CONCENTRATION

A. Methods

1. Experiment 5

The effect of adrenalectomy and acute administration of DOC on salivary sodium concentration was studied in female rats. The rats were subjected to either adrenalectomy or a sham operation while anesthetized with ether, and maintained on water and 0.25 *M* NaCl solution thereafter for a 2-week recovery period. During a subsequent 7-day intake period, oral samples were collected frequently for determination of sodium and potassium concentrations. Next, the rats were restricted from all fluids for 18 hours and salivary sodium concentration measured after 4, 12, and 18 hours of sodium deprivation. Following a 3-day recovery period the acute effect of sc administration of DOC (1 and 2 mg/kg) on salivary sodium concentration was determined.

2. Experiment 6

The effect of chronic treatment with an estrogen and a progestin, alone or combined, was studied in female rats. One group received ethynyl estradiol, one received norethynodrel, a third received both agents, and a fourth served as an untreated control group. The drugs were administered via silastic tubes implanted sc in the dorsal region of the neck. This procedure has been described in detail previously (Fregly and Thrasher, 1977). Briefly, drug dosages (μg/kg/day) were calculated by measuring the change in tube weight (before minus after implantation), divided by the body weight and the number of days the tubes were implanted. After implantation of the tubes, the rats were returned to their home cages and maintained on their normal diet and water for 5 weeks. During the sixth week of drug treatment, salivary samples were collected for determination of sodium and potassium concentrations. The rats were then offered a choice between water and 0.15 *M* NaCl solution for a 7-day intake period.

B. Results

1. Experiment 5

The adrenalectomized rats drank significantly ($p < 0.01$) more 0.25 *M* NaCl solution than controls (21.0 ± 1.7 [SE] versus 10.2 ± 2.0 ml/100 g body wt) as expected. Water intake by the adrenalectomized rats also differed significantly ($p < 0.05$) from controls (2.0 ± 0.7 versus 5.7 ± 0.4 ml/100 g body wt, respectively). However, body weights and food intakes of the two groups were not

TABLE IV

Effect of Salt and Water Deprivation on Relative Salivary Electrolyte Concentration in Intact and Adrenalectomized Rats

			Relative salivary concentration (mEq/liter)[a]			
Group	N	Ion	Predeprivation	4 Hours	12 Hours	18 Hours
Control	8	Na	0.17 ± 0.03	0.14 ± 0.02	0.15 ± 0.04	0.22 ± 0.04
		K	0.50 ± 0.06	0.42 ± 0.03[b]	0.62 ± 0.06	0.50 ± 0.09
Adrex	6	Na	0.52 ± 0.08[c]	0.38 ± 0.7[b,c]	0.32 ± 0.6[b,c,]	0.23 ± 0.03[b]
		K	0.56 ± 0.03	0.49 ± 0.05[b]	0.54 ± 0.05	0.45 ± 0.08

[a] Mean ± 1 S.E.
[b] Significantly different compared to predeprivation ($p < 0.05$).
[c] Significantly different compared to control at time indicated ($p < 0.01$).

different. Salivary sodium concentration in the adrenalectomized group was significantly ($p < 0.01$) higher than control in the salt replete state (Table IV). However, sodium concentration fell dramatically in the adrenalectomized group during sodium deprivation, and was no different from control levels after 18 hours of restriction. Salivary sodium levels of the control group were not affected significantly by 18 hours of sodium deprivation.

The effect of acute administration of either 1.0 or 2.0 mg DOC/kg (SC) on salivary sodium concentration in control and adrenalectomized rats is shown in Table V. No significant differences were observed between the effects of the two doses in the two groups; therefore these data were pooled. Prior to administration of DOC, the adrenalectomized group had a significantly higher salivary sodium concentration. Ten hours after DOC, sodium levels were significantly ($p < 0.05$) reduced in both groups. At 20 hours, sodium concentrations had returned to preadministration levels.

TABLE V

Effect of Acute Administration of DOC on Salivary Sodium Concentration of Control and Adrenalectomized Rats

		Salivary sodium concentration (mEq/liter)[a]		
Group	N	Before treatment	10 Hours[b]	20 Hours[b]
Control	9	0.19 ± 0.02	0.10 ± 0.02[c]	0.24 ± 0.06
Adrex	8	0.50 ± 0.09	0.29 ± 0.06[c]	0.39 ± 0.10

[a] Mean ± 1 S.E.
[b] After sc administration of DOC.
[c] Significantly different from pretreatment level ($p < 0.05$).

TABLE VI

Effect of Chronic Administration of Ethynyl Estradiol and Norethynodrel, Alone or Combined, on Intake of Food, Water, and 0.15 *M* NaCl Solution and on Salivary Sodium Concentration

Treatment	N	Mean body wt[a] (g)	Intake (ml or g/100 g body wt)[a] Food	Water	0.15 *M* NaCl	Salivary sodium concentration[b]
Control	9	298 ± 5	5.1 ± 0.3	3.1 ± 0.6	10.4 ± 1.5	0.14 ± 0.01
Norethynodrel	10	268 ± 6[d]	4.8 ± 0.1	2.7 ± 0.7	20.4 ± 1.6[d]	0.07 ± 0.01[d]
Ethynyl estradiol	10	262 ± 6[d]	6.2 ± 0.3[c]	2.9 ± 0.6	28.8 ± 2.0[d]	0.10 ± 0.02[d]
Combined	8	257 ± 6[d]	5.6 ± 0.3	3.8 ± 1.1	26.9 ± 1.9[d]	0.10 ± 0.01[d]

[a] Mean ± 1 S.E.
[b] After 5 weeks of treatment and before access to NaCl solution.
[c] Significantly different from control group ($p < 0.05$).
[d] Significantly different from control group ($p < 0.01$).

2. *Experiment 6*

Six weeks of treatment with either the estrogenic or progestational agent alone or combined, stimulated a significant ($p < 0.01$) salt appetite when compared to the control group (Table VI). Steroid treatment produced a significant reduction in salivary sodium concentration in all groups when compared to controls. No effect of treatment was seen on water intake, but body weight was reduced significantly ($p < 0.01$) below that of controls. Food intake was increased in the group receiving ethynyl estradiol alone. The dose of ethynyl estradiol and norethynodrel received was 27 μg/kg/day and 250 μg/kg/day, respectively.

C. Discussion

The sodium concentration in oral secretions of adrenalectomized rats maintained on 0.25 *M* NaCl solution is much higher than that of intact rats (Table IV). This agrees with observations on salivary sodium levels in Addisonian patients (Frawley and Thorn, 1951). During acute sodium restriction, sodium levels in saliva of the adrenalectomized rats fell dramatically, reflecting the rapid loss of body sodium. On the other hand, administration of DOC produced a significant reduction in salivary sodium concentration in both adrenalectomized and intact rats (Table V). These data show that the blood level of mineralocorticoids exerts a strong influence on the concentration of sodium in oral secretions.

Administration of oral contraceptives induced a significant salt appetite in accordance with previous reports (Fregly, 1973). Measurements of the salivary sodium concentration in treated rats showed that a significant reduction in sodium levels preceded the increased appetite for NaCl solution (Table VI). Whether the effect of these agents on saliva is direct or mediated by aldosterone is unknown. However, urinary excretion of aldosterone is elevated in women taking oral contraceptives, which suggests increased blood levels of the hormone (Crane *et al.*, 1966).

Conditions which stimulate a salt appetite in intact rats, e.g., sodium depletion, hypovolemia, or administration of DOC, are associated with increased blood levels of mineralocorticoids. Increased aldosterone secretion observed in sodium depletion and hypovolemia results from activation of the renal renin-angiotensin system (Davis, 1976). However, administration of exogenous mineralocorticoid depresses angiotensin levels due to sodium retention and subsequent volume expansion. On the other extreme, salt appetite after adrenalectomy occurs in the absence of aldosterone.

An explanation of these divergent observations has been proposed by Fregly (1967). He described a U-shaped dose-response relationship between blood levels of mineralocorticoids and intake of NaCl solution. In this model, the intact rat lies at the apex of the curve and the adrenalectomized rat is at the peak of the descending limb. Administration of graded doses of aldosterone to the adrenalectomized rat reduces NaCl intake, with maximal reduction being achieved at a dose of 100 μg/kg. This dose approximates the daily aldosterone secretion rate of the intact rat (Cade and Perenich, 1965), and thus returns the rat to the apex of the curve. Higher doses of aldosterone move the rat up the ascending limb of the curve, stimulating a salt appetite which approaches that of the untreated adrenalectomized control. Intact rats, subjected to salt depletion, hypovolemia, or exogenous DOC could also be considered to be on the ascending limb of the curve.

The results reported here suggest a U-shaped relationship between the concentration of sodium in saliva and intake of NaCl solution (Fig. 5). The intact sodium-replete rat is assumed to be near the apex of the curve relating sodium concentration to NaCl intake. The increased salt appetite induced by sodium depletion could then be explained in terms of reduced salivary sodium levels secondary to increased secretion of aldosterone. Administration of exogenous mineralocorticoid would also lower sodium in saliva, leading to increased NaCl intake even though total body sodium is elevated. According to this hypothesis, the adrenalectomized rat increases its intake of NaCl solution because of its high salivary sodium concentration (Table IV). The latter is the result of a reduction in the concentration of mineralocorticoid hormone in blood.

The acutely adrenalectomized rat, with continual access to NaCl solution, shows a gradual increase in NaCl intake (Richter, 1936; Epstein and Stellar, 1955). If the rate at which adrenalectomized rats lose sodium is taken into account, it seems reasonable to suggest that a decline in salivary sodium concentration could have preceded the increased intake. Conversely, adrenalectomized rats deprived of salt for a number of days postoperatively, show an immediate appetite for NaCl solution (Epstein and Stellar, 1955). Clearly, these animals

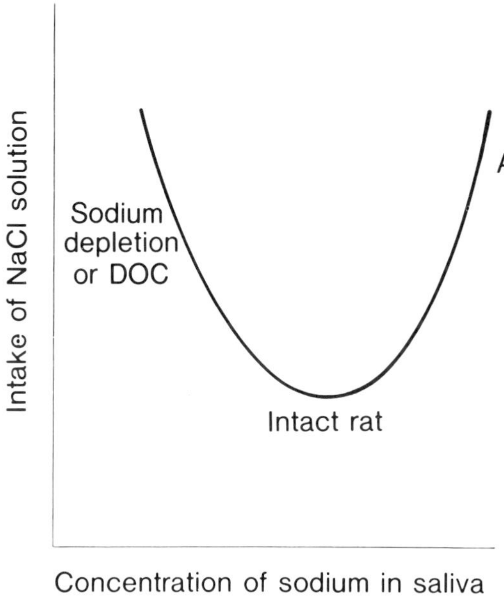

Fig. 5. Derived relationship between concentration of sodium in saliva and intake of NaCl solution. Proposed positions of intact rats, adrenalectomized rats, and sodium-deficient rats are illustrated on the curve.

would be severely depleted of sodium which would certainly be reflected in the level of sodium in saliva. However, maintenance of a high sodium intake by adrenalectomized rats may occur as a result of episodic changes in salivary sodium concentration. It is also possible that reduced salivary sodium concentration initiated the increased intake while maintained intake is due to learned responses as with other specific appetites (Rozin and Kalat, 1971).

The relationship between salivary sodium levels and preference threshold concentration (Fig. 3) is more easily reconciled with the data. Thus, a chronic reduction in salivary sodium levels regardless of cause, would allow recognition of the taste of sodium in solution at a concentration below that observed in sodium-replete rats. The reported experiments in which preference threshold was determined for adrenalectomized rats, all began with the choice between two bottles of water. Thus, it is likely that these rats suffered from sodium depletion producing very low levels of sodium in saliva. The reduced salivary sodium concentration would then be compatible with the observed reduction in preference threshold.

One possible way in which the levels of sodium in saliva could influence intake of NaCl solution is by affecting the neural output of the taste receptors. It has been shown that adrenalectomy does not alter the absolute level of sensitivity of the taste receptor to NaCl solution (Pfaffmann and Bare, 1950). However, the level of neural activity produced by a given concentration of sodium in solution is dependent on the adaptational state of the taste receptor (Pfaffmann, 1961). Thus, applying sodium to the tongue at the same concentration as in saliva does not alter integrated neural activity recorded from the chorda tympani. However, applying the same concentration of sodium to a tongue adapted to water produces a large increment in neural activity. Thus, the taste receptor response to a given NaCl solution may be constant, but the neural message represents the difference between the steady-state activity of the taste receptor, which is determined by the ambient environment provided by saliva, and the magnitude of the taste receptor response to that NaCl solution.

V. SUMMARY

The studies reported here suggest that the level of sodium bathing the taste receptors can influence preference for NaCl solution in the rat. Evidence has been presented which shows that systematically altering the sodium concentration of the fluid bathing the tongue affects both intake of NaCl solution and the ratio of NaCl to total fluid intake. Furthermore, data have been presented which indicate that the level of sodium in saliva is inversely related to the preference threshold for NaCl solution. It is proposed that the concentration of sodium in saliva is one factor which participates in the development of a salt appetite and that determines the preference threshold concentration for NaCl solution.

ACKNOWLEDGMENT

Supported by Grant HL-14526-07 from the National Heart, Lung and Blood Institute.

REFERENCES

Blair-West, J. R., Coghlan, J. P., Denton, D. A., Goding, J. R., and Wright, R. D. (1963). The effect of aldosterone, cortisol and corticosterone upon the sodium and potassium content of sheep's parotid saliva. *J. Clin. Invest.* **42,** 484–495.

Cade, J. E., and Perenich, T. (1965). Secretion of aldosterone by rats. *Am. J. Physiol.* **208,** 1026–1030.

Crane, M. G., and Harris, J. J. (1969). Plasma renin activity and aldosterone excretion rate. II. Effects of oral contraceptive agents. *J. Clin. Endocrinol. Metab.* **29,** 558–562.

Davis, J. O. (1976). Mechanisms regulating renin release. *Physiol. Rev.* **56,** 1–56.

Epstein, A. N., and Stellar, E. (1955). The control of salt preference in the adrenalectomized rat. *J. Comp. Physiol. Psychol.* **48,** 167–172.

Epstein, A. N., Spector, D., Samman, A., and Goldblum, C. (1964). Exaggerated prandial drinking in the rat without salivary glands. *Nature (London)* **201,** 1342–1343.

Falk, J. L. (1961). The behavioral regulation of water-electrolyte balance. *In* "Nebraska Symposium on Motivation" (M. R. Jones, ed.), pp. 71-108. Univ. of Nebraska Press, Lincoln.

Finger, F. W., and Mook, D. G. (1971). Basic drives. *Annu. Rev. Psychol.* **22,** 1-38.

Fitzsimons, J. T. (1969). The role of a renal thirst factor in drinking induced by extracellular stimuli. *J. Physiol. (London)* **201,** 349-369.

Frawly, P. F., and Thorn, G. W. (1951). The relation of the salivary Na/K ratio to adrenal cortical activity. *Proc. Clin. ACTH Conf., 2nd, 1950* Vol. I, pp. 115-123.

Fregly, M. J. (1967). The role of hormones in the regulation of salt intake in rats. *In* "The Chemical Senses and Nutrition" (M. R. Kare and O. Maller, eds.), pp. 115-138. Johns Hopkins Press, Baltimore, Maryland.

Fregly, M. J. (1973). Effect of an oral contraceptive on NaCl appetite and preference threshold in rats. *Pharmacol., Biochem. Behav.* **1,** 61-65.

Fregly, M. J., and Thrasher, T. N. (1977). Response of heart rate to acute administration of isoproterenol in rats treated chronically with norethynodrel, ethynyl estradiol, and both combined. *Endocrinology* **100,** 148-154.

Herxheimer, A., and Woodbury, D. M. (1960). The effect of deoxycorticosterone on salt and sucrose taste preference thresholds and drinking behavior in rats. *J. Physiol. (London)* **151,** 253-260.

Kissileff, H. R. (1967). Loss of saline preference in rats drinking prandially. *Am. Zool.* **7,** 352.

McBurney, D. (1963). Magnitude estimation of NaCl intensity after NaCl adaptation. *Proc. 4th Annu. Meet., Psychon. Soc., 1963* p. 000.

McBurney, D., and Pfaffmann, C. (1963). Gustatory adaptation to saliva and sodium chloride. *J. Exp. Psychol.* **65,** 523-529.

Nachman, M. (1962). Taste preferences for sodium salts by adrenalectomized rats. *J. Comp. Physiol. Psychol.* **55,** 1124-1129.

Pfaffmann, C. (1961). The sensory and motivating properties of the sense of taste. *In* "Nebraska Symposium on Motivation" (M. R. Jones, ed.), pp. 71-108. Univ. of Nebraska Press, Lincoln.

Pfaffmann, C., and Bare, J. K. (1950). Gustatory nerve discharges in normal and adrenalectomized rats. *J. Comp. Physiol. Psychol.* **43,** 320-324.

Richter, C. P. (1936). Increased salt appetite in adrenalectomized rats. *Am. J. Physiol.* **115,** 155-161.

Richter, C. P. (1939). Salt taste thresholds of normal and adrenalectomized rats. *Endocrinology* **24,** 367-371.

Rozin, P., and Kalat, J. W. (1971). Specific hungers and poison avoidance as adaptive specializations of learning. *Psychol. Rev.* **78,** 459-486.

Schneyer, L. H., Young, J. A., and Schneyer, C. A. (1972). Salivary secretion of electrolytes. *Physiol. Rev.* **52,** 720-777.

Spector, W. S. (1956). "Handbook of Biological Data," Pennsylvania. Philadelphia, p. 211. Saunders,

Stricker, E. M., and Wolf, G. (1966). Blood volume and tonicity in relation to sodium appetite. *J. Comp. Physiol. Psychol.* **62,** 275-279.

Vance, W. B. (1965). Observations on the role of salivary secretions in the regulation of food and fluid intake in the white rat. *Psychol. Monogr.* **79,** 1-22.

Yoshimura, H., Miyoshi, M., Matsumoto, S., Fujimoto, T., and Yamamoto, Y. (1963). Reflections of salt concentrations of blood upon those of saliva. *Jpn. J. Physiol.* **12,** 523-540.

Chapter 13

A Possible Role for Angiotensin in the Elicitation of Salt Appetite

R. W. BRYANT, A. N. EPSTEIN, AND S. J. FLUHARTY

I. INTRODUCTION

The appetite for sodium that is induced by disorders of sodium metabolism is a classic phenomenon of neuropsychology. It was first described by Richter (1936) in the adrenalectomized rat and is induced, we know now, by a variety of challenges (Denton and Sabine, 1961; Fregly and Waters, 1966; Falk, 1961; Stricker, 1973; Wolf, 1964), some of which occur naturally (adrenal insufficiency, sodium deprivation), others of which are inventions of the laboratory (intraperitoneal dialysis, parotid fistulation, subcutaneous trauma with formalin, treatment with furosemide and other diuretics), all of which have in common a reduction of plasma sodium. The ingestion of large amounts of sodium, even when offered at strong and normally avoided concentrations, by animals subjected to these challenges is an ideal example of self-regulatory behavior.

BIOLOGICAL AND BEHAVIORAL
ASPECTS OF SALT INTAKE

ISBN 0-12-397750-9

But the appetite does not appear to be a simple expression of sodium homeostatus. It can be produced by pharmacological doses of the mineralocorticoids (aldosterone and deoxycorticosterone) which maintain animals in positive sodium balance (Fregly and Waters, 1966; Wolf, 1964; Wolf and Handel, 1966), and it is not controlled by manipulations of plasma sodium (Beilharz *et al.*, 1962; Falk, 1961; Nachman and Valentino, 1966). Once it is established, decreases in the concentration of plasma sodium do not appear to be the direct cause of the appetite.

But, because hyponatremia is prominent in all causes of the appetite except the pharmacological doses of the mineralocorticoids, its arousal is associated with continuous and prolonged elevation of plasma angiotensin. If the hormone were causative in its arousal, as is suggested by the work of Chiaraviglio (1976), then intracranial injections of angiotensin should be effective in inducing an excess intake of strong salt solutions, and it should be most effective when infused into the brain continuously for several days. The experiments described here (Bryant *et al.*, 1979) and those reported by Avrith and Fitzsimons (1979) were undertaken in pursuit of this idea. They show that prolonged exposure of the brain to angiotensin II arouses a specific and persistent appetite for sodium.

II. GENERAL METHODS

Male, albino, Holtzman rats (280–487 g at the beginning of the experiment) were housed individually in temperature-controlled rooms with a light–dark cycle of 12-hours on 12-hours off. All animals were supplied freely with Purina Rat Chow (pelleted). Tap water and 3.0% (0.5 *M*) NaCl solution were usually available except when otherwise noted. The 3.0% NaCl solution is hereafter called salt.

Cannula guide shafts (23-gauge), cannulas (30-gauge), and obturator–dust cap assemblies (Plastic Products, Roanoke, Virginia, models C-313-G, C-313-I, C-313-DC, respectively) were prepared such that the tip of the cannula or the obturator was flush with its tip when inserted into the guide.

The chronic infusions required special modifications of the previously described cannulas and dust caps. First, the obturator was pulled out of the screw-on dust cap and a small hole was drilled in its center just wide enough to admit the injection cannula. PE-50 tubing (approximately 1.2 m in length) was fitted to the injection cannula. A 25-cm length of extension spring (Gardner–Barnes, Tulsa, Oklahoma #8E28C) was passed over the PE-50 tubing, one end of which was affixed to the modified dust cap–injection assembly with dental acrylic. The loose end of the PE-50 tubing was then passed through a modified plastic swivel (Epstein and Teitelbaum, 1962a) and attached to a 50 μl Hamilton microsyringe held in a Harvard syringe pump. With this chronic infusion apparatus the rats were allowed complete freedom to move about in their cages, with the spring protecting the PE tubing from damage. The rate of infusion in all experiments was 1 μl/hour.

A single guide shaft was implanted in each animal using a Kopf small-animal stereotaxic instrument (Model 1260). The surgery was performed under chloropent (Fort Dodge Laboratories, Fort Dodge, Iowa) anesthesia (0.3 ml/100 g body weight) administered intraperitoneally. The tip of the guide shaft was directed toward the most anterior ventral portion of the third ventricle. After surgery, all animals were allowed at least 5 days postoperative recovery before experimental manipulations were begun.

Angiotensin II (Ile_5-angiotensin II, Schwartz–Mann and Beckman) hereafter called AII, was dissolved in sterile 0.9% NaCl (saline). All doses are specified in terms of the peptide. Solutions of AII were divided into aliquots of 0.2–0.3 ml and immediately frozen at − 23°C. An aliquot was removed from the freezer and diluted (with sterile saline) if necessary just prior to loading of the infusion cannulas and was never reused.

All salt solutions (NaCl, KCl, NH_4Cl) were made using reagent grade salts dissolved in distilled water.

At the conclusion of the experiments rats were perfused with 10% formalin, the brain was removed and placed in 10% formalin for at least 5 days before being blocked and prepared for celloidin treatment. Once embedded in celloidin 40 μm sections were taken through the cannula track, stained with cresyl violet, and then mounted.

A. Experiment I: Chronic Infusion, Basic Phenomenon

1. Methods

Four male, albino, Holtzman rats were used. They were housed as previously described.

After the postoperative recovery period, the rats were placed on the following schedule. At approximately the same time each day (1200 hours), they were weighed, their food, water, 3.0% NaCl (salt) intakes recorded and the water and salt reservoirs (250- and 100-ml plastic graduated cylinders) refilled and replaced on the front of each cage. Positions of the water and salt were alternated daily. On infusion days the infusion system was checked, flushed with sterile, distilled, deionized water and refilled with AII solution (6 μg/μl). The rate of intraventricular infusion here and in all subsequent experiments was 1 μl/hour; thus in this experiment AII was infused at 6 μg/μl/hour or 100 ng/min.

The protocol for this experiment was as follows: animals were first given access to water and salt for 4 days as previously described but no intraventricular infusions were made (no infusion condition). On the fifth day, continuous intracranial infusion of AII began and continued for a total of 4 days. Then on the ninth day, infusion was terminated and the animals were returned to the no infusion condition for 4 more days.

2. *Results*

Continuous intraventricular infusion of AII evokes marked salt and water ingestion. The inset in the upper right of Fig. 1 shows that the pre-AII (no infusion condition) salt intake was virtually zero, and water intakes were in the usual range (30–50 ml/24 hour). The remainder of Fig. 1 shows that the water and salt intakes increased enormously for each rat on all 4 days of AII infusion. Rat CPR-13's salt intake increased from approximately 1 ml/24 hours to 62 ml for the first 24 hours of AII infusion and 400 ml/24 hours of water on the fourth day of AII infusion. Even the poorest responder, CPR-15, increased his 3.0% NaCl intake from 0 ml/24 hours to a maximum of 30 ml/24 hours.

It is emphasized that all rats, not only in this experiment, but in all experiments described below, showed excessive salt intake as well as water intake in response to continuous infusion of AII. There have been no exceptions in a total of thirty-five cases at this writing.

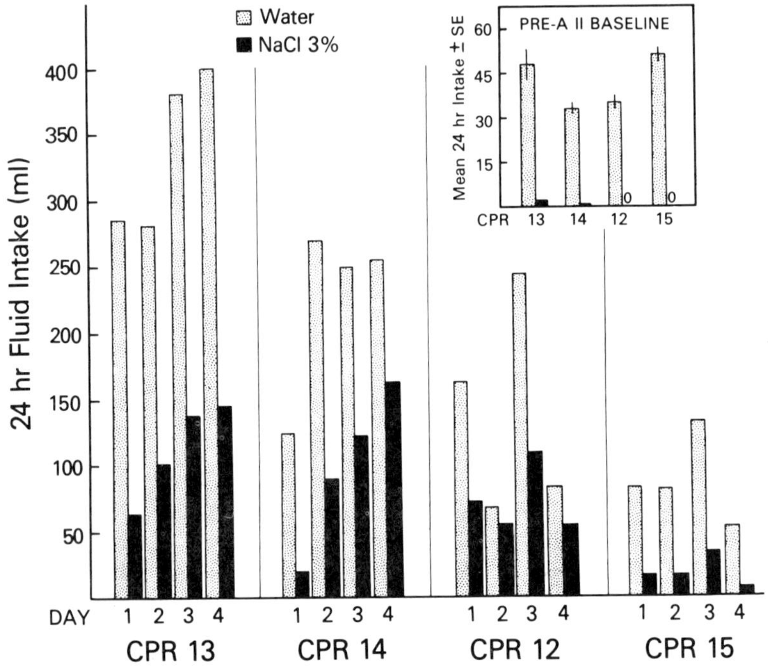

Fig. 1. Individual daily intakes for 4 days during AII infusion (6 μg/μl/hour) into the anterior ventral third ventricle. Inset (upper right) shows mean 24 hr water (stippled bars) and 3% (0.5 *M*) NaCl (solid bars) intakes for the 4 days preceding AII infusion in rats CPR 13, 14, 12, 15.

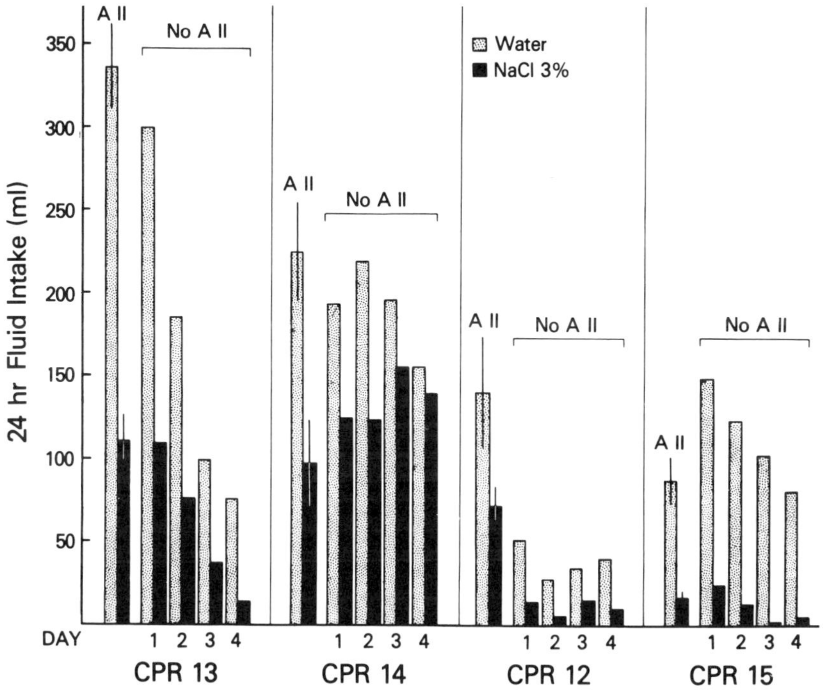

Fig. 2. Comparison of 24-hr water and 3% (0.5 *M*) NaCl intakes during 4 days of AII infusion (first pair of bars show mean intakes and S.E.'s for each rat) and for the 4 days after termination of AII infusion (designated "No AII"). Same animals as in Fig. 1.

Figure 2 shows that the excessive salt and water intake persists after termination of intraventricular infusion. Although Fig. 2 shows representative data of four rats for only the first 4 days after termination of AII infusion, we observed CPR-12, -13, and -14 and one other animal for 2 months after termination of the AII infusion, during which time they continued to consume from 10 to 125 ml of 3.0% NaCl/day. Throughout the course of the experiments reported in this chapter, no animal has stopped drinking the salt immediately after termination of AII infusions. Four rats slowly reduced their salt intake to 0–4 ml during at least 7 days postinfusion, and one rat reduced salt intake to 1 ml after 3 days postinfusion. All other rats continued to consume substantial volumes of salt for the usual postinfusion period of 4 days.

Serial coronal sections from the brains of all the rats in this experiment as well as those in the following four experiments showed that the tips of the guide cannulas opened into the anterior third ventricle and nearby parenchyma. They were positioned to assure rapid intraventricular distribution of infused solutions.

B. Experiment II: Dose Response

After establishing that chronic infusion of a large dose of AII evokes massive intake of salt and water, the following study was undertaken to delineate the dose-response characteristics of the phenomenon.

1. Methods

Seventeen male, albino, Holtzman rats were used in this experiment and were housed and equipped with intraventricular cannulas as previously described.

The protocol for this experiment was identical to Experiment I, except that the dose of AII was varied across the range 0 (0.9% NaCl), 6, 60, 600, or 6000 ng/μl/hr AII. At least 3 rats were in each group and no rat received more than one dose of AII; thus we are comparing "between animal" responsiveness. This was necessary because of the persistence of salt drinking after termination of AII infusion (Experiment I, Fig. 2).

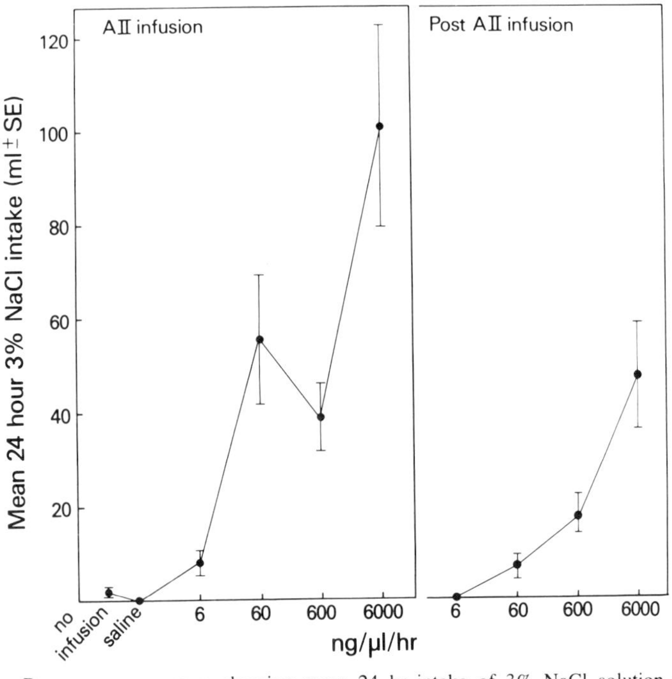

Fig. 3. Dose-response curves showing mean 24 hr intake of 3% NaCl solution during no infusion, 0.9% saline infusion, and the last 2 days of a 4-day infusion of AII at 6, 60, 600, or 6000 ng/μl/hour (left panel, AII infusion). The right panel (post AII infusion) shows mean salt intake for the 4 days following termination of AII infusion in same animals arranged according to previous dose of AII. (From Bryant *et al.*, 1979)

2. *Results*

The left panel of Fig. 3 shows that there is no salt ingestion during saline infusion, but at 6 ng/μl/hr a small (mean 7.8 ml), but statistically insignificant amount of salt is consumed. At the 60, 600, and 6000 ng/μl/hour doses, marked ingestion of salt occurred (means: 58.1, 39.0, 100.9 ml, respectively). The 6 ng/μl/hour dose appears to be very close to threshold, 3 out of 5 rats on at least 2 days during AII infusion did not drink any salt, although excessive water intake was observed. It is interesting to note that there was no significant difference between the intakes evoked by the 60 and 600 ng/μl/hour doses. The 6000 ng/μl/hour dose was significantly more potent than all other doses ($p < 0.01$). The right panel of Fig. 3 presents data showing that the persistence of the salt drinking after termination of AII infusion (previously described in Experiment I) is also dose dependent; that is, the magnitude of the drinking response increases concomitantly with the AII dose.

Figure 4 shows that the dose–response curve for water intake is quite similar to

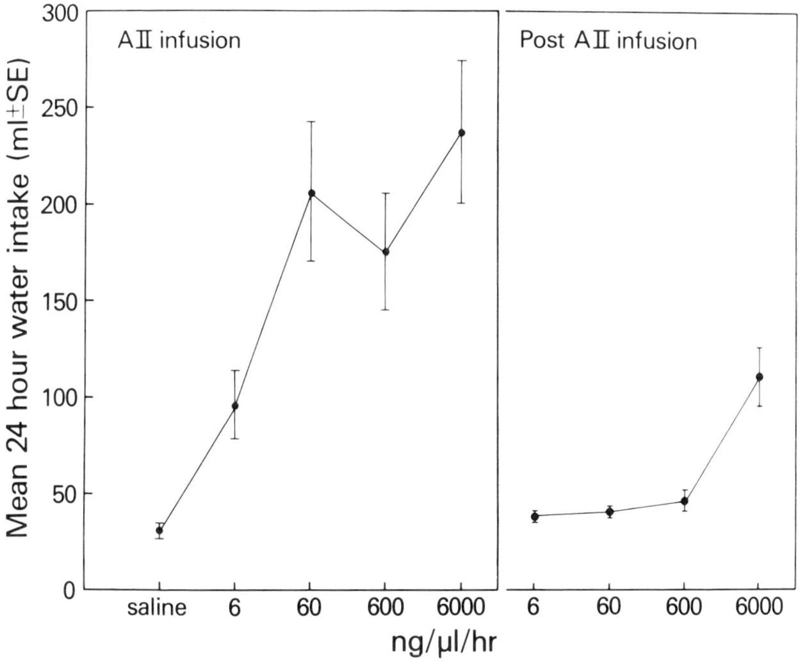

Fig. 4. Dose–response curves showing mean 24 hr water intake during the last 2 days of 0.9% saline infusion and AII infusion at 6, 60, 600, 6000 ng/μl/hour (left panel, AII infusion). The right panel (post AII infusion) shows mean water intake for the 4 days following termination of AII infusion in the same animals arranged according to previous dose of AII. (From Bryant *et al.*, 1979)

the salt intake curve (Fig. 3). The lowest AII dose (6 ng/μl/hour), however, did evoke a proportionally larger increase in water intake than salt intake. Also, there was less difference between the 6000 ng dose and the 60 and 600 ng/μl/hour doses of AII. Nonetheless, the highest intakes of water were observed at the 6000 ng dose (e.g., 334, 380, 400 ml/24 hours).

It should be noted that rats given AII at any dose usually exhibited normal food intake and weight gains throughout the experiment. Rats were healthy and showed no signs of malaise during or after the chronic intraventricular infusions of AII.

C. Experiment III: Specificity of Phenomenon

An important question is whether the "salt" appetite evoked by chronic intraventricular infusions of AII is specific for the sodium ion. This experiment sought to answer that question by substituting other salts in place of NaCl.

1. Methods

Eight male, albino, Holtzman rats were used in this experiment and were housed as previously described.

The protocol for this experiment was identical to Experiment I, except that the rats were given a choice between water and KCl (0.5 *M*) or water and NH_4Cl (0.5 *M*) to drink before, during, and after intraventricular AII infusion. All animals received AII at the highest dose of 6 μg/μl/hour to maximize the possibility of unmasking any nonspecific fluid intake that may be generated by this procedure.

2. Results

Table I (lower half) shows that very little ingestion of 0.5 *M* KCl was observed during AII infusion although water intakes were substantially elevated. The NH_4Cl data are presented in the upper half of Table I showing that no rat consumed any 0.5 *M* NH_4Cl during AII infusion, but again water intakes increased markedly.

These data show that the observed salt appetite is primarily a sodium appetite. Some KCl was consumed, but as reported previously (Falk, 1965; Richter, 1956), KCl ingestion is sometimes observed in sodium-depleted rats, which is not surprising considering the similarity of taste between NaCl and KCl.

D. Experiment IV: Independence of Water Intake

One possible explanation of the sodium appetite evoked by chronic infusion of AII is that the salt intake is secondary to the massive water intake produced by intracranial AII. In the following experiment, that question was explored using two different approaches. First, rats were subjected to passive overhydration

TABLE I

Fluid Intakes of Rats Given Either NH_4Cl (0.5 *M*) and Water or KCl (0.5 *M*) and Water to Drink during Chronic Angiotensin II (6 μg/μl/hour) Infusion

	CPR-26		CPR-27		CPR-28	
Day	NH_4Cl	Water	NH_4Cl	Water	NH_4Cl	Water
1	0	72	0	198	0	66
2	0	175	0	146	0	—
3	0	224	0	260	0	172
4	0	194	0	274	0	164
	0	166.2±28.5[a]	0	219.5±25.5	0	134±27.8

	BA-4		BA-5		BA-6	
Day	KCl	Water	KCl	Water	KCl	Water
1	0	74	0	41	0	70
2	5	117	0	210	5	104
3	9	114	0	108	13	174
4	0	166	0	100	2	74
	3.5±1.8	117.7±16.3	0	114.7±30.3	5±2.4	105.5±20.8

[a] Mean ± S.E.

using a nasopharyngeal-gastric tube, and second, rats were given a single bottle of salt without water.

1. Methods

Eight male, albino, Holtzman rats were used in this experiment and housed as previously described. Three rats were assigned to the overhydration group and five to the single-bottle group.

IG Infusion. Three large (400–450 g) rats were equipped with nasopharyngeal-gastric tubes under chloropent anesthesia. A length of PE-50 tubing was passed through the nares into the stomach and was fixed to the skull by connection to a piece of bent metal tubing (for details, see Epstein, 1960; Epstein and Teitelbaum, 1962b). After food and water intakes returned to preoperative levels, the animals were given continuous access to water, salt, and Purina pellets. Three days later direct intragastric infusions of tap water were begun (delivered, as described previously, by continuous peristaltic pump at rates from 5.3 to 26.9 ml/hour) resulting in the total daily infusion volumes shown in Table II. Water and salt intakes were measured daily. No intracranial infusions were made.

Single Bottle. All rats in this experiment had access to both tap water and salt for 2 days prior to intracranial AII infusion. As a first condition during infusion,

TABLE II

Water and Salt Intakes of Rats Receiving Large Volumes of Water by Continuous Gavage

	CPR-30			CPR-31			CPR-32		
Day	IG water	Water intake	3% NaCl intake	IG water	Water intake	3% NaCl intake	IG water	Water intake	3% NaCl intake
1	0	32	0						
2	0	29	2	0	40	5	0	29	5
3	121	11	0	220	5	0	150	0	0
4	205	0	0	534	0	0	225	6	0
5	182	20	0	620	0	0	210	9	1
6	370	27	0	350	0	0	0	46	1
7	360	5	0	0	33	1	0	47	1
8	0	49	0						
9	0	69	0						

three rats had access to salt as the sole available fluid (CPR-17, -19, -20) and two rats had access only to water (CPR-22, -23). Rats in the salt only condition were given access to water without salt present for 2 hours during the day (1200–1400 hr). This was necessary since rats cannot survive solely on 3.0% NaCl solution; this salt concentration is beyond the concentrating capability of the rat kidney (Adolph, 1943; Barker and Adolph, 1953; Schmidt-Nielsen, 1964). Purina rat chow was always available to all animals. Intraventricular AII infusion was at the usual 6 $\mu g/\mu l$/hour dose.

2. Results

Table II shows first (above upper dashed line) that there was very little spontaneous salt intake in these three rats. When intragastric (IG) infusion began (between upper and lower dashed lines) salt intake did not increase and in fact was zero, except for day 4 when rat CPR-32 drank 1 ml of salt. The column under IG water presents the amount of water infused intragastrically. Thus, rats receiving 24-hour gastric infusions of 121–620 ml did not drink any salt. The animals remained in excellent health throughout. They continued to eat, and, surprisingly, drank variable amounts of water.

The left panel of Table III shows that AII infusion evoked substantial salt intake when salt was the only available fluid. In all five rats salt intake increased over the 4-day infusion period. Rats continued to drink the salt after termination of infusion (left panel, lower half). Two rats, CPR-17 and -20, decreased their salt intake over the 4 days of no infusion, whereas CPR-19's intake dropped immediately after termination of AII infusion but then increased during the next 3 days, CPR-22 reduced its salt intake to zero in 3 days, whereas CPR-23 reduced its salt intake but did not go below 20 ml/day. All five rats showed the previously described persistence phenomenon.

The right panel of Table III shows that AII infusion produced a marked increase in water intake which did not persist after termination of AII infusion.

In this experiment, gastric infusions of massive volumes of water comparable to the intakes observed during intraventricular AII infusion, did not result in salt intake. It seems clear, therefore, that the observed salt appetite during AII infusion is not secondary to large water turnovers. The data obtained from the salt-only experiment show that water intake is not necessary for the exhibition of AII-induced salt appetite during intracranial infusion with AII. When it was absent, rats drank large volumes of salt. Moreover, the salt intakes persisted in the absence of large water intakes when the infusions were terminated.

E. Experiment V: Drinkometer Analysis of Pattern of Onset

In this experiment a drinkometer was used to determine the pattern of the onset of salt drinking after the beginning of intraventricular AII infusion. In addition,

TABLE III

Fluid Intakes during Access to Either a Single Bottle of Water or 3% NaCl during AII Infusion or No Infusion

		Rats given only 3% NaCl					Rats given only water	
	Day	CPR-17	CPR-19	CPR-20	CPR-22	CPR-23	CPR-22	CPR-23
AII	1	5	1	15	22	5	44	96
Infusion	2	7	9	24	42	11	138	200
6 μg/μl/hour	3	15	25	25	33	27	152	187
	4	29	39	50	41	45	—	140
		14 ± 4.7[a]	18.5 ± 7.3	28.5 ± 6.5	35.5 ± 4	22 ± 7.7	111.3 ± 2.7	155.7 ± 20.5
NO	5	35	8	18	45	48	42	48
INFUSION	6	12	12	2	2	21	62	48
	7	6	22	7	0	20	36	45
	8	16	25	7	—	—	29	52
		17.2 ± 5.4	16.7 ± 3.4	8.5 ± 2.9	15.6 ± 11.9	29.6 ± 7.4	42.2 ± 6.1	48.2 ± 1.2

[a] Mean ± S.E.

the drinkometer records were used to reveal the temporal relationships between the water and salt drinking during intraventricular infusion of AII.

1. Methods

Five male, albino, Holtzman rats were used in this experiment and were housed and equipped as previously described.

After the usual postoperative recovery period each rat was given access to tap water and salt for at least 2 days before intraventricular AII infusion began. At the beginning of AII infusion every twelfth lick for both water and salt was recorded by means of Grason–Stadler drinkometers and standard relay programming equipment. A four-pen event recorder was used to record licks graphically. For all five animals AII infusion continued and drinkometer records were kept for at least 2 days. The dose of AII used was 6 μg/μl/hour.

2. Results

Representative drinkometer records (Fig. 5) illustrate three main points. First, the onset of salt drinking after the start of AII infusion varied from animal to animal. Some rats, such as CPR-24, began drinking the salt immediately, while others did not drink the salt for several hours. CPR-25 did not even sample the salt until over 6 hours into the first day and did not start drinking copiously until almost 14 hours after the start of AII infusion. Figure 5 also shows that on the second (CPR-48) or third (CPR-24, CPR-25) day of AII infusion, salt intake began immediately or within the first 45 min (CPR-25) of the renewal of the solutions and re-insertion of the injector, and this was typical of the larger group of all infused animals. Once initiated, salt drinking was slow and sporadic in some animals and rapid in others. In addition, there seemed to be no consistent relationship between a rat's predisposition to drink hypertonic salt solutions spontaneously and the onset of salt drinking after the start of AII infusion. It should also be noted that although the animals were infused continuously until 1200 hr, at which time they were weighed, infusion system refilled and so on, they drank very little water or salt within the several hours before noon. As soon as the new infusion began, however, all rats began drinking avidly. This may have been a result of degradation of the AII which was at room temperature for the infusion period.

Second, salt drinking is not temporally linked to water ingestion, although this does occur occasionally. All three rats depicted in Fig. 5 show that there is a great deal of salt drinking without concomitant water ingestion (for example, CPR-48, Day 2). Rats do not appear to be mixing an "isotonic cocktail." An animal may alternate between salt and water (CPR-24, Day 3, 2100 hr) but there are long bouts of salt drinking without water and vice versa (CPR-25, Day 1, 3; CPR-48, Day 2).

The third main point illustrated by the drinkometer records in Fig. 5 is that

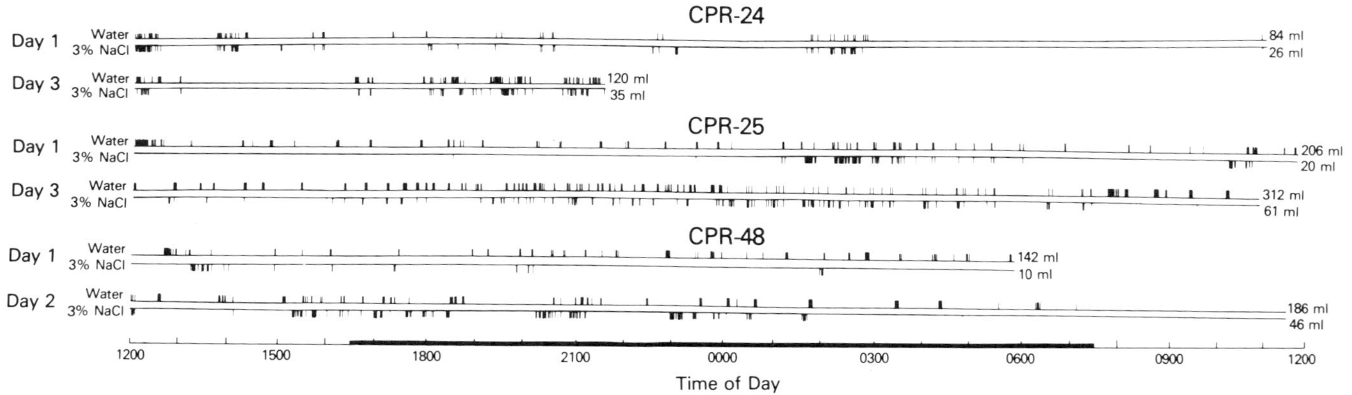

Fig. 5. Representative drinkometer records from CPR-24, -25, -48. Time of day is indicated at the bottom with the dark line representing the dark phase of the day. Each pen excursion represents 12 licks. The total amount of water (upper record of each pair) and 3% NaCl (lower record of each pair) drunk in 24 hours is presented at the right of each day's records. The truncated records of CPR-24 (day 3), CPR-25 (day 3), and CPR-48 (day 1) are a result of recorder failure. Water and salt intakes are nevertheless for the entire 24-hr period. (From Bryant *et al.*, 1979)

most drinking, of both salt and water, occurs during the dark period of the nychthemeron even though the animals are continuously infused throughout both light and dark periods. Thus, the nocturnal drinking pattern of the rats is maintained despite chronic AII infusion.

III. DISCUSSION

These experiments show clearly that prolonged exposure of the brain to angiotensin II produces an appetite for sodium. When the hormone was infused continuously into the anterior cerebral ventricles, the appetite occurred in all animals without exception, was never less (on a volume intake/day basis) than that seen after adrenalectomy, and in some rats was expressed in massive intakes of 3.0% NaCl. At doses of 60 ng/μl/hr to 6 μg/μl/hour, 46% of the animals drank at least 100 ml/day and 76% drank at least 59 ml/day. Furthermore, all animals at these doses drank at least 20 ml/day after the first day of AII infusion and for as long as the infusions continued. These are the largest daily intakes of strong salt solution to be reported in the 42-year history of the salt appetite phenomenon (Richter, 1936). The brain mechanisms for the appetite are clearly responsive to angiotensin and can be driven by it to extremes of excess.

The appetite induced by intracranial angiotensin has the essential characteristics of the natural phenomenon. First, it is specific for sodium. Our rats did not drink NH_4Cl and only an occasional animal drank increased amounts of KCl, as is the case after adrenalectomy (Richter, 1956) and intraperitoneal dialysis (Falk, 1965), but in even the most extreme of these the intake was less by an order of magnitude than the amount of NaCl ingested during infusion with comparable doses of angiotensin. Second, in these experiments the intake of strong salt solution is persistent. Once initiated by AII infusion the appetite continued after the termination of the treatment. A majority of our animals continued to drink 3.0% NaCl in the postinfusion period usually in progressively diminishing amounts. Several animals drank it in large amounts indefinitely for as long as their intake was monitored. Although considerably less than the massive intakes induced by the infusion, the intakes in the period of spontaneous persistence were nevertheless the equivalent of those seen after pathological disturbances of sodium balance. And, third, the appetite was accompanied by increased water intake.

Being a potent dipsogen, especially when given intracranially, the angiotensin as used here generated very large daily water intakes, sometimes exceeding the animals' body weights. These however were not the cause of the sodium appetite. Animals that were passively infused with volumes of water that equaled or exceeded the amounts that were drunk during angiotensin infusion ignored 3.0% NaCl. Nor were the animals drinking the salt in order to ingest an isotonic mixture of water and hypertonic salt; first because the infusions induced excess salt solution intake when it was the only fluid offered, and, second, because records of the animals' drinking behavior revealed that ingestion of the water and of salt solution were not concurrent.

It is impossible with the present evidence to offer a credible statement of the effective dose of angiotensin for induction of the appetite. We have infused the hormone at an unknown distance from unknown receptors and have utilized, as medium, the CSF which is very likely an artifactual route of access to the brain for angiotensin. But we can point out that our doses are not larger than those used to elicit thirst by intraventricular injection of the hormone. At our lowest effective dose (6 ng/μl/hour) the animals were receiving only 100 pg/min which is not an excessive dose for production of the dipsogenic response. Nor can we specify the portions of the brain that may harbor receptors for the induction of sodium appetite by angiotensin, and we cannot comment on how they may be related to the forebrain structures that have been implicated in the mediation of the appetite by Covian and Antunes-Rodrigues (1963) and by Wolf (1967, 1968, 1971). All of our infusions were made through cannulas that opened into the anterior cerebral ventricles and the hormone was therefore broadcast widely in the brain, undoubtedly gaining access to the circumventricular organs and to the ECF and parenchyma of the brain wherever the cannulas penetrated the ependyma.

We can conclude however that a role for angiotensin in the arousal of the sodium appetite is likely from the evidence presented here and from the prior work of Chiaraviglio (1976). This conclusion is supported by Avrith and Fitzsimons (1979) who also find that continuous intracerebral infusion of AII produces excessive intake of hypertonic salt solution in rats that are in positive sodium balance. Such a role for the hormone is most reasonable when it is recalled that with the exception only of pharmacological doses of the mineralocorticoids, all known causes of the appetite are associated with decreases in plasma sodium and with prolonged elevations of plasma angiotensin, and it is an appealing simplification to think of angiotensin as mediating both the conservation of sodium by the kidney and the urge for salt ingestion by the brain. But, the hormone cannot be the sole cause of the appetite because it survives nephrectomy (Bott *et al.*, 1967), is produced by pharmacological doses of DOCA and aldosterone (both of which severely depress plasma renin) as well as by treatment with ACTH (Denton *et al.*, 1977; Weisinger *et al.*, 1978) and because it persists long after the withdrawal of angiotensin treatment. The appetite is clearly a complex phenomenon that may require an interaction of angiotensin and aldosterone for its natural arousal and it may be sustained in the absence of endocrinological determinants by a conditioning process during which the taste of strong salt solution is associated with the benefits of salt ingestion.

REFERENCES

Adolph, E. F. (1943). Do rats thrive when drinking sea water? *Am. J. Physiol.* **140,** 25–32.

Avrith, D., and Fitzsimons, J. T. (1979). Induction of delayed sodium appetite in the rat by intracranial administration of components of the renin–angiotensin system. *J. Physiol. (London)* (in press).

Barker, J. P., and Adolph, E. F. (1953). Survival of rats without water and given seawater. *Am. J. Physiol.* **173,** 495–502.

Beilharz, S., Denton, D. A., and Sabine, J. R. (1962). The effect of concurrent deficiency of water and sodium on the sodium appetite of sleep. *J. Physiol. (London)* **163,** 378–390.

Bott, E., Denton, D. A., and Weller, S. (1967). The effect of angiotensin II infusion, renal hypertension and nephrectomy on salt appetite of sodium-deficient sheep. *Aust. J. Exp. Biol. Med. Sci.* **45,** 595–612.

Bryant, R. W., Epstein, A. N., Fitzsimons, J. T., and Fluharty, S. J. (1979). Arousal of a specific and persistent sodium appetite with continuous intracerebroventricular infusion of angiotensin II. *J. Physiol. (London)* (in press).

Chiaraviglio, E. (1976). Effect of renin–angiotensin system on sodium intake. *J. Physiol. (London)* **255,** 57–66.

Covian, M. R., and Antunes-Rodrigues, J. (1963). Specific alterations in sodium chloride intake after hypothalamic lesions in the rat. *Am. J. Physiol.* **205,** 922–926.

Denton, D. A., and Sabine, J. R. (1961). The selective appetite for Na^+ shown by Na^+ deficient sheep. *J. Physiol. (London)* **157,** 97–116.

Denton, D. A., McKinley, M. J., Nelson, J. F., and Weisinger, R. S. (1977). Pregnancy, lactation, and hormone-induced mineral appetite. *In* "Food Intake and Chemical Senses" (Y. Katsuki *et al.*, eds.), pp. 247–261. Univ. Park Press, Baltimore, Maryland.

Epstein, A. N. (1960). Water intake without the act of drinking. *Science* **131,** 497–498.

Epstein, A. N., and Teitelbaum, P. (1962a). A watertight swivel joint permitting chronic injection into moving animals. *J. Appl. Physiol.* **17,** 171–172.

Epstein, A. N., and Teitelbaum, P. (1962b). Regulation of food intake in the absence of taste, smell, and other oropharyngeal sensations. *J. Comp. Physiol. Psychol.* **55,** 753–759.

Falk, J. L. (1961). The behavioral regulation of water–electrolyte balance. *In* "Nebraska Symposium on Motivation" (M. R. Jones, ed.), pp. 1–33. Univ. of Nebraska Press, Lincoln.

Falk, J. L. (1965). Limitations to the specificity of NaCl appetite in sodium-depleted rats. *J. Comp. Physiol. Psychol.* **60,** 393–396.

Fregly, M. J., and Waters, I. W. (1966). Effect of mineralocorticoids on spontaneous sodium chloride appetite of adrenalectomized rats. *Physiol. Behav.* **1,** 65–74.

Nachman, M., and Valentino, D. A. (1966). Roles of taste and postingestional factors in the satiation of sodium appetite in rats. *J. Comp. Physiol. Psychol.* **62,** 280–283.

Richter, C. P. (1936). Increased salt appetite in adrenalectomized rats. *Am. J. Physiol.* **115,** 155–161.

Richter, C. P. (1956). Salt appetite in mammals—its dependence on instinct and metabolism. *In* "L'instinct" (M. Autouri, ed.), pp. 577–629. Masson, Paris.

Schmidt-Nielsen, K. (1964). "Desert Animals." Oxford Univ. Press, London and New York.

Stricker, E. M. (1973). Thirst, sodium appetite and complementary physiological contributions to the regulation of intravascular fluid volume. *In* "The Neuropsychology of Thirst" (A. N. Epstein, H. R. Kissileff, and E. Stellar, eds.), pp. 73–98. Holt, New York.

Weisinger, R. S., Denton, D. A., McKinley, M. J., and Nelson, J. F. (1978). ACTH-induced sodium appetite in the rat. *Pharmacol., Biochem. Behav.* **8,** 339–342.

Wolf, G. (1964). Sodium appetite elicited by aldosterone. *Psychon. Sci.* **1,** 211–212.

Wolf, G. (1967). Hypothalamic regulation of sodium intake: Relations to preoptic and tegmental function. *Am. J. Physiol.* **213,** 1433–1438.

Wolf, G. (1968). Thalamic and tegmental mechanisms for sodium intake: Anatomical and functional relations to lateral hypothalamus. *Physiol. Behav.* **3,** 997–1002.

Wolf, G. (1971). Neural mechanisms for sodium appetite: Hypothalamus positive-hypothalamofugal pathways negative. *Physiol. Behav.* **6,** 381–389.

Wolf, G., and Handel, P. J. (1966). Aldosterone-induced sodium appetite: Dose-response and specificity. *Endocrinology* **78,** 1120–1124.

Chapter 14

The Physiological Basis of Sodium Appetite: A New Look at the "Depletion–Repletion" Model

EDWARD M. STRICKER

I. INTRODUCTION

Sodium appetite is a strong motivation to seek, obtain, and ingest sodium that apparently is innate, at least in rats (see reviews by Denton, 1966; Wolf, 1969). It does not seem to be associated readily with some peripheral cue, as dry mouth is with thirst and gastric filling is with hunger, nor does it commonly occur in Western societies due to the abundance of salt in our foods. Thus, sodium appetite usually is not recognized and reported by most human subjects during sodium deficiency (Thorn *et al.*, 1942). Perhaps for these reasons sodium appetite has received relatively little experimental attention since the pioneering work

BIOLOGICAL AND BEHAVIORAL
ASPECTS OF SALT INTAKE

ISBN 0-12-397750-9

of Richter (1936), in contrast with the long history of research and interest in thirst and hunger. Consequently, the physiological basis of sodium appetite remains obscure.

In attempting to elucidate the stimuli for sodium appetite, experimental evidence usually has been interpreted from the perspective of the "depletion-repletion" model. That is to say, ingested sodium is presumed to satisfy putative biological needs that result from sodium deficiency and stimulate sodium appetite. This general approach also has been popular in considering the physiological origins of hunger and thirst. However, we have recently concluded that it may not provide an appropriate perspective for viewing hunger after all, because metabolic fuels remain available to tissues in amounts that are adequate for their function even when food deprivation is prolonged (Friedman and Stricker, 1976). These deliberations have prompted us to reevaluate the depletion-repletion models of thirst and sodium appetite.

The model is clearly satisfactory in consideration of the most common basis for water consumption, "osmoregulatory thirst." Here, body fluid osmolality is elevated by dehydration and restored to normal by ingested water. Of more relevance to the present discussion are the thirst and sodium appetite that result following the isosmotic loss of body fluids. From the perspective of a depletion-repletion model, these ingestive behaviors are easily understood because the extracellular space is contracted by the loss of what is essentially an isotonic NaCl solution and is reexpanded only when both water and NaCl are consumed.

These facts encouraged us to consider as important in formulating the physiological basis of sodium appetite the same factors that evidently provide the physiological basis of thirst. Although the precise stimulus for thirst during simple dehydration still is unsettled (e.g., Andersson, 1978), an increase in the effective osmolality or the sodium concentration of extracellular fluid appears to be critical. The basis for "volume-regulatory thirst" may be more complex. A reduction of intravascular fluid volume appears to activate cardiovascular baroreceptors that stimulate thirst (e.g., Hosutt *et al.*, 1978; Stricker, 1966), and associated increases in circulating angiotensin may provide an additional dipsogenic stimulus (see reviews by Epstein, 1978; Fitzsimons, 1978; but see also Stricker, 1978). Consequently, we believed that changes in body fluid osmolality or sodium concentration, in plasma volume, and in the renin-angiotensin-aldosterone system should also be considered in describing the stimulus for sodium appetite. The following section considers the model of sodium appetite that was derived according to these principles.

II. THE MODEL

Richter (1936) first demonstrated the sodium appetite of rats in response to uncontrolled losses of sodium after adrenalectomy. This finding has been replicated and extended in many laboratories, perhaps most elegantly in a series of experiments by Denton and his colleagues that integrate studies of sodium appetite with research on the control of aldosterone secretion in intact sodium-deficient sheep (see review by Denton, 1965). In these and other investigations it has been observed repeatedly that animals suffering negative external sodium balances develop a sodium appetite.

Sodium need can also be produced without external loss. For the past 15 years we have been studying the adaptive behavioral and physiological responses of rats to a benign procedure for redistributing extracellular fluid that induces hypovolemia. Subcutaneous injections of hyperoncotic colloidal solutions disrupt the Starling equilibrium across local capillaries and lead to a gradual withdrawal of isosmotic protein-free plasma fluid into the interstitium, with increased fluid accumulation and plasma deficits proportional to the administered dose of colloid (Stricker, 1968; Stricker and MacArthur, 1974). The progressive hemoconcentration that results after administration of a 30% solution of polyethylene glycol (PEG) is illustrated in Fig. 1. In response to the effective loss of extracellular fluid, PEG-treated rats increase renal conservation of water and sodium and thereby minimize further fluid loss. This results both from decreases in glomerular filtration rate (Brenner *et al.*, 1968) and exponential increases in the secretions of antidiuretic hormone (ADH) (Dunn *et al.*, 1973) and aldosterone (Fig. 2). Comparable increases also occur in renin release (Leenen and Stricker, 1974; Stricker *et al.*, 1979), and associated changes in angiotensin levels presumably contribute to the secretion of the antidiuretic and antinatriuretic hormones.

Complementing these physiological responses are ingestive behaviors motivated by thirst and sodium appetite. Water intake increases within the first hour or two after PEG treatment and rises steadily in parallel with developing plasma volume deficits (Fig. 3). After a delay of at least 6–10 hours, rats begin to drink hypertonic saline as well (Fig. 3) and thereby obtain a fluid mixture approximating the isotonic NaCl solution that is optimal for restoring plasma volume (Stricker and Jalowiec, 1970). Hypovolemic rats remain oliguric and retain virtually all ingested sodium until plasma volumes are restored, after which renin and aldosterone secretions return to normal (Fig. 4), urine sodium concentrations rise abruptly, and sodium balances stabilize despite continued sodium intake.

There are two additional aspects of these findings that deserve comment. First, water intake during hypovolemia correlates highly both with plasma volume deficits and with plasma renin activities (Stricker, 1968; Leenen and Stricker, 1974). Nevertheless, only a small fraction of the ingested water remains in the circulation because it is distributed by osmosis in proportion to existing volumes of the body fluid compartments (note the unchanged hematocrits and plasma protein concentrations in Fig. 1). It is the consumption of NaCl that restores plasma volume (Fig. 5). Second, when only water is available, rats stop drinking

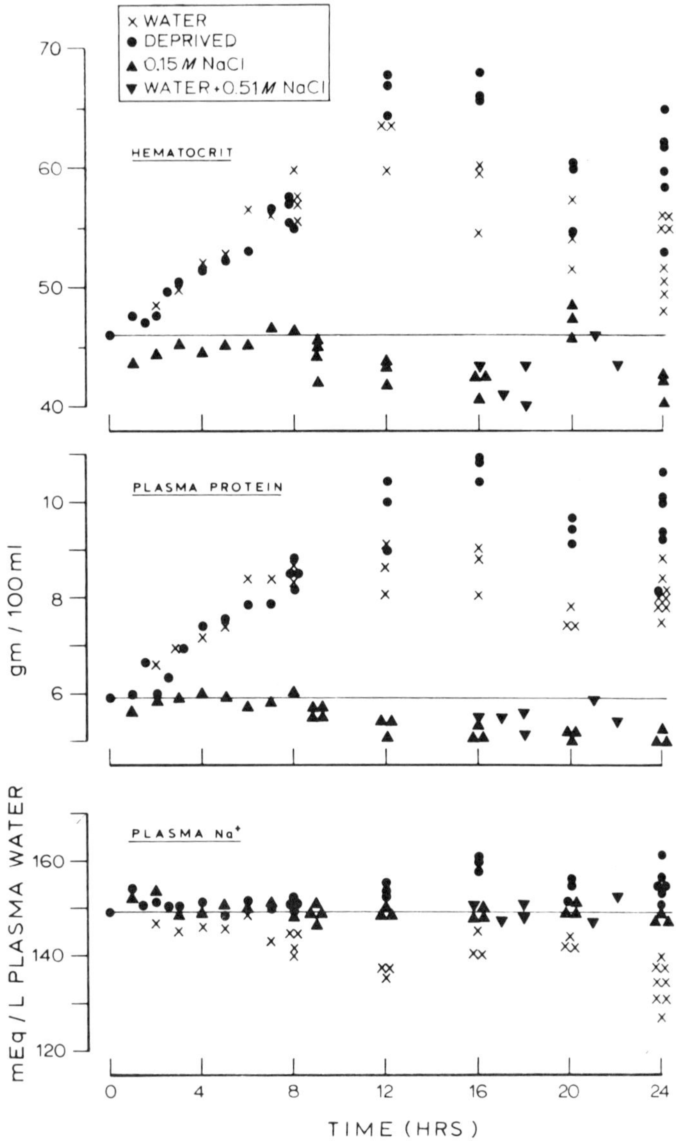

Fig. 1. Hematocrit, plasma protein concentration, and plasma sodium concentration of rats after 30% PEG treatment. Rats were given water, 0.15 *M* NaCl, water and 0.51 *M* NaCl, or nothing to drink. Each point represents a value from one animal. Mean values from nine untreated rats are presented as control values for purposes of comparison (0 hr). Reprinted from Stricker and Jalowiec (1970) with permission.

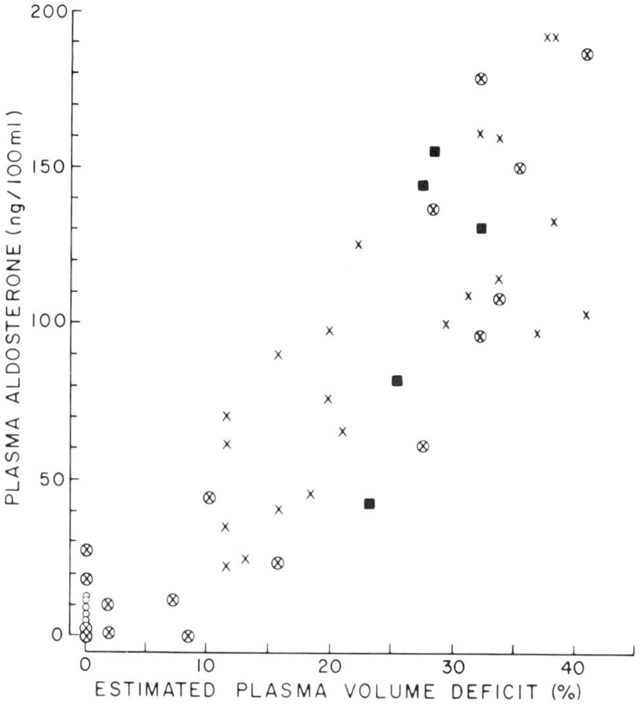

Fig. 2. Plasma aldosterone concentration at various times (2–16 hr) after treatment with 30% PEG solution, as a function of estimated plasma volume at each time. PEG-treated rats were allowed nothing to drink (■), water alone (X), or water and 0.5 *M* NaCl (encircled X). Values from control animals also are given (○). Each point represents a value from one animal. Reprinted from Stricker *et al.* (1979) with permission.

despite the continued presence of plasma volume deficits (Stricker, 1969, 1971a). This inhibition of hypovolemic thirst is associated with dilution of body fluids that may reach 8–10% (note the progressive hyponatremia in Fig. 1). However, when hypertonic NaCl solution is also available, rats drink it and thereby avoid prolonged osmotic dilution and inhibition of thirst (Fig. 3).

These findings illustrate the important interaction between thirst and sodium appetite and their combined contribution to volume regulation. As indicated previously, thirst appears to be stimulated by osmotic concentration of body fluids, by hypovolemia, and by angiotensin. If analogous factors serve as stimuli for sodium appetite, then osmotic dilution of body fluids, hypovolemia, and some hormone involved in sodium metabolism should be considered as candidates. A schematic representation of control systems involving such parameters is presented in Fig. 6.

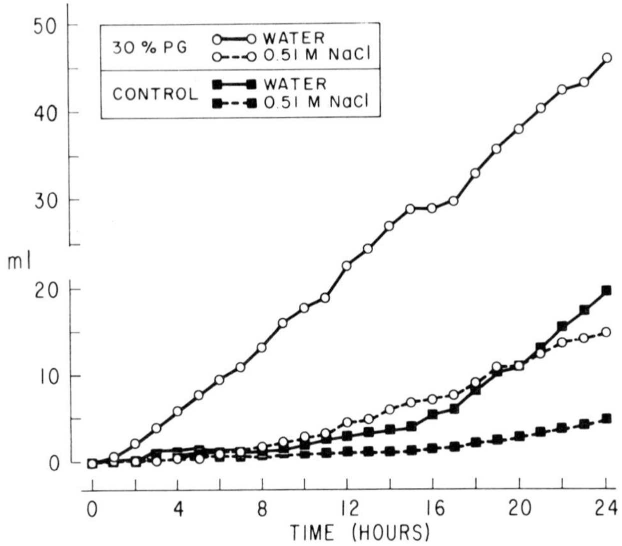

Fig. 3. Cumulative mean volumes of water and 0.51 *M* NaCl ingested by rats during food deprivation (control) and after subcutaneous injection of 30% PEG solution ($N = 8$ in each group). Data from Stricker, 1971b.

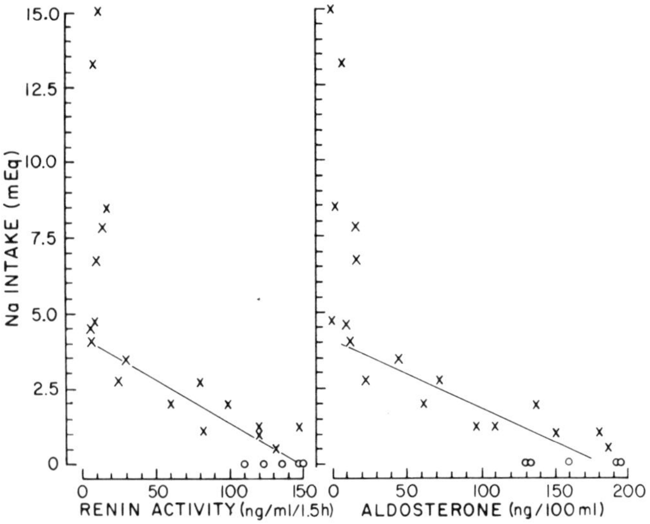

Fig. 4. Effect of sodium intake on plasma renin activity and aldosterone concentration in rats 16 hours after 30% PEG treatment. Rats were allowed to drink water alone (O) or together with either 0.5 *M* NaCl or 0.15 *M* NaCl (X). Each point represents a value from one animal. Reprinted from Stricker *et al.* (1979) with permission.

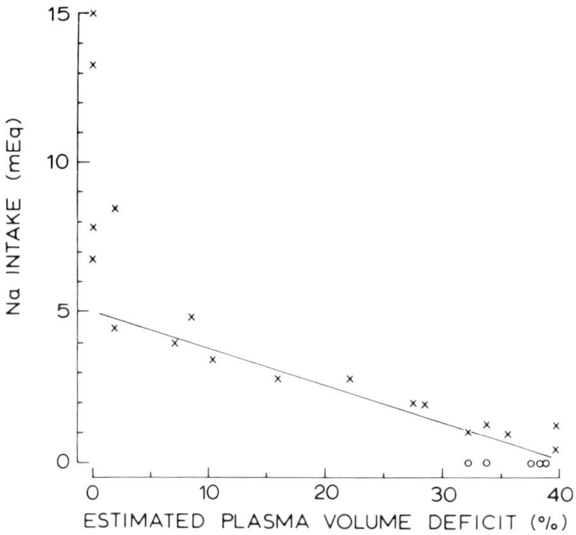

Fig. 5. Effect of sodium intake on estimated plasma volume deficit in rats 16 hours after 30% PEG treatment. Symbols as in Fig. 4. Reprinted from Stricker *et al.* (1979) with permission.

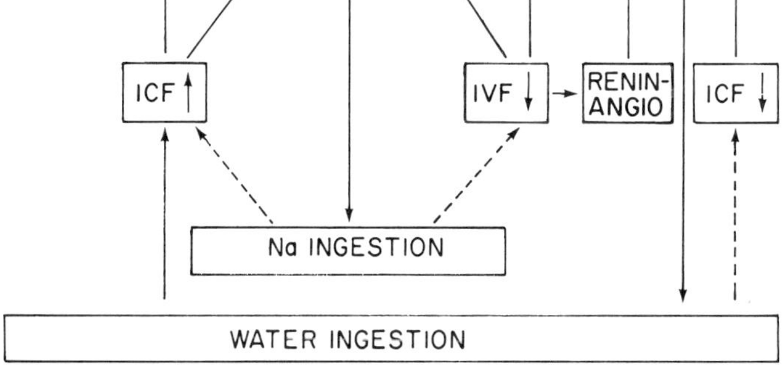

Fig. 6. Schematic representation of some physiological mechanisms that might control thirst and sodium appetite. (The stimulation of sodium appetite by aldosterone is not shown). Solid arrows indicate stimulation; dashed lines indicate inhibition; ICF indicates intracellular fluid volume; and IVF indicates intravascular fluid volume.

This speculative model highlights the interdependent roles of water and NaCl ingestion in regulating the volumes of the intracellular and intravascular fluid compartments. The identification and arrangement of variables is consistent with the perspective provided by the depletion-repletion model. It also accords well with known facts and widely accepted conjecture with one important exception—the anomalous delay in appearance of sodium appetite. Since sufficient hypovolemia evidently is present to stimulate thirst, why don't afferent signals from baroreceptors stimulate sodium appetite concurrently?

One possible explanation is that the delayed acceptance of 0.5 *M* NaCl solution by rats after 30% PEG treatment is an artifact of the testing conditions. It is conceivable that sodium appetite actually developed as rapidly as thirst, but that animals avoided the unpalatable saline solution until their motivation became great. However, we tested this hypothesis and found that saline intake did not increase for 6-10 hours after 30% PEG treatment even when palatable 0.15 *M* NaCl solution was offered with water (Stricker, 1971b).

What then is responsible for the delay? Working within the context of Fig. 6, three possibilities come to mind. (1) Time may be required for the plasma volume deficits to reach threshold levels for the stimulation of sodium appetite (i.e., the levels may be greater than those required to stimulate thirst). (2) Alternatively, time may be required for some direct consequence of the progressive hypovolemia, such as the increase in circulating levels of angiotensin or aldosterone, to reach threshold levels for the stimulation of sodium appetite. (3) Finally, time may be required for some indirect consequence of the progressive hypovolemia, such as osmotic dilution resulting from the renal retention of ingested water, to reach threshold levels for the stimulation of sodium appetite. The following section describes recent experimental evidence regarding each of these possibilities.

III. EVALUATION OF THE MODEL

A. Hypovolemia

Plasma volume deficits reach 25% by 6 hours after 30% PEG treatment in rats (Stricker, 1968; see Fig. 1). If this level of hypovolemia represents the critical threshold for the stimulation of sodium appetite, then PEG treatments that do not produce such large plasma volume deficits should not elicit sodium appetite. This prediction was examined by comparing the thirst and sodium appetite after 30% PEG treatment with the intakes of water and 0.5 *M* NaCl solution by adult rats injected subcutaneously with 5 ml of 10 or 20% PEG solutions. Plasma volume deficits of 25% developed by 8-9 hours after 20% PEG was given, but they never reached that level after the smallest PEG treatment. Nevertheless, sodium appe-

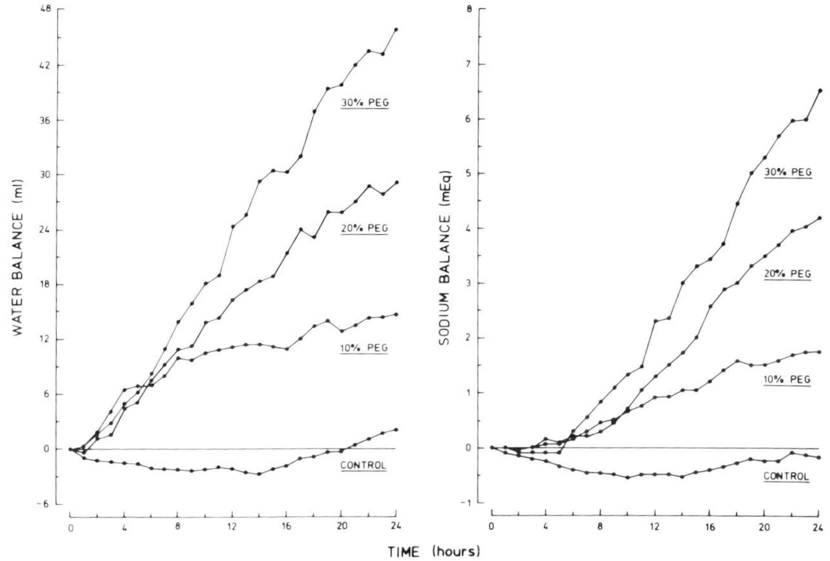

Fig. 7. Cumulative mean water balances (i.e., total fluid intake minus urine volume) and sodium balances (i.e., sodium intake minus urine sodium) of rats during control test or after subcutaneous injection of 10, 20, or 30% PEG solution ($N = 5$ in each group). Data from Stricker and Jalowiec (1970), and E. M. Stricker, unpublished observations.

tite was observed in all three groups beginning 6–10 hours after PEG was injected (Fig. 7).*

The rate of saline intake was proportional to the PEG treatment and was reflected in the rate at which positive sodium balance increased (Fig. 7). The impact of sodium appetite was also evidenced in each group by the progressive rise towards isotonicity of the fluid that was retained. Thirst persisted throughout the 24-hour test period and contributed to a positive water balance in these oliguric animals that ultimately paralleled the changes in sodium balance (Fig. 7). These volumes of retained fluid far exceeded actual plasma deficits of 2–4 ml. In fact, most of the fluid was sequestered at the injection site and formed a large local edema. In accordance with the Starling equilibrium, plasma volume in

*Sodium appetite usually is defined operationally as the intake of hypertonic NaCl solutions in amounts greater than those consumed normally. After PEG or other experimental treatments, however, it is possible that sodium appetite begins even before the intakes of saline reach control values. If so, then the developing positive sodium balance would be a more sensitive index of sodium appetite than an increse in saline intake. Accordingly, I have presented data on sodium balance rather than sodium intake throughout this essay. (N.b., basal intakes of hypertonic saline were low in these experiments, so the difference in onset of sodium appetite according to the two indices was only a few hours at most.)

the three groups of rats was restored gradually and at similar rates despite the conspicuous differences in saline consumption.

These results suggest that plasma volume deficits of 25% do not represent a critical threshold for the stimulation of sodium appetite. In an alternative approach to this issue, we determined whether treatments producing such deficits in less time than 6 hours would elicit sodium appetite that much sooner. This hypothesis was tested first by giving adult rats two injections (i.e., 10 ml) of 30% PEG solution subcutaneously. Plasma volume deficits of 25% developed within 3 hours and rats consumed 8–10 ml of water during this time. However, sodium appetite did not appear then or later in the 24-hour test period. Rather than facilitating sodium appetite, administration of more colloid abolished saline consumption. These unexpected results were traced to the anuria produced by the extreme hypovolemia; other procedures eliminating urine excretion also abolished sodium appetite in PEG-treated rats (Table I), even when 0.15 *M* NaCl solution was available with water (Stricker, 1971b, 1973). Although the absence of sodium appetite in these animals remains a mystery (see also Fitzsimons and Stricker, 1971; Fitzsimons and Wirth, 1978), it is noteworthy that hypovolemic thirst appeared normally during anuria.

In order to produce a large plasma volume deficit rapidly without compromising the renal circulation, a rubber band was wound tightly around one hind limb and left there for 5 hours (Ashworth *et al.*, 1944; Andree *et al.*, 1957). When it was removed, protein-rich plasma fluid was lost into the interstitial space of the affected limb and plasma volumes decreased by 40% within 2 hours. Plasma electrolyte concentrations did not change nor did rats become anuric. They drank water rapidly after the tourniquet was removed but did not begin to drink 0.5 *M*

TABLE 1

Effects of Anuria on Thirst and Sodium Appetite Elicited by 30% PEG Treatment in Rats[a]

Treatment	N	Water (ml)	0.5 *M* NaCl (ml)	Urine (ml)
30% PEG	10	46.4±3.6[b]	11.3±1.4	17.0±2.7
30% PEG	13	28.7±1.7	Absent	7.5±1.4
30% PEG + nephrectomy	7	21.6±1.6	0.0±0.0	0.0±0.0
30% PEG + ureter ligation	5	23.9±2.0	0.2±0.2	0.0±0.0
30% PEG + bladder puncture	5	27.0±3.6	0.4±0.1	0.0±0.0
30% PEG + cava ligation	5	31.8±3.1	0.0±0.0	0.0±0.0
30% PEG + 30% PEG	5	36.3±1.6	0.6±0.2	0.0±0.0

[a] *Note:* Intakes and urine volumes were recorded 24 hr after the treatments. Food was not available. $p < .001$ for all values in comparison with intact rats given a single subcutaneous injection of 5 ml 30% PEG solution and ad libitum access to water and 0.5 *M* NaCl solution. Data from Stricker, 1973.

[b] Mean ± S.E.

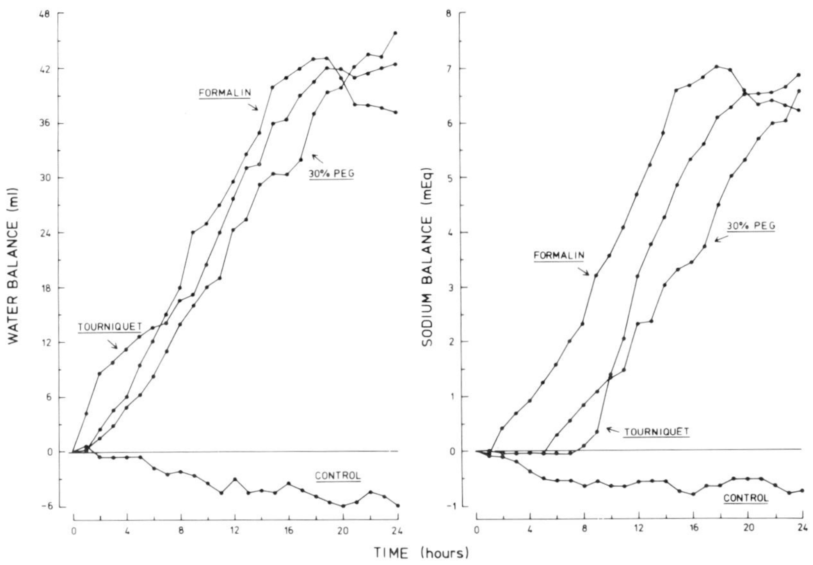

Fig. 8. Cumulative mean water balances and sodium balances of rats during control test or after subcutaneous injection of 30% PEG or 1.5% formalin solution, or release of a tourniquet from a hind limb ($N = 5, 12, 7$, respectively). Data from Jalowiec and Stricker (1970a), Stricker and Jalowiec (1970), and E. M. Stricker, unpublished observations.

NaCl solution for 8–10 hours. Cumulative water and sodium balances thereafter resembled those seen after 30% PEG treatment (Fig. 8). This experiment dissociates onset of pronounced hypovolemia from onset of saline consumption and again offers no support to the hypothesis that baroreceptors provide a critical stimulus for sodium appetite.

B. Renin–Angiotensin–Aldosterone

During the first 8 hours after 30% PEG treatment, there is an exponential relation between plasma volume deficit and plasma renin activity (Leenen and Stricker, 1974; Stricker *et al.*, 1979). The increase in circulating angiotensin during hypovolemia has many useful functions, including the maintenance of blood pressure and the stimulation of aldosterone and ADH secretions. Fitzsimons (1969) has proposed that angiotensin additionally provides an important stimulus for thirst. Although there is no question that exogenous angiotensin reliably augments water consumption, Fitzsimons' hypothesis remains controversial because it is still unclear how much the elevated angiotensin levels contribute to thirst observed during hypovolemia and experimental hypotension; available evidence suggests that it is responsible for 20–30% of the drinking after such treatments in rats (Stricker, 1977; Stricker *et al.*, 1976). Recent observations (Avrith and Fitzsimons, 1978; Bryant *et al.*, 1978) that angiotensin injected into the brain provokes saline consumption in rats raise the possibility that the hormone also participates in sodium appetite, although previous reports had indicated that sodium appetite was not induced when large amounts of renin or angiotensin were administered systematically (Fitzsimons and Stricker, 1971; Fitzsimons and Wirth, 1978). The mechanism by which intracerebrally applied angiotensin stimulates salt intake, and the relevance of this phenomenon to saline consumption after PEG treatment or other procedures, remains to be elucidated.

The appropriate increase in saline consumption by rats after adrenalectomy (Jalowiec and Stricker, 1973; Richter, 1936) indicates that aldosterone is not a necessary stimulus for sodium appetite. Mineralocorticoids may provide a sufficient stimulus for this drive, however, because rats increase NaCl intake after deoxycorticosterone or aldosterone is administered (Rice and Richter, 1943; Wolf and Handal, 1966). It is not yet known whether circulating levels of mineralocorticoid achieved after exogenous treatment compare well with the levels observed when sodium appetite is elicited by hypovolemia. As an alternative approach to this issue, we decided to enhance the aldosterone secretion provoked by hypovolemia and determine whether sodium appetite was similarly increased. It was. Maintenance of rats on a sodium-deficient diet for 4 days prior to 30% PEG treatment increased circulating aldosterone to 300–500 ng/100 ml, levels several times greater than those seen in PEG-treated rats that had been maintained normally (cf. Fig. 2). Rats were allowed 0.5 *M* NaCl and water 4 hours after the injection and they began drinking large amounts of both fluids so rapidly that within 4 hours their positive sodium and water balances equalled those seen in normally maintained rats 24 hours after PEG treatment (Stricker *et al.*, 1979).

At this early onset of sodium appetite, plasma volume deficits and renin activities were only slightly greater in the PEG-treated rats than usual and plasma sodium concentrations were unchanged. Thus, among the variables being considered that might be responsible for the marked increase in saline intake, only aldosterone levels were conspicuously elevated. In order to determine whether this was the critical stimulus for sodium appetite, NaCl intake was studied in rats given a different treatment that produced a comparable secretion of aldosterone. Total ligation of the inferior vena cava, below the liver and above the kidneys, drops blood pressure for several hours until a collateral circulation restores the venous return to normal (Fitzsimons, 1969; Stricker, 1977). Renin secretion remains elevated long afterward (Leenen and Stricker, 1974), however, presumably because blood flow through the renal artery remains low due to the chronic increase in renal venous pressure caused by the ligation. Aldosterone secretion increases in parallel with plasma renin activity (Stricker *et al.*, 1979). Despite elevations of aldosterone to 75–150 ng/100 ml (cf. Fig. 2), caval ligated rats did not show a sodium appetite whether 0.5 *M* NaCl or 0.15 *M* NaCl was offered with water (see also Fitzsimons, 1969; Stricker, 1971b). After maintenance of rats for 4 days on a sodium-deficient diet, aldosterone levels reached 350–400 ng/100 ml after caval ligation; yet rats still did not show a sodium appetite (Stricker *et al.*, 1979). These results suggest that aldosterone does not provide the stimulus for sodium appetite in rats after PEG treatment.

C. Osmotic Dilution of Body Fluids

During the first 6 hours after 30% PEG treatment, rats drink and retain approximately 10 ml of water and thereby dilute body fluids by about 5%. It is conceivable that some aspect of the dilution was responsible for stimulating sodium appetite. A preliminary experiment gave results that were consistent with this hypothesis. If dilution was prevented by withholding drinking fluids for 8 hours, PEG-treated rats showed little initial interest in saline when the fluids became available (Stricker and Wolf, 1966).

In order to further explore the relation between osmotic dilution and sodium appetite, we decided to investigate the increase in saline consumption that occurs following acute sodium loss. Subcutaneous injection of formalin (2.5 ml of 1.5% solution, phosphate buffered) produces sodium deficiency as a result of extensive local damage to cellular and capillary membranes at the injection site (Stricker, 1966). By disrupting cellular metabolism, diffused sodium is no longer extruded from cells and extracellular sodium concentrations are thereby reduced. By damaging capillary walls, considerable plasma protein leaks out into the interstitium and reduced plasma oncotic pressure results in a rapid extravasation of plasma fluid.

Within a few hours after formalin treatment, plasma volume decreased by 25% and plasma sodium concentrations dropped by 6% (Jalowiec and Stricker, 1970a). Increased intake of water also began then and net fluid retention ultimately was comparable to that seen after 30% PEG treatment or tourniquet injury (Fig. 8). However, unlike the delay observed after those procedures, formalin treatment elicited sodium appetite quite rapidly. Indeed, sodium balance rose almost as quickly as it did when thirsty rats were allowed to drink 0.15 *M* NaCl and promptly restore their plasma volume deficits (Fig. 9), and the consumption of hypertonic saline kept pace with water intake so that the fluid retained always approximated isotonicity (Fig. 10).

The importance of hyponatremia to sodium appetite also was suggested by two related experiments. In one, formalin-treated rats evidenced immediate sodium appetite even when drinking fluids had been withheld for 8 hours, in contrast with PEG-treated rats having comparable hypovolemia (Stricker and Wolf,

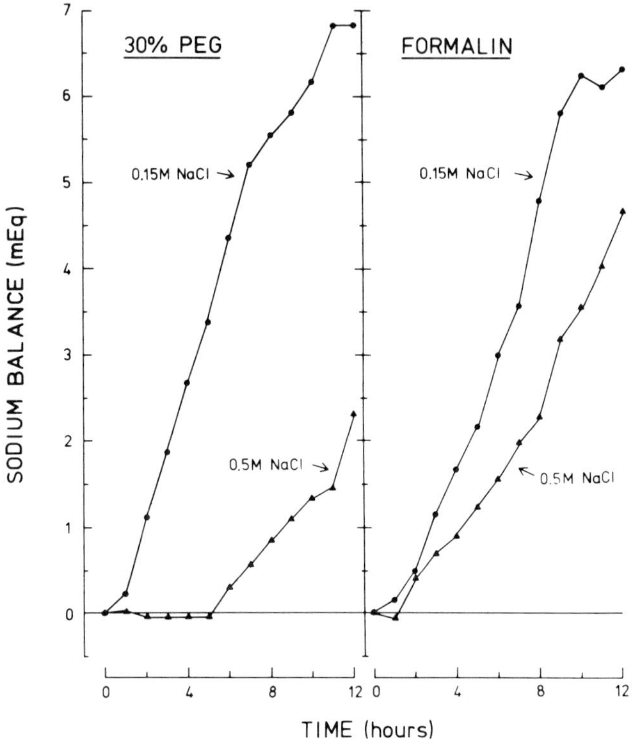

Fig. 9. Cumulative mean sodium balances of rats drinking either 0.15 *M* NaCl or water plus 0.5 *M* NaCl after subcutaneous injection of 30% PEG ($N = 6, 5$, respectively) or 1.5% formalin solution ($N = 8, 12$, respectively). Data from Jalowiec and Stricker (1970a) and Stricker and Jalowiec (1970).

1966). In another study, formalin-treated rats given water but not 0.5 *M* NaCl for 24 hours became much more hyponatremic than usual and showed a greater sodium appetite when saline became available (Jalowiec and Stricker, 1970b). On the other hand, two other investigations suggested the need for caution in interpreting these findings. In one, PEG-treated rats denied access to water and hypertonic saline for 24 hours (and therefore not hyponatremic) drank both fluids as soon as they were offered and in such proportion as to concoct a solution that was isotonic with extracellular fluid (Stricker and Wolf, 1966). Finally, it has been found that acute osmotic dilution produced by a water load does not provoke the ingestion of NaCl (Stricker and Wolf, 1966). Collectively, these results indicate that although osmotic dilution of body fluids may potentiate saline consumption, it is neither a necessary nor a sufficient stimulus for sodium appetite in rats.

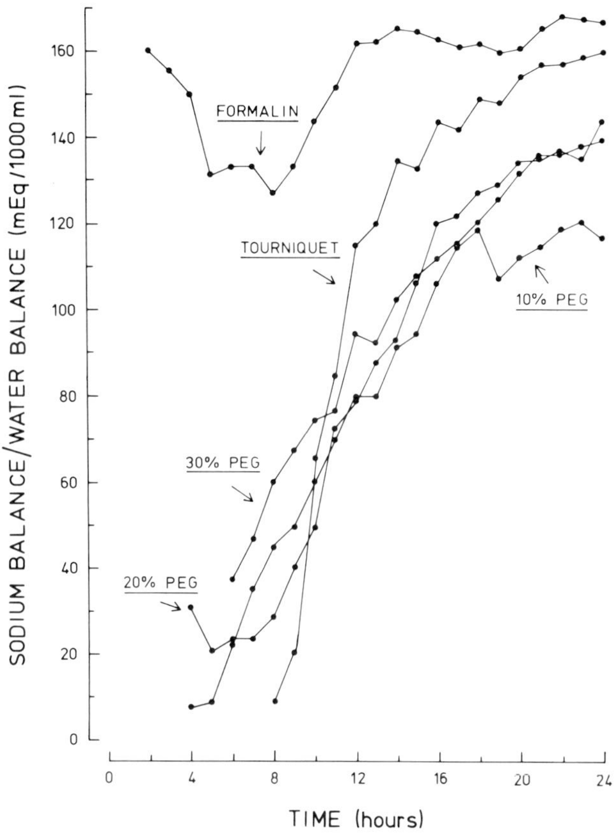

Fig. 10. Mean ratios of cumulative sodium balance to cumulative water balance of rats after subcutaneous injection of 10, 20, or 30% PEG, or 1.5% formalin solution, or release of a tourniquet from a hind limb. Data replotted from Figs. 7 and 8.

IV. IMPLICATIONS

The work just described was designed to analyze sodium appetite from the same perspective as contemporary views of thirst. Three factors are mentioned prominently in discussions of the physiological basis of water intake: hypovolemia, osmotic concentration of body fluids, and angiotensin. Like ADH secretion, drinking is promptly stimulated by remarkably small decreases in intravascular or intracellular hydration or increases in circulating angiotensin levels (Fitzsimons, 1963; Hsaio *et al.*, 1977; Stricker, 1968). These three variables are not so readily associated with sodium appetite, however. Treatments that produce simple hypovolemia usually enhance saline consumption but only after considerable delay. Osmotic dilution does seem to potentiate the effects of hypovolemia on sodium appetite but is neither necessary for the drive nor capable of stimulating it independently. Circulating levels of both angiotensin and aldosterone are elevated in association with sodium deficiency but neither hormone seems responsible for the sodium appetite that is then observed.

The same conclusions are reached when thirst and salt appetite are studied during sodium depletion in sheep, the only other species in which these motivations have been investigated extensively. For example, when acute sodium deficiency is produced by administration of the natriuretic agent furosemide, NaCl consumption begins to increase many hours after hypovolemic thirst appears (Zimmerman *et al.,* 1978). Moreover, the saline consumption of sodium-deficient sheep is not diminished by sudden increases either in plasma volume (Denton *et al.,* 1971) or in plasma sodium concentration (Beilharz *et al.,* 1965; see also Beilharz *et al.,* 1962; Beilharz and Kay, 1963). Nor do angiotensin or aldosterone stimulate sodium appetite in sheep (Bott *et al.,* 1967; Denton *et al.,* 1969). When taken together with the findings in rats, these results suggest that baroreceptors, osmoreceptors (or sodium receptors), and receptors for angiotensin or aldosterone are not the sites at which the signal for sodium appetite originates in either species.

If the important contribution of NaCl consumption to volume regulation does not provide the basis for sodium appetite, what does? Thus far we have been preoccupied with the effects of PEG treatment on plasma volume and the sequelae of hypovolemia. Paralleling these changes—indeed, underlying them—is the gradual sequestration of extracellular fluid in an edema local to the injection site. This accumulation includes interstitial fluid that has been drawn into the circulation from other extravascular sites due to the elevation in plasma oncotic pressure. In other words, the effective volume of extracellular fluid is reduced by PEG treatment even though total extracellular fluid volume is not changed. The magnitude of fluid accumulated by the colloid when drinking fluids are withheld is considerable; the 20–25 ml found after 5 ml of 30% PEG was administered intraperitoneally (Stricker and MacArthur, 1974; see also Fitzsimons, 1961) represents about one-third of the entire extracellular fluid volume of a 300-g rat.

A sizable reduction in the availability of sodium throughout the body should ultimately affect normal cellular function. Such effects in the brain may serve to trigger sodium appetite. This possibility conforms with a depletion–repletion model despite the change in orientation from that considered at the beginning of this chapter. In some ways it resembles the "sodium reservoir" hypothesis that Wolf and I proposed 10 years ago (Stricker and Wolf, 1969; Wolf and Stricker, 1967). At that time we imagined a special depot of sodium (such as the skeleton) gradually gave up the ion during sodium deficiency and in so doing triggered sodium appetite. I now view the stimulus as originating from neurons that are specialized only in their ability to affect NaCl ingestion (and perhaps other aspects of sodium metabolism), much like osmoreceptors are believed to be special not in their ability to detect changes in the effective osmolality of body fluids but in their location and their neural connections with various effector systems.

Dilution of extracellular sodium concentration by water ingestion and/or sodium depletion should further reduce the availability of sodium and thereby enhance the stimulus for salt appetite. This proposal is consistent with obtained data. However, it is less obvious how a mechanism of the sort proposed could account for the other experimental findings. Some insights may be obtained when we finally learn how osmotic dilution inhibits thirst during hypovolemia. But if sodium appetite is not closely analogous to thirst, then our speculations must include new variables and relationships (see also Denton, 1966). I believe that a rationale developed in this way is necessary to stimulate the experiments that ultimately will reveal the physiological basis of sodium appetite.

V. CONCLUSIONS

Sodium depletion reduces the effective osmolality of extracellular fluid and causes a contraction in its volume. The consumption of NaCl restores this deficit. Because the metabolisms of water and sodium are closely intertwined, it is tempting to consider sodium appetite from the same perspective as thirst. However, recent experiments do not support a model of sodium appetite based on changes in the volume of body fluid compartments and the levels of related hormones in the blood, critical variables in the physiology of thirst. I believe that further preoccupation with the contribution of sodium to the maintenance of plasma volume will not be helpful in illuminating the basis of sodium appetite. I suggest that new rationales be developed and propose, as an example, that reduced availability of sodium to the brain be considered as a stimulus for sodium appetite.

ACKNOWLEDGMENTS

I am grateful to my students and associates who have contributed so importantly to the work described in this chapter: E. Blaine, J. Hosutt, J. Jalowiec, F. Leenen, R. McDonald, N. Rowland, A. Vagnucci, G. Wolf, J. Yen, and M. Zimmerman. Our research has been supported, in part, by a grant from the United States National Institute of Mental Health (MH-25140). I also thank Dr. Paul McHugh for making the facilities of the Phipps Psychiatric Clinic at the Johns Hopkins University School of Medicine available to me for my sabbatical leave from the University of Pittsburgh, during which this chapter was written, and Dr. James B. Wirth for his continued interest and helpful comments regarding the ideas expressed herein.

REFERENCES

Andersson, B. (1978). Regulation of water intake. *Physiol. Rev.* **58,** 582–603.

Andree, R. A., Wingard, D. W., and Koletsky, S. (1957). Saline therapy in tourniquet shock. *Am. J. Phys.* **190,** 517–521.

Ashworth, C. T., Jester, A. W., and Guy, E. L. (1944). Local loss of fluid and protein in experimental shock: Relation to decrease of plasma volume and total circulating protein. *Am. J. Phys.* **141,** 571–574.

Avrith, D., and Fitzsimons, J. T. (1978). Intracranial angiotensin II stimulates sodium appetite. *J. Physiol. (London)* **282,** 40P–41P.

Beilharz, S., and Kay, R. N. B. (1963). The effects of ruminal and plasma sodium concentrations on the sodium appetite of sheep. *J. Physiol. (London)* **165,** 468–483.

Beilharz, S., Denton, D. A., and Sabine, J. R. (1962). The effect of concurrent deficiency of water and sodium on the sodium appetite of sheep. *J. Physiol. (London)* **163,** 378–390.

Beilharz, S., Bott, E., Denton, D. A., and Sabine, J. R. (1965). The effect of intracarotid infusions of 4 *M* NaCl on the sodium drinking of sheep with a parotid fistula. *J. Physiol. (London)* **178,** 80–91.

Bott, E., Denton, D. A., and Weller, S. (1967). The effect of angiotensin II infusion, renal hypertension and nephrectomy on salt appetite of sodium-deficient sheep. *Aust. J. Exp. Biol. Med. Sci.* **45,** 595–612.

Brenner, B. M., Bennett, C. M., and Berliner, R. W. (1968). The relationship between glomerular filtration rate and sodium reabsorption by the proximal tubule of the rat nephron. *J. Clin. Invest.* **47,** 1358–1374.

Bryant, R. W., Fluharty, S. J., and Epstein, A. N. (1978). Excessive drinking of sodium solutions by rats receiving continuous intracranial infusion of angiotensin. *Fed. Proc., Fed. Am. Soc. Exp. Biol.* **37,** 323.

Denton, D. A. (1965). Evolutionary aspects of the emergence of aldosterone secretion and salt appetite. *Physiol. Rev.* **45,** 245–295.

Denton, D. A. (1966). Some theoretical considerations in relation to innate appetite for salt. *Cond. Reflex* **1,** 144–170.

Denton, D. A., Nelson, J. F., Orchard, E., and Weller, S. (1969). The role of adrenocortical hormone secretion in salt appetite. *Olfaction Taste, Proc. Int. Symp., 3rd, 1968,* pp. 535–547.

Denton, D. A., Orchard, E., and Weller, S. (1971). The effect of rapid change of sodium balance and expansion of plasma volume on sodium appetite of sodium-deficient sheep. *Commun. Behav. Biol.* **6,** 245–258.

Dunn, F. L., Brennan, T. J., Nelson, A. E., and Robertson, G. L. (1973). The role of blood osmolality and volume in regulating vasopressin secretion in the rat. *J. Clin. Invest.* **52,** 3212–3219.

Epstein, A. N. (1978). Consensus, controversies, and curiosities. *Fed. Proc., Fed. Am. Soc. Exp. Biol.* **37,** 2711–2716.

Fitzsimons, J. T. (1961). Drinking by rats depleted of body fluid without increase in osmotic pressure. *J. Physiol. (London)* **159,** 297–309.

Fitzsimons, J. T. (1963). The effects of slow infusions of hypertonic solutions on drinking and drinking thresholds in rats. *J. Physiol. (London)* **167,** 344–354.

Fitzsimons, J. T. (1969). The role of a renal thirst factor in drinking induced by extracellular stimuli. *J. Physiol. (London)* **201,** 349–368.

Fitzsimons, J. T. (1978). Angiotensin, thirst, and sodium appetite: Retrospect and prospect. *Fed. Proc., Fed. Am. Soc. Exp. Biol.* **37,** 2669–2675.

Fitzsimons, J. T., and Stricker, E. M. (1971). Sodium appetite and the renin–angiotensin system. *Nature (London), New Biol.* **231,** 58–60.

Fitzsimons, J. T., and Wirth, J. B. (1978). The renin-angiotensin system and sodium appetite. *J. Physiol. (London)* **274,** 63-80.

Friedman, M. I., and Stricker, E. M. (1976). The physiological psychology of hunger: A physiological perspective. *Psychol. Rev.* **83,** 409-431.

Hosutt, J. A., Rowland, N., and Stricker, E. M. (1978). Hypotension and thirst in rats after isoproterenol treatment. *Physiol. Behav.* **21,** 593-598.

Hsaio, S., Epstein, A. N., and Camardo, J. S. (1977). The dipsogenic potency of peripheral angiotensin II. *Horm. Behav.* **8,** 129-140.

Jalowiec, J. E., and Stricker, E. M. (1970a). Restoration of body fluid balance following acute sodium deficiency in rats. *J. Comp. Physiol. Psychol.* **70,** 94-102.

Jalowiec, J. E., and Stricker, E. M. (1970b). Sodium appetite in rats after apparent recovery from acute sodium deficiency. *J. Comp. Physiol. Psychol.* **73,** 238-244.

Jalowiec, J. E., and Stricker, E. M. (1973). Sodium appetite in adrenalectomized rats following dietary sodium deprivation. *J. Comp. Physiol. Psychol.* **83,** 66-77.

Leenen, F. H., and Stricker, E. M. (1974). Plasma renin activity and thirst following hypovolemia or caval ligation in rats. *Am. J. Physiol.* **226,** 1238-1242.

Rice, K. K., and Richter, C. P. (1943). Increased sodium chloride and water intake of normal rats treated with deoxycorticosterone acetate. *Endocrinology* **33,** 106-115.

Richter, C. P. (1936). Increased salt appetite in adrenalectomized rats. *Am. J. Physiol.* **115,** 155-161.

Stricker, E. M. (1966). Extracellular fluid volume and thirst. *Am. J. Physiol.* **211,** 232-238.

Stricker, E. M. (1968). Some physiological and motivational properties of the hypovolemic stimulus for thirst. *Physiol. Behav.* **3,** 379-385.

Stricker, E. M. (1969). Osmoregulation and volume regulation in rats: Inhibition of hypovolemic thirst by water. *Am. J. Physiol.* **217,** 98-105.

Stricker, E. M. (1971a). Inhibition of thirst in rats following hypovolemia and/or caval ligation. *Physiol. Behav.* **6,** 293-298.

Stricker, E. M. (1971b). Effects of hypovolemia and/or caval ligation on water and NaCl solution drinking by rats. *Physiol. Behav.* **6,** 299-305.

Stricker, E. M. (1973). Thirst, sodium appetite, and complementary physiological contributions to the regulation of intravascular fluid volume. *In* "The Neuropsychology of Thirst" (A. Epstein, H. R. Kissileff, and E. Stellar, eds.), pp. 73-98. Holt, New York.

Stricker, E. M. (1977). The renin-angiotensin system and thirst: A reevaluation. II. Drinking elicited in rats by caval ligation or isoproterenol. *J. Comp. Physiol. Psychol.* **91,** 1220-1231.

Stricker, E. M. (1978). The renin-angiotensin system and thirst: Some unanswered questions. *Fed. Proc., Fed. Am. Soc. Exp. Biol.* **37,** 2704-2710.

Stricker, E. M., and Jalowiec, J. E. (1970). Restoration of intravascular fluid volume following acute hypovolemia in rats. *Am. J. Physiol.* **218,** 191-196.

Stricker, E. M., and MacArthur, J. P. (1974). Physiological bases for different effects of extravascular colloid treatments on water and NaCl solution drinking by rats. *Physiol. Behav.* **13,** 389-394.

Stricker, E. M., and Wolf, G. (1966). Blood volume and tonicity in relation to sodium appetite. *J. Comp. Physiol. Psychol.* **62,** 275-279.

Stricker, E. M., and Wolf, G. (1969). Behavioral control of intravascular fluid volume: Thirst and sodium appetite. *Ann. N.Y. Acad. Sci.* **157,** 553-567.

Stricker, E. M., Bradshaw, W. G., and McDonald, R. H., Jr. (1976). The renin-angiotensin system and thirst: A reevaluation. *Science* **194,** 1169-1171.

Stricker, E. M., Vagnucci, A. H., McDonald, R. H., Jr., and Leenen, F. H. (1979). Renin and aldosterone secretions during hypovolemia in rats: Relation to NaCl intake. *Am. J. Physiol.* **237,** R45-R51.

Thorn, G. W., Dorrance, S. S., and Day, E. (1942). Addison's disease: Evaluation of synthetic deoxycorticosterone acetate therapy in 158 patients. *Ann. Intern. Med.* **16,** 1053–1096.

Wolf, G. (1969). Innate mechanism for regulation of sodium appetite. *Olfaction Taste, Proc. Int. Symp., 3rd, 1968,* pp. 548–553.

Wolf, G., and Handal, P. J. (1966). Aldosterone-induced sodium appetite: Dose-response and specificity. *Endocrinology* **78,** 1120–1124.

Wolf, G., and Stricker, E. M. (1967). Sodium appetite elicited by hypovolemia in adrenalectomized rats: Reevaluation of the "reservoir" hypothesis. *J. Comp. Physiol. Psychol.* **63,** 252–257.

Zimmerman, M. B., Stricker, E. M., and Blaine, E. H. (1978). Water and NaCl intake after furosemide treatment in sheep (*Ovis aires*). *J. Comp. Physiol. Psychol.* **92,** 501–510.

Chapter 15

Rapid Sodium Depletion and Salt Appetite Induced by Intraperitoneal Dialysis

JOHN L. FALK and MAISY TANG

I. INTRODUCTION

The companionship of salt and water in the regulation of body fluid balance is basic to the analysis of the internal environment. As behaviorists we can be forgiven, perhaps, for our primary interest in the mechanisms controlling the *intake* of these substances, rather than their output. Given even a modicum of renal function, large variations in the ingestion of water are compensated for by differential reabsorption and excretion. But here, in terms of probable long-term consequences, the companionship ends. While a persistent overingestion of water under these conditions leads to only minor inconveniences, salt overindulgence can produce more serious results. Given particular pre-existing factors,

BIOLOGICAL AND BEHAVIORAL
ASPECTS OF SALT INTAKE

ISBN 0-12-397750-9

excess NaCl ingestion has been implicated in edematous accumulation, cardiovascular pathological changes, and chronic hypertension.

As a too liberal intake of NaCl is correlated with the development of various health problems, the mechanisms controlling an inappropriate and persistent NaCl appetite are of potential clinical interest. Animals besides man can exhibit spontaneous salt intakes that are far in excess of bodily need. For example, it is well known that laboratory rats show preferences for saline solution over water and high levels of saline acceptance under a variety of conditions (Bare, 1949; Richter, 1939; Weiner and Stellar, 1951; Young and Chaplin, 1949; Young and Falk, 1956). Not only do a number of species exhibit this overzealous response to opportunities to indulge in ingestion of NaCl solution when they are ostensibly in sodium balance, but also chronic overdrinking of saline after an acute episode of sodium depletion yields further evidence that elevated salt intake may continue long after sodium balance has been restored. We shall describe some of the conditions under which a persistent overindulgence in highly hypertonic NaCl solution occurs in spite of putative sodium repletion.

II. THE DEPLETION OF SODIUM BY TRANSPERITONEAL DIALYSIS

Following studies on the changes that occur in the composition of various fluids when they are injected intraperitoneally (Schecter *et al.*, 1933), the technique of intraperitoneal dialysis with isotonic glucose was used to investigate problems in body water–electrolyte redistribution (Darrow and Yannet, 1936; Elkinton *et al.*, 1946; Woodbury, 1956; Yannet, 1940), renal function (Baker *et al.*, 1961; Cizek and Huang, 1951; Frieden *et al.*, 1952), bone sodium mobilization (Bergstrom, 1955; Bergstrom and Ruva, 1960; Bergstrom and Wallace, 1954; Munro *et al.*, 1957), and water intake (Darrow and Yannet, 1936; Cizek *et al.*, 1951; Remington *et al.*, 1941). The intraperitoneal injection of a load of isotonic glucose produces a rapid depletion of extracellular electrolytes without a concomitant removal of body water (see Fig. 1). In a typical experiment, a load (10% of body weight) of isotonic (5%) glucose solution at body temperature is injected intraperitoneally and allowed to remain for 4 hours. During the dialysis, extracellular electrolytes move into the peritoneal pool and water moves from the extracellular into the intracellular compartment (Fig. 1). There is no net exchange of water between the peritoneal and extracellular fluids. At the end of the 4-hour dialysis, ascitic fluid in an amount equivalent to 10% of body weight can be withdrawn from the peritoneal cavity by paracentesis with a needle (13-gauge) attached to a syringe. This removes approximately one-quarter of the animal's body sodium without decreasing body water (the injected solution and the dialysate removed are both isotonic). The absolute salt depletion produced by this

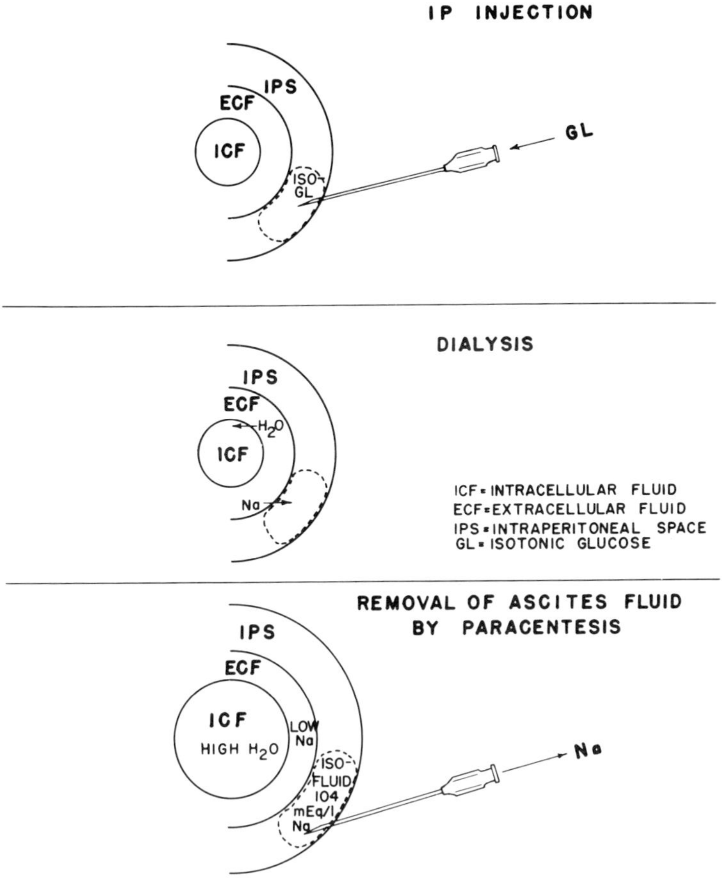

Fig. 1. Water-electrolyte changes produced by intraperitoneal dialysis.

method can be contrasted with the mixed salt and water decrement produced from a local pooling of extracellular fluid by the subcutaneous injection of polyethylene glycol or formalin, or the intraperitoneal injection of hyperoncotic colloid (Cort, 1952; Stricker, 1966).

In an initial series of experiments, the postdialysis intake of water and of NaCl solution were determined independently (Falk, 1961; Falk, 1965a). Rats were allowed a feeding and drinking period from 9 AM until 12 noon daily during which Purina Laboratory Chow and water were available. From 8 PM until 9 AM daily either water or 3% (0.5 *M*) NaCl solution was available without food (the fluid test period). The overnight fluid test period allowed the effect of salt-depletion dialysis on fluid intake to be evaluated independently of any influence on food intake. The highly hypertonic 3% NaCl was employed to be certain that any increased intake of NaCl observed was not simply due to an increase in water turnover occasioned by the dialysis. After measurement of intakes of water and 3% NaCl solution during separate fluid test periods following sham dialyses, rats were dialyzed by injecting the dialyzing solution at 12 noon and withdrawing it at 4 PM, with either water or 3% NaCl solution being the available fluid during the ensuing overnight fluid test period. During the following 2 days the same schedule of food and water availability was maintained, with water the fluid available during the fluid test period. A second dialysis was performed on the next day. Animals which were given water overnight after the first dialysis had 3% NaCl solution available after the second dialysis; animals given 3% NaCl solution after the first dialysis had water available after the second dialysis. These orders of postdialysis fluid presentation are denoted as the W–S and S–W orders, respectively (Fig. 2). The figure shows that animals increased their fluid intakes during the fluid test period after the first dialysis (IPD I), but that the increases were much greater after the second dialysis (IPD II). The increased water intake is of interest insofar as it throws light on the conditions necessary and sufficient for stimulating water intake. However, they will not be discussed here as they are not germane to our present concern. The progressive increase in the intake of 3% NaCl solution after the second dialysis is of interest because this augmented NaCl ingestion occurs even after animals have taken in much more

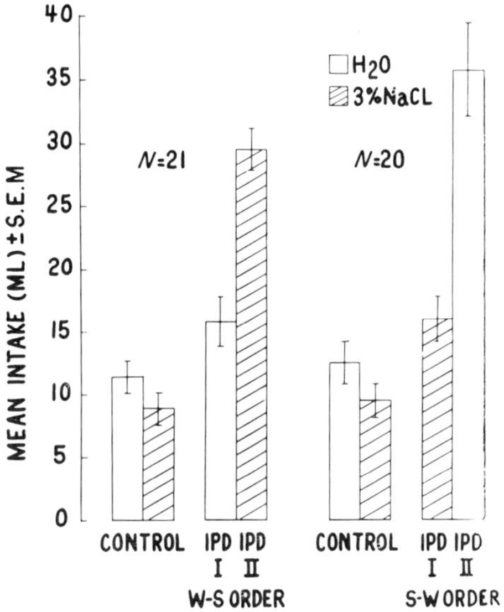

Fig. 2. Intakes of water and 3% (0.5 *M*) NaCl solution during fluid test periods under control and postdialysis conditions during water–salt (W–S) and salt–water (S–W) orders of fluid presentation after the first (IPD I) and second (IPD II) dialyses.

sodium than is necessary to replete the amount removed after the first dialysis. Recall that the animals ate the rather NaCl-rich diet (Purina Laboratory Chow contains about 0.5% NaCl) for two feeding periods before the second dialysis. But better evidence for persistence of an NaCl appetite despite putative repletion is contained in most of the following figures. Before this theme is developed, however, a few technical points should be clarified.

First, the 41 animals whose results are shown in Fig. 2 were not all dialyzed with 5% glucose. The results shown are actually from 3 combined groups. As indicated in Fig. 3, one group was dialyzed against isotonic glucose solution, the dialyzing solution for a second group was isotonic glucose plus 90 mEq/liter Cl^- (ammonium chloride) to prevent anion depletion, while a third group was dialyzed against a solution of isotonic glucose to which 5 mEq/liter K^+ (potassium chloride) had been added to prevent the possible removal of some potassium. Figure 3 shows the mean pre- and postdialysis intakes for these 3 groups during the overnight fluid test periods. The post-IPD columns combine the results of the two orders (W–S and S–W). The 3 dialyzing solutions yielded essentially the same results, indicating that the important factor removed by dialysis which produced the increases in intake was apparently sodium.

In the above experiments only one fluid was offered during any particular fluid test period. In order to determine whether the increased intake of water or of 3%

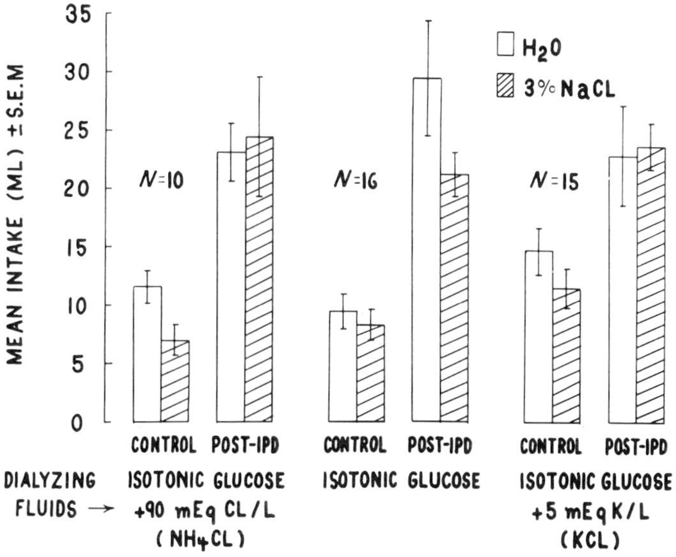

Fig. 3. Intakes of water and 3% NaCl solution during fluid test periods under control and postdialysis conditions for three dialyzing solutions. Only one of the two fluids was presented during a test period.

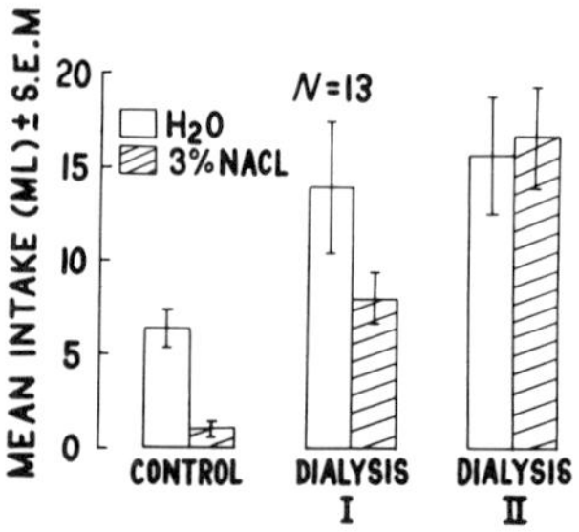

Fig. 4. Intakes of water and 3% NaCl solution for fluid test periods when both fluids were simultaneously available under control and postdialysis conditions.

NaCl solution was the primary effect, an additional experiment used the same dialysis schedule (5% glucose) but both fluids were available during the fluid test periods following each of the two dialyses. After IPD I the intake of 3% NaCl solution increased (Fig. 4). The increase in water intake would be difficult to interpret since this could be simply due to the NaCl increase. However, after IPD II water intake failed to show any further significant increase while NaCl solution ingestion increased significantly over the post-IPD I level. Thus, when given concurrent access to both fluids NaCl seems to dominate the ingestion picture.

III. POSTDIALYSIS NaCl APPETITE—IS IT LEARNED?

It is possible that the greater effect of IPD II on ingestion occurs because animals learn compensatory intake behavior following IPD I and then perform more effectively after IPD II. To test this possibility one group of rats was dialyzed against isotonic glucose and allowed to drink 3% NaCl solution during the fluid test period. A second group was stomach-loaded with the mean amount of 3% NaCl solution ingested by the first group at the time of dialysate withdrawal and allowed to drink only water during the fluid test period. After the usual 2-day interval, both groups were given IPD II and allowed to drink 3% NaCl solution during the overnight fluid test period (Fig. 5). Both groups drank a comparable, elevated amount after IPD II indicating that, although the first group was denied an opportunity to learn compensatory NaCl ingestion after IPD I, such a history was not necessary for IPD II to produce an augmented effect (Falk, 1966).

But what happens during the fluid test period after IPD I when animals first begin to ingest an increased amount of 3% NaCl solution? Is this a function of drive reduction learning in which ingesting some NaCl produces a beneficial, repletional effect which then reinforces further intake of this substance? To test this notion rats were trained to make brief-taste choice runs on a two-choice

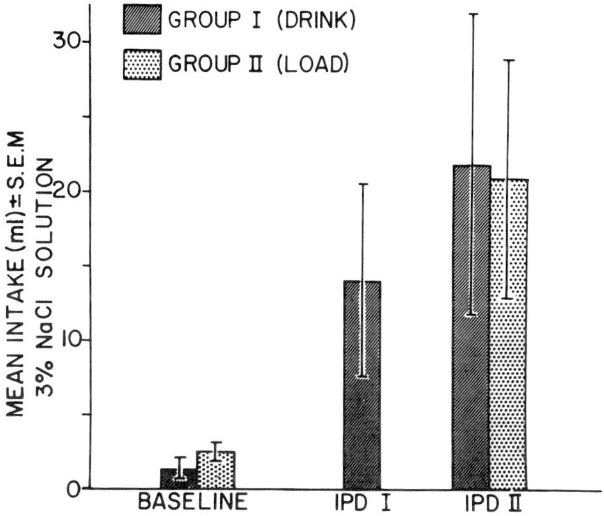

Fig. 5. Intake of 3% NaCl solution during fluid test period before (baseline) and after dialysis (IPD). Group I drank NaCl solution after IPD I and IPD II. Group II was stomach-loaded with 14.1 ml of 3% NaCl after IPD I and drank NaCl solution after IPD II.

preference apparatus. Animals were given choices between 3% NaCl solution and water and were run until they demonstrated a significant preference sequence of trials for one of the fluids. Under water-deprivation conditions, rats soon learned to go to the side displaying water where they were allowed a few licks of fluid on each trial. After IPD, animals all ceased showing a water preference. They either became indiscriminate, adopting a position habit so that they tasted salt on half the trials and water on the other half, or else they demonstrated a rapidly significant sequence of NaCl preference choices (Falk and Herman, 1961). The mean time to complete a significant number of NaCl choices at the 0.01 level was 23.8 minutes, with the total fluid ingested amounting to only 1–2 ml. The brief time taken for the behavioral change to occur and the small amount of NaCl solution animals were permitted to ingest indicate that the preference change is not attributable to a postingestional sodium repletion effect.

IV. POSTDIALYSIS NaCl APPETITE—IS IT SPECIFIC?

It is all well and good to deplete an animal of sodium and demonstrate that now a quite hypertonic NaCl solution will be ingested. But, in his scrupulously designed studies, Dr. Curt Richter taught us decades ago not to constrain the testing situation so as to force the animal to yield us only one kind of answer. To this end, it is interesting to ask what will happen if the dialyzed animal is offered KCl during the fluid test period rather than NaCl. Rats were dialyzed against an isotonic glucose solution to which ammonium chloride and KCl were added (as described above) to prevent K^+ and Cl^- depletion. Both water and a 0.3 *M* KCl solution were simultaneously available during the fluid test period (Falk, 1965b). Pilot work had shown that a 0.3 *M* KCl solution was about as acceptable to water-deprived rats as a 3% NaCl (0.5 *M*) solution. After IPD II, KCl solution intake increased greatly and was preferred to water. While this indicates that the post-IPD solution appetite is not absolutely specific to NaCl, perhaps the test for specificity was not entirely appropriate as the proper repletion substance (sodium) was not offered as a choice. Consequently, further studies offered rats a choice between 0.5 *M* NaCl and 0.3 *M* KCl solutions. This work showed that in over half the instances of this postIPD choice, animals strongly preferred either one solution or the other. Mean group intakes for the two were approximately equal. Again, this hardly indicates great specificity of the postIPD appetite. An additional experiment showed that if the choice was between 0.5 *M* NaCl and 0.5 *M* KCl solutions, then the NaCl solution is preferred overwhelmingly. But this last experiment is not a legitimate test of specificity since 0.5 *M* NaCl solution is much more acceptable to rats than 0.5 *M* KCl in preIPD baseline measures.

One commentator has found these studies puzzling and has speculated that IPD would produce potassium depletion followed by hyperkalemia and also a dilution of intracellular potassium as extracellular water moves into the cells (Michell, 1978). However, we found that urinary loss of potassium was no greater in dialyzed animals than in sham-dialyzed controls (Falk and Tang, 1973), a result which agrees with research on the dialyzed dog (Gann and Wright, 1966). We did observe the development of hyperkalemia and the cells are undoubtedly overhydrated, but these factors would scarcely form the basis for a potassium appetite. To our knowledge, efforts to induce a potassium appetite by potassium depletion have not been successful. For the present, we conclude that the IPD procedure does not produce a potassium depletion. Nor does it produce water-electrolyte changes which could be expected to increase KCl ingestion. The KCl ingestive increases observed, then, remain to be explained and must limit any claim that the postIPD NaCl solution intake is a highly specific appetite.

V. THE POSTREPLETIONAL PERSISTENCE OF NaCl INTAKE

At first blush, studies showing an increased ingestion of NaCl resulting from sodium depletion appear to fit the conventional depletion-repletion homeostatic model. The KCl ingestion studies constitute a minor embarrassment for this model, but could be overlooked as an artifact. After all, KCl as a salt or hypertonic solution is not present in quantity in environments to which animals have become adapted, so that some uncertainty of choice under contrived laboratory conditions is perhaps not entirely surprising. Yet, even a cursory look at the degree of sodium depletion and its subsequent intake fails to support a simple input–output model of adjustment. For example, in one of the studies previously described (Falk, 1966), about 3.2 mEq of sodium were removed by each dialysis. After IPD I, however, animals drank a mean of 7.1 mEq of sodium. In spite of this ingestive "hyperreplacement" of sodium and 2 recovery days during which the animals ate Purina Laboratory Chow (0.5% NaCl), IPD II produced an intake of 10.9 mEq of sodium. The dialysis depletion of sodium seems to occasion a quite excessive NaCl appetite.

Now if the above result is viewed from a traditional gain–loss homeostatic framework, then something rather curious is happening. Sodium ingestive replacement fails to terminate NaCl appetite. At this point it was reasoned that if much more NaCl is drunk than is depleted, then it should be difficult to prevent NaCl intake by a postdialysis repletional stomach load of NaCl. In fact, almost twice the amount of sodium depleted was loaded at the time of dialysate removal after both IPD I and II (Falk and Lipton, 1967). A 4% body-weight load of 0.5 *M* NaCl solution was loaded into the load group while a sham load was given to a control group. Figure 6 shows that although given massive NaCl loads after both IPD I and II, the load group drank volumes of 0.5 *M* NaCl solution comparable to the control group during the fluid test periods. Only the time course of the ingestive response to dialysis differed for the load group after IPD II. The maximal NaCl intake occurred a day later for the load group than for the control

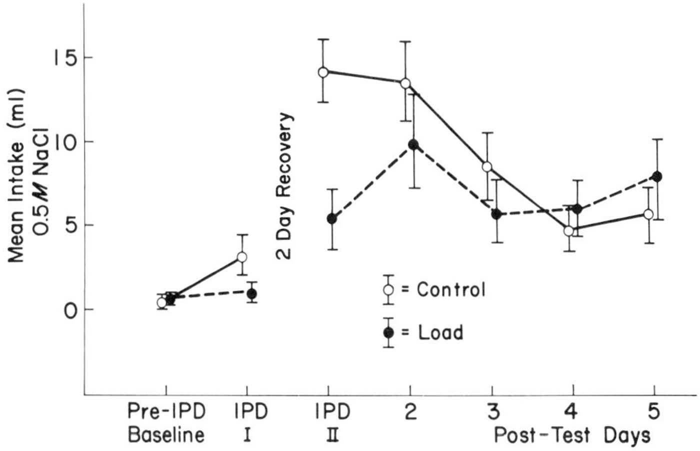

Fig. 6. Intake of 0.5 *M* NaCl solution during the fluid test periods preIPD, after IPD I, and for 5 days after IPD II. Load group received 4% body-weight load of 0.5 *M* NaCl solution at start of IPD I and II, while control group was sham-loaded.

group and the difference between these peaks was not statistically significant. Figure 7 shows that the fluid test period NaCl intake failed to return down to the preIPD baseline level in both groups for the 30 days they were observed.

It is apparent that once sodium depletion dialysis has operated for a few hours, even massive NaCl loading cannot counteract the major part of the ensuing NaCl appetite. In order to evaluate this phenomenon further, it was reasoned that if the massive NaCl load were given at the *start* of the 4-hour dialysis, rather than at the end, then the NaCl appetite should be blocked. The procedure would prevent even a short-term sodium sequestration from occurring. This result was obtained (Falk and Lipton, 1967). Further, Fig. 8 shows once again that the group which received standard dialyses remained above the preIPD NaCl intake baseline level for 30 days, while the group loaded at the start of both dialyses remained at the baseline level.

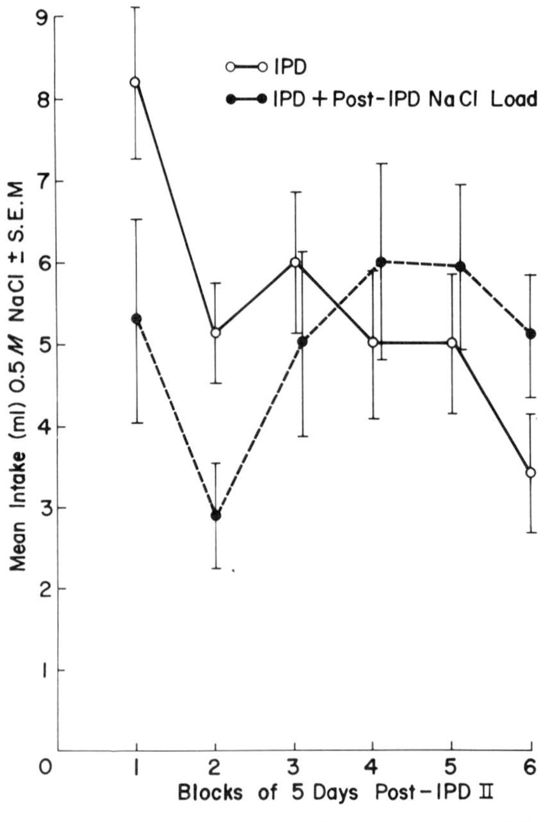

Fig. 7. Intakes of 0.5 *M* NaCl solution during fluid test periods for six 5-day means (30 days) after IPD II for group NaCl-loaded at end of each IPD and control group.

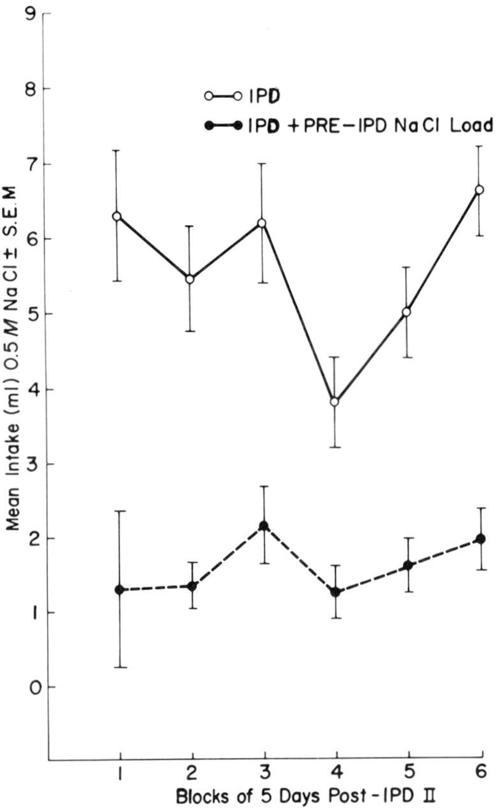

Fig. 8. Intakes of 0.5 *M* NaCl solution during fluid test periods for six 5-day means (30 days) after IPD II for group NaCl-loaded at start of each IPD and control group.

The sequestration of sodium in the peritoneal cavity for a few hours seemed sufficient for the production of a NaCl appetite that was rather resistant to alleviation by NaCl loading. Hence, the question arises: Is it necessary to remove the dialysate in order to produce a full-fledged NaCl appetite? The reabsorption of the unremoved dialysate should take place too late to prevent the NaCl appetite. This possibility was investigated by giving different groups of rats either 2, 4, 8, or 10% body-weight IPD injections of isotonic glucose without withdrawal of the dialysate (Tang and Falk, 1979). Fluid test period intakes of water and 0.5 *M* NaCl solution were followed for 3 days, a second glucose injection was given to each group (same percentage body weight load) and intakes were measured for 3 more days. Figure 9 shows that the 2 and 4% loads were ineffective in producing a NaCl appetite. At 8 and 10% loads, a graded increase occurred after IPD I. This was further exaggerated by IPD II. These results indicate that a temporary

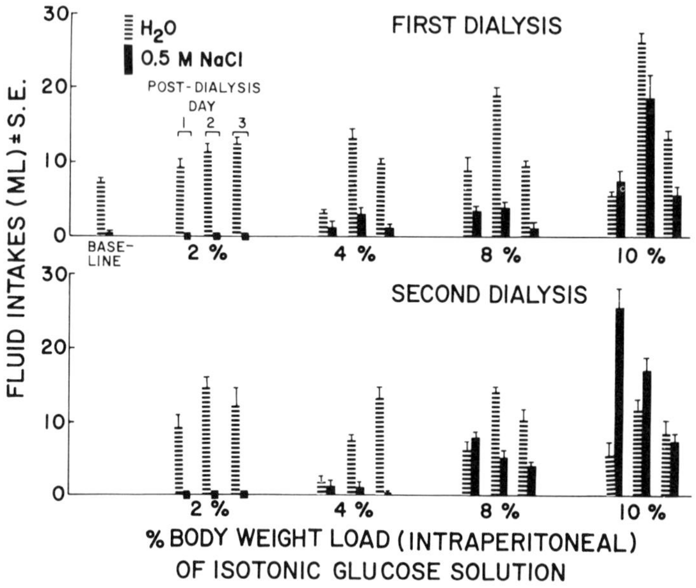

Fig. 9. Mean 0.5 *M* NaCl solution and water intakes during fluid test periods for preIPD baseline and for 3 consecutive days after IPD I and II. Group given either 2, 4, 8, or 10% body-weight IPD loads after both dialyses.

sequestration of about 20% of body sodium in the peritoneal cavity is a sufficient condition for the production of a persistent NaCl appetite.

VI. THE POSTREPLETIONAL RENAL CONSERVATION OF SODIUM

When humans maintained on a low sodium diet (Black *et al.*, 1950) and dialyzed dogs (Frieden *et al.*, 1952) were infused with hypertonic NaCl solutions, they reabsorbed greater than normal amounts of sodium. This effect outlasted the reconstitution of blood volume and serum sodium.

In order to determine if the unusual persistence of the NaCl appetite was also mirrored by a persistence in renal sodium saving, the postdialysis urinary response to NaCl loading was investigated. Rats housed in individual metabolism cages were divided into two groups fed either Purina Laboratory Chow (denoted as "Meal") or low sodium diet (ICN Nutritional Biochemical Corp. #1165B). Food and water were made unavailable for a 10-hour period each day (9 AM–7 PM). This permitted 4 hours of deprivation to precede a 6-hour excretion observation period which on occasion was initiated with an NaCl load. After 17 days adaptation to this regimen, the two diet groups were subdivided further into four groups ($N = 6$): (a) low sodium-IPD, (b) low sodium-control, (c) meal-IPD, and (d) meal-control. On day 18, the IPD groups were injected at 1 PM with a 10% body-weight load of dialyzing solution (5% glucose plus 5 mEq/liter potassium), the dialysate being withdrawn at 4 PM. The control groups were given sham dialyses in which light ether anesthesia and needle insertion occurred at 1 and 4 PM, but no solution was injected or withdrawn. Thereafter, on every second day, beginning 24 hours after the dialysis injection, animals were loaded at 1 PM with a 3% body-weight stomach load of 0.5 *M* NaCl solution. Six loads were given (days 19, 21, 23, 25, 27, and 29).

Figure 10 shows that, in terms of sodium input-output, the meal-control group excreted the same amount after each load. Both the low sodium-control group and the meal-IPD group excreted a constant amount by the second load. The low sodium-IPD group attained a constant excretion response to loading only by the third load. Figure 11 reveals the same general picture, with urine volume excreted remaining rather constant and sodium concentration mirroring the sodium output pattern shown in Fig. 10.

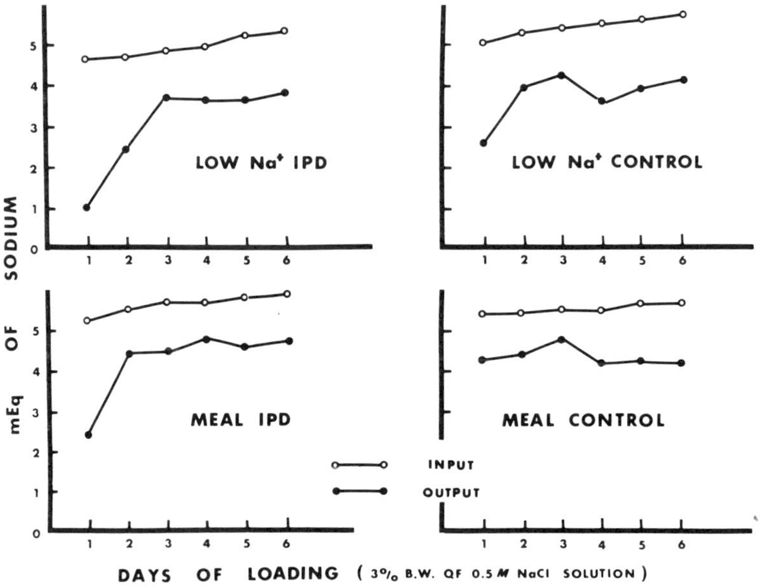

Fig. 10. Sodium input (3% body weight loads of 0.5 *M* NaCl) and 6-hour urinary sodium outputs for groups loaded every second day (6 loads).

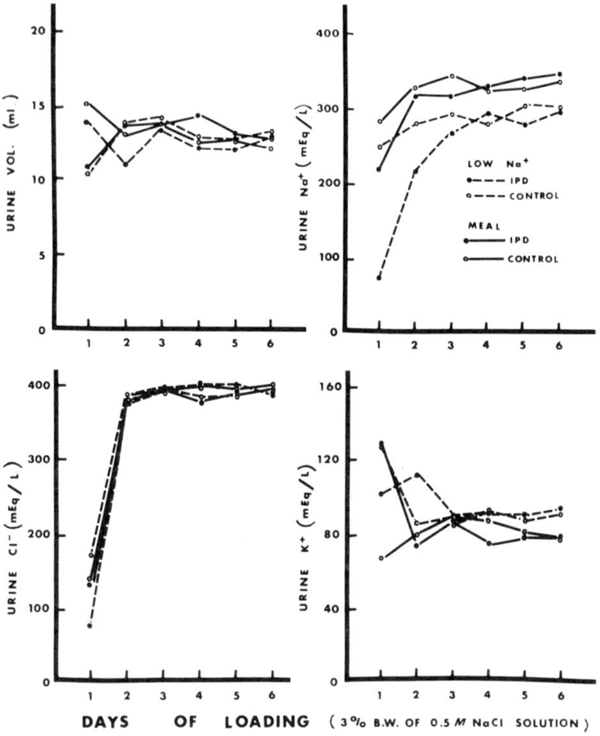

Fig. 11. Urine values for groups represented in Fig. 10.

VII. SUMMARY

Intraperitoneal dialysis (IPD) against a large load of isotonic glucose solution is a simple procedure for the production of a persistent NaCl appetite. The appetite is not only persistent, but is excessive in that intake is much greater than the sodium removed in the dialysate. Furthermore, a temporary sequestration of body sodium in the peritoneal cavity is sufficient for production of a persistent appetite. The dialysate need not be removed. The postrepletional maintenance of a long-lasting NaCl appetite is mirrored by a lag in the cessation of renal sodium saving despite excessive NaCl loads.

ACKNOWLEDGMENT

Part of this research and the preparation of this chapter was supported by Grant HL-19612 from the National Institutes of Health.

REFERENCES

Baker, G. P., Levitin, H., and Epstein, F. H. (1961). Sodium depletion and renal conservation of water. *J. Clin. Invest.* **40,** 867–873.

Bare, J. K. (1949). The specific hunger for sodium chloride in normal and adrenalectomized white rats. *J. Comp. Physiol. Psychol.* **42,** 242–253.

Bergstrom, W. H. (1955). The participation of bone in total body sodium metabolism in the rat. *J. Clin. Invest.* **34,** 997–1004.

Bergstrom, W. H., and Ruva, F. D. (1960). Changes in bone sodium during acute acidosis in the rat. *Am. J. Physiol.* **198,** 1126–1128.

Bergstrom, W. H., and Wallace, W. W. (1954). Bone as a sodium and potassium reservoir. *J. Clin. Invest.* **33,** 867–873.

Black, D. A. K., Platt, R., and Stanbury, S. W. (1950). Regulation of sodium excretion in normal and salt-depleted subjects. *Clin. Sci.* **9,** 205–221.

Cizek, L. J., and Huang, K. C. (1951). Water diuresis in the salt-depleted dog. *Am. J. Physiol.* **167,** 473–484.

Cizek, L. J., Semple, R. E., Huang, K. C., and Gregersen, M. I. (1951). Effect of extracellular electrolyte depletion on water intake in dogs. *Am. J. Physiol.* **164,** 415–422.

Cort, J. H. (1952). The renal response to extrarenal depletion of the blood volume. *J. Physiol. (London)* **116,** 307–319.

Darrow, D. C., and Yannet, H. (1936). Metabolic studies of the changes in body electrolyte and distribution of body water induced experimentally by deficit of extracellular electrolyte. *J. Clin. Invest.* **15,** 419–427.

Elkinton, J. R., Danowski, T. S., and Winkler, A. W. (1946). Hemodynamic changes in salt depletion and in dehydration. *J. Clin. Invest.* **25,** 120–129.

Falk, J. L. (1961). The behavioral regulation of water-electrolyte balance. *In* "Nebraska Symposium on Motivation" (M. R. Jones, ed.), pp. 1–33. Univ. of Nebraska Press, Lincoln.

Falk, J. L. (1965a). Water intake and NaCl appetite in sodium depletion. *Psychol. Rep.* **16,** 315–325.

Falk, J. L. (1965b). Limitations to the specificity of NaCl appetite in sodium-depleted rats. *J. Comp. Physiol. Psychol.* **60,** 393–396.

Falk, J. L. (1966). Serial sodium depletion and NaCl solution intake. *Physiol. Behav.* **1,** 75–77.

Falk, J. L., and Herman, T. S. (1961). Specific appetite for NaCl without postingestional repletion. *J. Comp. Physiol. Psychol.* **54,** 405–408.

Falk, J. L., and Lipton, J. M. (1967). Temporal factors in the genesis of NaCl appetite by intraperitoneal dialysis. *J. Comp. Physiol. Psychol.* **63,** 247–251.

Falk, J. L., and Tang, M. (1973). Nonuremic hyperosmolality produced by sodium depletion. *Physiol. Behav.* **10,** 793–799.

Frieden, J., Lester, R., and Elisberg, E. I. (1952). Renal tubular sodium metabolism in sodium deficiency states. *Am. J. Physiol.* **168,** 93–96.

Gann, D. S., and Wright, H. K. (1966). Increased renal sodium reabsorption after depletion of the extracellular or intravascular fluid volumes. *J. Surg. Res.* **6,** 196–204.

Michell, A. R. (1978). Salt appetite, salt intake, and hypertension: A deviation of perspective. *Perspect. Biol. Med.* **21,** 335–347.

Munro, D. S., Satoskar, R. S., and Wilson, G. M. (1957). The exchange of bone sodium with isotopes in rats. *J. Physiol. (London)* **139,** 474–488.

Remington, J. W., Parkins, W. M., and Hays, H. W. (1941). Influence of prolonged electrolyte deprivation and final restoration on fluid intake, balance and distribution. *Proc. Soc. Exp. Biol. Med.* **47,** 183–187.

Richter, C. P. (1939). Salt taste thresholds for normal and adrenalectomized rats. *Endocrinology* **24,** 367–371.

Schechter, A. J., Cary, M. K., Carpentieri, A. L., and Darrow, D. C. (1933). Changes in composition of fluids injected into the peritoneal cavity. *Am. J. Dis. Child.* **46,** 1015–1026.

Stricker, E. M. (1966). Extracellular fluid volume and thirst. *Am. J. Physiol.* **211,** 232–238.

Tang, M., and Falk, J. L. (1979). Temporary peritoneal sequestration of NaCl and persistent NaCl appetite. *Physiol. Behav.* **22,** 595–597.

Weiner, I. H., and Stellar, E. (1951). Salt preference of the rat determined by a single-stimulus method. *J. Comp. Physiol. Psychol.* **44,** 394–401.

Woodbury, D. M. (1956). Effect of acute hyponatremia on distribution of water and electrolytes in various tissues of the rat. *Am. J. Physiol.* **185,** 281–286.

Yannet, H. (1940). Changes in the brain resulting from depletion of extracellular electrolytes. *Am. J. Physiol.* **28,** 683–689.

Young, P. T., and Chaplin, J. P. (1949). Studies of food preference, appetite, and dietary habits. X. Preferences of adrenalectomized rats for salt solutions of different concentrations. *Comp. Psychol. Monogr.* **19,** 45–74.

Young, P. T., and Falk, J. L. (1956). The relative acceptability of sodium chloride as a function of concentration and water need. *J. Comp. Physiol. Psychol.* **49,** 569–575.

Chapter 16

Salt in Processed Foods

RICHARD H. FORSYTHE and RALPH A. MILLER

I. INTRODUCTION

Salt has been a valuable food ingredient since the dawn of civilization. Numerous biblical references could be cited to show the high value placed on this common material by earlier cultures. Whether salt was first used for flavor or for food preservation is unknown, but undoubtedly the human desire for salt was an evolutionary process. As with most foods and food ingredients, availability always played an important role in the growth of its popularity. In the case of salt, its unique property of inhibiting microbiological spoilage was a significant development in the earliest recorded food technology. Indeed, if not wars, certainly skirmishes were fought over the control of salt. Fortunes were made in the salt trade in colonial times before suitable sources were located in this country. In any event, whether the desire for salt resulted from its flavoring properties, its preserving properties or just because of its occasional lack of availability, its presence in today's foods is considered essential by most consumers. The fact that it may be consumed in quantities larger than those dictated by physiological

BIOLOGICAL AND BEHAVIORAL
ASPECTS OF SALT INTAKE

ISBN 0-12-397750-9

requirements (like some other nutrients, i.e., calories, fats and proteins) is undisputed.

The study of the role of palatability in food acceptance is, as sciences go, relatively new. It began during World War II when foods of great stability and compactness were required, often at the expense of eating quality. But no quartermaster or soldier has to be convinced that food has to be acceptable to be eaten. It should also be noted that palatability is not just a concern of food processors, but of all those who prepare food, whether it be the gourmet chef or the "harried" homemaker. This chapter will primarily consider only one of the factors involved in palatability, namely taste or flavor, but will touch on those other properties, such as texture and appearance, which are influenced by salt.

In earlier times, when food was not so plentiful, flavor was used to encourage the consumption of nutrients and to add variety to bland or monotonous diets, for example, sauces with rice dishes in the Orient. It was also used to encourage the consumption of food that might otherwise be wasted, such as sausage from meat by-products in Germany. Once established, these foods became embedded in the social patterns of the cultures. Dr. Zotterman (1977), in opening the International Symposium on Food Intake and Chemical Senses in Japan in 1976, cited Brillat Savarin's introductory remarks in his 1825 *Physiologie du Gout,* "The pleasures of the table are of all times and all ages; they go hand in hand with all other pleasures, outlast them and in the end console us for their loss."

What we need to emphasize is that the use of salt in food preparation is, indeed, not new, nor, as we will discuss, is the use of salt by food processors significantly different when preparing the more convenient processed counterparts of our traditional diet. It is recognized that increased use of some foods traditionally containing higher levels of salt may have increased overall salt intake in selected portions of the population. What is new is the developing body of information on relating excess salt consumption (along with many other factors) and hypertension. Indeed, this issue is not clear, but it is beyond the scope of this presentation to review it here. SCOGS-102 (Life Sciences Research Office, 1978) states, "For at least 80 percent of the population of the United States, present salt intake has not been demonstrated to be harmful."

II. SALT INTAKE

Salt in the human diet comes from drinking water, that occurring naturally in foods, that added to food during processing, and that added by the consumer at the table. Total daily intake is estimated at 10–12 g (Life Sciences Research Office, 1978) and is divided approximately one-third from naturally occurring sources, one-third from that added in processing, and one-third from that added just prior to eating, as shown in Table I.

TABLE I

Estimates of Adult Daily Salt Intake

Source	NaCl, g
Discretionary addition to food by the consumer	3–4
Naturally occurring	3–4
Food processing	3–4
Total	10–12

Small quantities of sodium, other than from NaCl, are found in nature and used in some processing operations, but this probably constitutes less than 10% of the total resulting from salt.

In comparing per capita disappearance of salt used in food processing in 1970 and 1975 (Filer, 1978a), usage appears to have decreased from 10.9 to 8.4 g per day. It should be pointed out that not all this is consumed, as a considerable portion is discarded in brines. It is too early to predict if this 23% reduction is a real trend and the public is responding to their increased information on potential health benefits that might result from reducing salt consumption.

Salt is found in a wide variety of food categories and at widely varying levels as shown in Table II.

An additional source of salt intake data is from the FDA Market Basket studies carried out in 1972–1973 and again in 1976 (Life Sciences Research Office,

TABLE II

Average Adult Daily Intake of Salt by Food Categories[a]

Food category	Percentage salt	Daily intake, g[b]
Baked goods	1.3	1.8
Breakfast cereals	1.1	0.2
Grain products	0.7	0.2
Milk products	0.5	0.2
Cheese	1.0	0.1
Processed juices, fruits	0.5	0.6
Meat products	2.5	1.9
Condiments, relishes	3.2	0.3
Soups	1.0	0.3
Snacks	2.1	1.2[c]

[a] Adapted from Life Sciences Research Office, 1978.
[b] 2–65 year olds.
[c] From Filer, 1978a.

TABLE III

Calculated Salt Content of 1976 FDA Market Basket Survey[a]

Food category	Salt (g/3900 kcal)[b]
Grain and cereal products	5.1
Meat, fish, and poultry	2.5
Dairy products	1.8
Oils and fats	1.0
Garden fruits	0.7
Legumes	0.6
Discretionary	4.6
Total	17.0

[a] From Filer, 1978a.
[b] Salt intake per 1000 kcal equals 4.35.

1978). Each collection (117 individual food items) consists of retail purchases for a 3900 kcal daily diet for a 15- to 20-year-old male. For the purposes of the survey, the amount of salt consumed daily under discretionary control is added to the food composite for analysis. Filer has adapted these data as shown in Table III.

It is obvious from the above, that an individual's daily salt intake is controlled by his choice of food categories, by the amount of food consumed, and by his usage of discretionary salt. Guidance in these choices has come from many sources, the most notable of which is the McGovern Committee's Dietary Goals for the United States which has recommended no more than 5 g of salt added in processing or the home, which added to the approximately 3 g occurring naturally, leads to an acceptable intake some 2–4 g less than that now estimated.

III. SALT ADDED TO ENHANCE FLAVOR

It is easily recognized and understood that individual preferences for salt taste vary widely with cultural backgrounds, and perhaps with age, sex, and race. The control of the satisfaction for the salt taste by the consumer is directly related to his proximity to the point of salt addition. The mother of small children salts foods with little or no feedback from the consumer. The individual who cooks for himself has direct control to achieve the salt taste he desires. As more food is processed in commercial operations, the distance between consumer and "salter" is increased and the feedback mechanism becomes more complicated. This has led food processors to monitor consumer salt desires carefully and to respond to these preferences in the marketplace. Filer (1978b) showed that preschool children preferentially selected a salted beef stew over an unsalted one. Lauer and co-workers (1976) studying salt preferences in children 11–16 years of age, found that these children added salt to unsalted beef broth or tomato juice to levels only slightly below that found in commercial products and posed the question—"Is freshly added salt more readily perceived as being salty than salt added to a product that is further processed and stored?"

Tests in our laboratories with Chicken and Rice Soup, using both "in-house" and consumer panels, indicated an optimal salt preference at approximately 0.8% as served. The equivalent commercial product contains 0.87% salt. In other tests, using Chicken Vegetable and Beef Vegetable soups experimentally prepared with no added salt, panelists were asked to salt to their own taste and the remaining soup was analyzed for salt content. The results indicated that the optimal added salt level in these soups was approximately 0.6%, while the comparable commercial soups contained slightly less than 1.0%. The difference between the level added just prior to eating and that in the commercially heat processed product is believed to be due to the fact that the broth retains much of the salt in the unprocessed soup, while the salt is uniformly distributed between broth and garnish in the heat processed and stored products. The initial taste is mostly from the broth and so, in fact, similar effective salt levels were in the broths of the experimental and commercial processed soups. This effect may also be active in other processed and stored foods where uniform saltiness may not be achieved with the addition of fresh discretionary salt by the consumer.

Campbell Soup Company for several years has marketed a number of "Low Sodium Soups" with sodium levels of 30–75 mg Na/7.5 oz serving (15–35 mg Na, or 36.75–85.75 mg salt/per 100 g). A variety of other processed foods with similar salt levels have recently been brought to the market.

It is reasonable to assume that the levels of salt shown in Table II are a close approximation of what the consumer expects in "salt taste."

IV. SALT AS A FUNCTIONAL INGREDIENT

As indicated earlier, salt is usually thought of as a flavor or flavor enhancer in foods, but in several food categories it plays an essential role in food processing. These were discussed in some detail at the recent conference on Sodium and Potassium in American Foods organized by the American Medical Association, but will be reviewed here.

Some product categories, as shown in Table II, contain relatively high levels of salt and, as they are consumed in larger quantities, contribute significantly to the daily intake of salt. In several of these products, salt is used as a functional ingredient in addition to its role as a flavor enhancer.

Salt in bakery products obviously contributes to their flavor and palatability, but plays other important functional roles as well. Salt controls yeast activity in the fermentation of dough for bread, aiding in the prevention of objectionable bacterial action and "wild yeast fermentations." Salt also has a strengthening effect on gluten, enabling it to hold water and carbon dioxide and permits even expansion of the dough. Crust color is improved in the presence of salt. Sodium is added to chemically leavened bakery products through the use of baking acids and sodium bicarbonate. In some products, such as cookies, as much as 40% of the sodium may come from sodium bicarbonate, but in the high-use products, such as bread, most comes from salt. Bread is an important component of the American diet. If an unacceptable product results from reduced salt, it could have a significant effect on reducing the overall nutrient intake of consumers.

Americans consume about ten billion pounds of processed meats each year, which according to Marsden (1978) contain salt levels from 1.8% in fresh pork sausage to 10.6% in chipped beef. Salt is a basic ingredient in all processed meat. Salt acts as a preservative by lowering water activity (a_w) and limiting microbial growth. Salt also performs an important function by solubilizing certain muscle proteins which aid in developing gel structure and color. Salt is a necessary ingredient in most meat emulsions. One of the USDA approved processes for destroying live trichinae is treatment of pork with 3.3% sodium chloride. Additional sodium-containing ingredients in meat processing include phosphates, nitrates, nitrites, caseinates, hydrolyzed vegetable proteins, soy isolates, and monosodium glutamate. These can contribute significant quantities of sodium in some products, but clearly, most comes from common salt.

Among dairy products, salt plays an important functional role in the manufacture of butter (and margarine) and cheese products. Cheese and cheese products are among the fastest growing food categories at present. Salt added to butter at levels of 2–3% inhibits bacterial growth (15–20% in the aqueous phase) and prolongs shelf life. Unsalted butter is available for those who need or desire it but usually must be marketed frozen. Salt plays a significant role in the control of ripening, flavor development, and texture of all cheese. The inhibition of proteolytic bacteria by salt during ripening decreases the rate of formation of protein decomposition products. In the case of Cheddar cheese, one of the most popular varieties, too low a salt level causes a weak and pasty body, abnormal ripening, and increased shrinkage during curing. Many cheeses must contain at least 1.75–2.0% salt to accomplish these purposes.

In a variety of fermented foods, such as sauerkraut, pickles, soy sauces, and other condiments, salt plays an essential role in controlling the microbiological flora and giving a desirable fermentation. Brining of pickles is a common practice to preserve the product until it can be further processed or marketed. Much of the salt used in this process is discarded with the brine and so is not consumed.

Elimination or significant reduction of salt usage would remove most of these processed foods from the market.

V. THE FUTURE SITUATION

The degree of controversy surrounding the need for establishing guidelines for salt consumption at this time makes it almost impossible to predict the course of future actions. Filer (1978b) has concluded,

> On the basis of current knowledge, it seems safe to conclude that a dietary intake of less than 0.6 g of salt (per day) will lower the incidence of hypertension in a population and that intakes of 11.4 g of salt will probably increase the incidence of hypertension. It is not known whether or not moderate changes in dietary salt between these two extremes will actually affect the incidence of hypertension.

On the basis of our review, any practical changes the food industry could make would be within these extremes.

Dr. R. Gaurth Hansen (1979), Chairman of the National Academy of Sciences Committee for the Revision of the RDA's, suggested that the Ninth Edition of the RDA's may contain a provisional listing for sodium and potassium. These would be a daily allowance of 1.2 g/1000 kcal/day for potassium and 1.5 for sodium. On the basis of a 2500 kcal/day intake, this equates to a daily salt intake from all sources of 9.4 g.

Dr. C. F. Gastineau (1979), of the Mayo Clinic, at a recent Nutrition Foundation Conference, concluded that

> some small proportion of the population is susceptible to hypertension and that consumption of generous amounts of salt will permit emergence of the disorder. The balance of the population is thought to have little or perhaps varying susceptibility to the hypertensive effects of generous sodium ingestion. Whether sodium restriction should be urged on our general population has become more of a political than a scientific issue.

The Center for Science in the Public Interest has filed two separate petitions with the Food and Drug Administration, one requesting the FDA to require all processed food labels to show the sodium content and the other proposes that FDA limit the amounts of sodium-containing additives manufacturers add to processed foods. The FDA has not publicly responded to these petitions at this time.

While the Food and Drug Administration has made no formal announcements regarding the salt issue, it is expected they will announce a program to include sodium and perhaps potassium content as part of the voluntary nutritional labeling program. No action is expected on guidelines or salt content regulation.

Several industry spokesmen, including one for a large trade association, have gone on record favoring the labeling of sodium content on foods. This could be of value if one accepts the premise that sodium restriction is desirable for everyone. This may not be true. Dr. Gastineau suggested that sodium labeling may have some problems. He stated, "Foods may be assigned a 'good' or 'bad' character, depending on minor differences of sodium content and foods with otherwise desirable nutritional qualities may be avoided." In any event, the control of salt intake will not be accomplished through labeling alone, but only when accompanied by appropriate food selection.

VI. CONCLUSION

Regardless of other actions, the food processing industry will continue to monitor its customers and processes, and, as in the past, respond to changes that appear to be in the best interests of the public.

REFERENCES

Filer, L. J. (1978a). Are suitable low-salt foods available in the market? Presented at International Symposium—Primary Prevention in Childhood of Atherosclerotic and Hypertensive Disease, Chicago, 1978 (personal communication).

Filer, L. J. (1978b). Appropriate consumption of sodium and potassium. Presented at American Medical Association Symposium on Sodium and Potassium in American Foods, Washington, 1978 (personal communication).

Gastineau, C. F. (1979). "Salt: The Medical Viewpoint" (presented at Nutrition Foundation, Food and Nutrition Liaison Committee, Naples, Florida). Nutrition Foundation, New York.

Hansen, R. C. (1979). Unpublished comments at Nutrition Foundation, Food and Nutrition Liaison Committee, Naples, Florida, 1979.

Lauer, R. M., Filer, L. J., Jr., Reiter, M. A., and Clarke, W. C. (1976). Blood pressure, salt preference, salt threshold and relative weight. *Am. J. Dis. Child.* **130,** 493.

Life Sciences Research Office, Federation of American Societies for Experimental Biology (1978). "Tentative Evaluation of the Health Aspects of Sodium Chloride and Potassium Chloride as Food Ingredients," SCOGS-102. Prepared for Bureau of Foods, Food and Drug Administration, Department of Health, Education and Welfare, Washington, D.C.

Marsden, J. L. (1978). Sodium containing additives in processed meats—A technological overview. Presented at American Medical Association Symposium on Sodium and Potassium in American Foods, Washington, 1978.

Zotterman, Y. (1977). Introductory remarks. *In* "Food Intake and Chemical Senses" (Y. Katsuki *et al.*, eds.), p. xvi. Univ. Park Press, Baltimore, Maryland.

Chapter 17

The Influence of Reproductive Processes on Salt Appetite

D. A. DENTON and J. F. NELSON

I. INTRODUCTION

The hunger for salt exhibited by wild animals in many regions of the world has been reported over the centuries. It was first shown by the scientific teams of our Institute, and Myers of the Wildlife Division of the Commonwealth Scientific and Industrial Research Organizations, that creatures behaving in this fashion were indeed severely depleted of sodium (Bott *et al.,* 1964; Myers, 1967; Blair-West *et al.,* 1968). The investigations were made on wild native and introduced species of animals in the alpine areas of Australia and in the interior of the continent. Basic to the fact that large areas of the earth have vegetation in which Na is very scarce is the decrease of Na content of rain water with distance from the ocean (Eriksson, 1952; Hutton, 1958). Our field observations have been confirmed on other continents (Weir, 1972; Jordan *et al.,* 1973). We have observed also that specific sodium appetite, as tested with cafeterias of various salts, is most avid in pregnant and lactating animals. Pregnancy involves sequestration of Na in the tissues of the developing young *in utero,* and the

BIOLOGICAL AND BEHAVIORAL
ASPECTS OF SALT INTAKE

ISBN 0-12-397750-9

adnexa. Na loss occurs in lactation. Thus a Na-deficient environment would be predicted to be a stress on the biologically critical process of reproduction. A Na-deficient environment has been verified to impair reproductive efficiency (Aumann and Emlen, 1965; Myers, 1970). Against this background, the following laboratory investigations have been made. They have centered on the wild rabbit [*Oryctolagus cuniculus* (L.)] since this animal was the focus of initial field studies in the Australian alps. It has seemed important also to extend the knowledge of salt appetite by systematic and extensive investigation of species other than the sheep and the inbred laboratory white rat on which most experimental investigation has been made to date.

II. SATIATION OF SALT DEFICIENCY IN THE WILD RABBIT

A. Methods

Wild rabbits of both sexes weighing 1150–1900 g were used for this study. The methods of housing, provision, and measurement of intake of food, water, and NaCl solution, of collection and analysis of urine, and measurement of sodium balance have been described (Denton and Nelson, 1970), except that in this and subsequent studies reported here the animals were kept in an air conditioned room maintained at 20°C. The technique of adrenalectomy and the maintenance requirements of adrenal steroid hormones have also been described (Blaine *et al.*, 1975).

Sodium deficiency was produced in these animals by withdrawal of mineralocorticoid support and removal of NaCl solution for 24, 48, or 72 hours. On the day of test, a maintenance dose of adrenal steroids was administered 2 hours prior to the commencement of measurements. This ensured that at the time of test and in the ensuing hours no urinary loss of sodium attributable to adrenal insufficiency occurred. The maintenance dose of adrenal steroids itself had no appetite-inducing effects. NaCl was presented as a 0.50 *M*/liter solution. Measurements were made 2, 4, 6, 9, 12, and 24 hours after commencement of the test.

B. Results and Discussion

A series of thirty-five tests were carried out on five adrenalectomized rabbits with sodium deficits ranging between 3.8 and 14.2 m*M*. The relationship between degree of deficit and degree of correction for each observation period is shown in Fig. 1, and the time course of correction for all tests in Fig. 2. These show that there is a close correlation between the degree of correction and extent

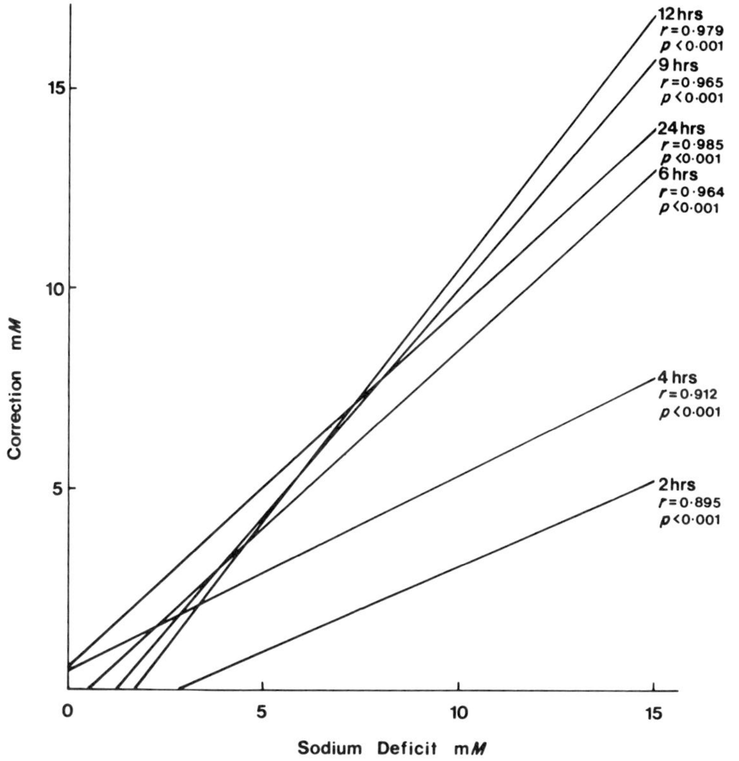

Fig. 1. Relationship between the degree of sodium deficit and its extent of correction 2, 4, 6, 9, 12, and 24 hours after presentation of 500 m*M*/liter NaCl solution. The data were obtained from thirty-five tests in five adrenalectomized rabbits.

of deficit at all stages ($r > 0.89$ and $p < 0.001$). The rate of correction is very much slower than in the sheep (Denton *et al.*, 1969a) and the rat (Jalowiec and Stricker, 1973). A period of about 8 hours elapsed before a 90% correction of sodium deficits was achieved, compared with a few minutes in the sheep or the rat. The results also show that in the rabbit there is a remarkable precision in this correction. There is no evidence of drinking beyond need, a finding similar to that obtained usually with sheep, but differing markedly from the rat in which, as pointed out by Jalowiec and Stricker, overcompensation is frequently observed. The strictly linear nature of the relation between rate of intake and initial deficit suggests that the central drive so induced is preeminent in governing intake over the whole time course of consummatory action with no feedback from any sequelae of ingestion.

Jalowiec and Stricker (1970) also reported that 0.51 *M* NaCl was too unpalatable to rats for sodium ingestion to proceed as rapidly as when 0.15 *M* NaCl was

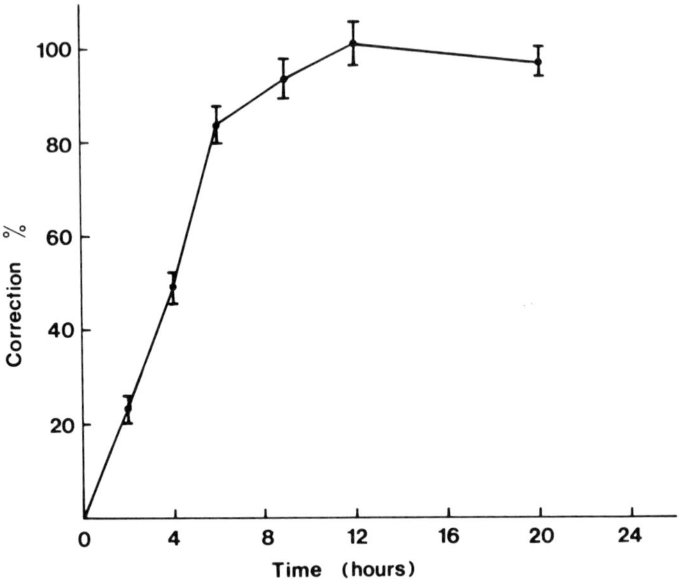

Fig. 2. Time course of correction of sodium deficit in adrenalectomized rabbits after presentation of 500 m*M*/liter NaCl solution ± S.E.M. ($n = 35$).

available. As correction in the rabbit was very much slower than in sheep or rats, it was considered that a similar aversion to high NaCl concentration might also occur in this species. Accordingly a second experiment involving six tests was carried out using 24-hour sodium-deficient animals offered 0.15 *M* NaCl during correction. The range of deficits obtained was 3.6–5.8 m*M* and the rate of correction was even slower than with 0.5 *M* NaCl. Correction was 6.6% at 2 hours, 18% at 4 hours, 29% at 6 hours, 45% at 9 hours, 61% at 12 hours, and 92% at 24 hours. Thus the slow correction in the first study was not due to aversion to the higher concentration. It could not be due to the necessity to consume large volumes, as during the period between 2 and 12 hours after commencing the test, when the rate of drinking was almost constant and most rapid, the volume drunk/hour was only 1.9 ml. This approximates insensible water loss in these animals.

III. SALT APPETITE IN PREGNANCY AND LACTATION

Richter and Barelare (1938) made a detailed study of the nutritional requirements of domesticated rats during pregnancy and lactation. They found, *inter alia*, that on a salt-free diet, the intake of 3% NaCl solution increased soon after mating and remained high until the end of pregnancy. The mean intake during the second half of gestation was three times as high as before conception. Intake was further augmented during lactation, reaching four times the control level and it fell to basal within 7 days of weaning. They pointed out that, since the increase in salt appetite occurred within the first few days of mating, when the embryos were still minute, the salt appetite of pregnancy probably had a maternal rather than a fetal origin, i.e., it was not a consequence of provision of sodium to the developing embryo. Since external sodium balance studies were not carried out, they were not able to provide other evidence to support this thesis.

We have investigated the effects of pregnancy and lactation on the electrolyte intakes of wild rabbits (Denton and Nelson, 1971). The animals had continuous access to 500 m*M*/liter solutions of NaCl and KCl, 250 m*M*/liter solution of $MgCl_2$ and $CaCl_2$, pelleted food, and water. The food contained adequate Na^+, K^+, Mg^{2+}, and Ca^{2+} to meet metabolic needs. Measurement of intakes and sodium balance were made daily.

An increase in NaCl intake commenced on about the fifth day of gestation and for the first 14 days of pregnancy intake was approximately doubled (Fig. 3). The intake reached a peak mean value of 9.5 m*M*/day just prior to parturition. During the second half of gestation the mean intake was five times as high as the mean control level. Intake rose rapidly immediately after parturition and reached a maximum on the fourteenth day of lactation when the mean daily intake was 31 m*M*. Intake averaged 22 m*M*/day for the first 3 weeks of lactation. This reflected daily turnover of about half the Na content of the extracellular fluid. A rapid fall

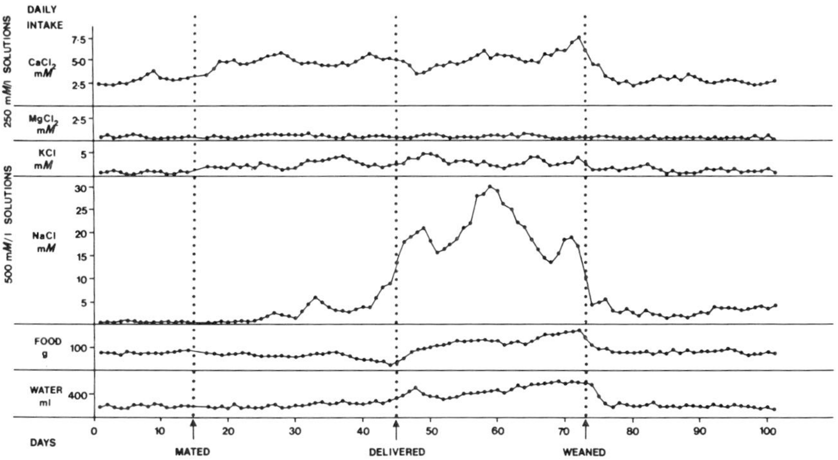

Fig. 3. Mean daily food, water and electrolyte intakes by seven rabbits during a control period, during pregnancy, during lactation, and subsequent to weaning. Reprinted from Denton and Nelson (1971) with permission.

occurred on weaning but it remained above prepregnancy levels for the rest of the study. At no stage of the study, i.e., during early pregnancy or with the big rise of intake at the onset of lactation, was there a preceding fall of urinary Na excretion in individual animals, suggestive of some onset of deficit in the dam by virtue of metabolic need. After making allowance for maternal weight gain during pregnancy, or growth of the young during lactation, no appreciable alteration of sodium balance from the prior control period was observed during either of these phases. The data strongly support the initial idea of Richter and Barelare that the increased appetite during pregnancy was not a consequence of sodium sequestration by the developing young, and in our eyes strongly suggested a hormonal origin.

Increases in KCl and $CaCl_2$ intakes were also present throughout pregnancy and were maintained during lactation. These too fell rapidly on weaning. Both the mean (Fig. 4) and maximal intakes of NaCl were related to litter size, but no

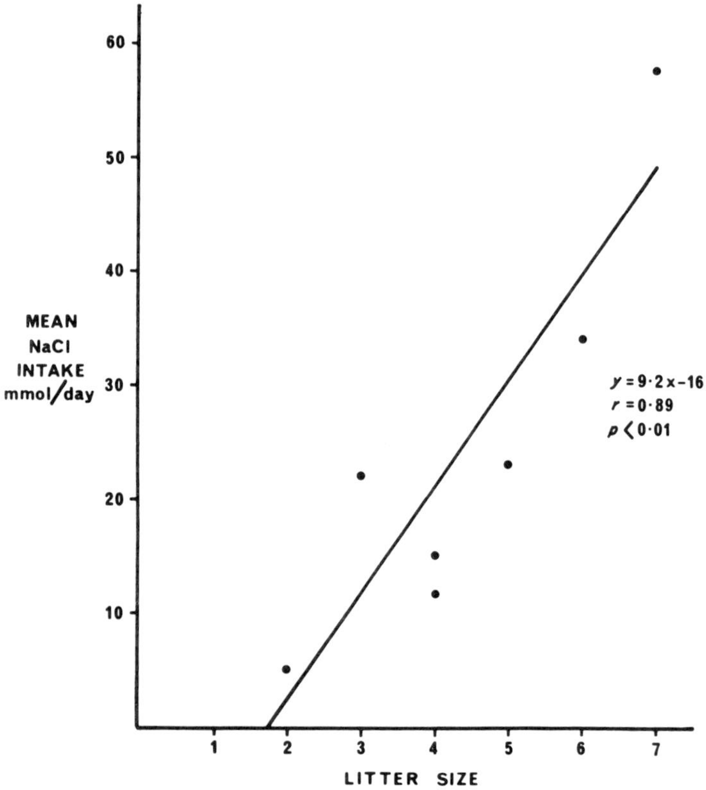

Fig. 4. Relationship between number of babies in individual litters and the mean daily NaCl intakes of the respective mothers during lactation.

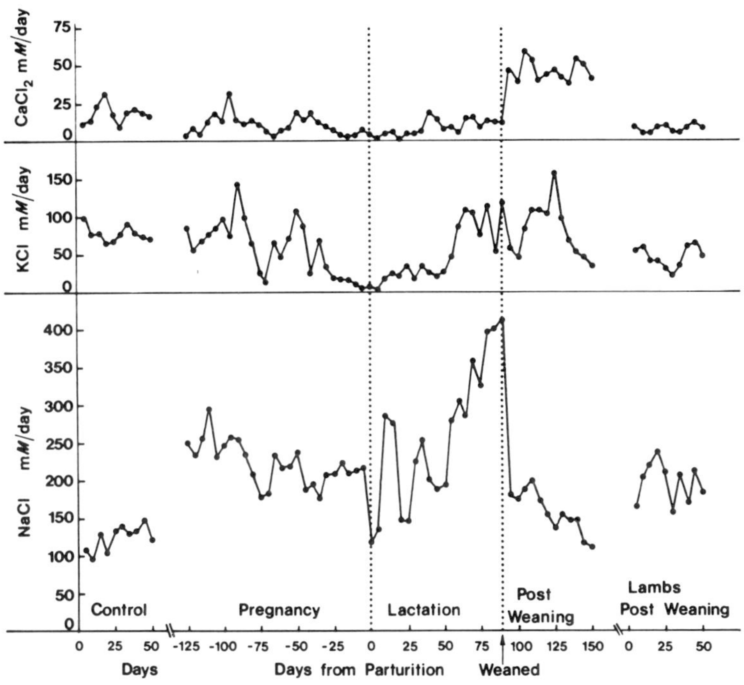

Fig. 5. Mean daily intake of NaCl, KCl, and $CaCl_2$ of five ewes during a control period, during pregnancy, during lactation, and after weaning. Also mean daily electrolyte intake of their five lambs after weaning. Each point represents the mean of the previous 5 days' observations.

such correlation was found with either KCl or $CaCl_2$ intakes. It was suggested that hormonal, pheromone or sensory factors may be responsible for the correlation between litter number and salt intake.

A similar study has recently been carried out with five sheep, each bearing a single lamb, in which intakes of 500 m*M* solutions of NaCl, KCl, and 250 m*M* $CaCl_2$ were measured during pregnancy and lactation. The mean intakes for 5-day periods are shown in Fig. 5. Mean NaCl intake increased early in pregnancy from a control level of 123 m*M*/day to 208 m*M*/day, and then remained fairly constant. There was little change in KCl or $CaCl_2$ intakes until the last month of pregnancy, when both fell to levels below those observed during the control period.

The mean intake of NaCl during the first 50 days of lactation was maintained at the high level recorded in pregnancy, but wide variations, both from day to day and between animals, make this value not significant. During this phase of lactation, the KCl and $CaCl_2$ intakes remained low. After this time, increases in intakes of NaCl and KCl occurred. At this stage the lambs were eating some solid food, drinking some water, and were occasionally seen taking small amounts of electrolyte solutions.

After the lambs were weaned, the intake of NaCl by the mothers fell to control levels in about 30 days, KCl intake was unaltered, and $CaCl_2$ intake rose. The electrolyte intake of the lambs was also measured after weaning. The results show that most, if not all, of the increases in NaCl and KCl intakes during the later stages of lactation could be attributed to the developing appetites of the lambs.

This experiment confirms the findings of increased NaCl intake previously made in rats and rabbits during pregnancy. It also indicates that when suckling a single offspring, the sheep behaves differently than the other two species suckling larger numbers of babies.

In a further experiment with rabbits (Denton and Nelson, 1978), seven pregnant animals were kept in cages with a 2.5 cm mesh base, and no nesting sites were available at parturition. When the young were born they were either removed immediately, or in their first movements crawled through the mesh to a tray 5 cm below and were then removed. Under these conditions the offspring were not able to suckle at any time. The average litter size, its range and the gestation period were similar to those of the previous study.

The changes in electrolyte intakes during pregnancy were the same as those observed earlier. Similarly the rapid postpartum rise in NaCl intake occurred (Fig. 6) despite the fact that the litters were not present. From the fifth day after birth, NaCl intakes were significantly lower than during lactation and by the twelfth day had returned to control levels.

The rate of fall was much slower than that seen after normal weaning where a precipitous fall occurred on the first day. $CaCl_2$ and KCl intakes fell immediately after the young were born and had returned to control levels in a few days. Thus, a clear-cut dissociation between Na appetite and that for $CaCl_2$ occurred. There was again a correlation between NaCl intake and litter size (Fig. 7).

The somewhat surprising observations that, in rabbits not subjected to stimulated lactogenic hormone secretion as a consequence of suckling, the NaCl intake still rises as rapidly as in normal lactation and still correlates well with the number of young born, shows that the increase in NaCl intake after parturition is not due to sensory stimuli associated with the presence of the litter. It appears that the rise is due, at least in part, to the continued secretion of lactogenic hormones superimposed on the residual changes due to steroid hormone secretion during pregnancy. It indicates that the birth process has an important, previously unrecognized influence on NaCl intake after parturition. Even in nonsuckling rabbits the NaCl intake after the young are born is much higher than that observed at the end of pseudopregnancy (Covelli *et al.*, 1973) when milk is also produced (Hammond and Marshall, 1914) and the hormone secretion patterns are

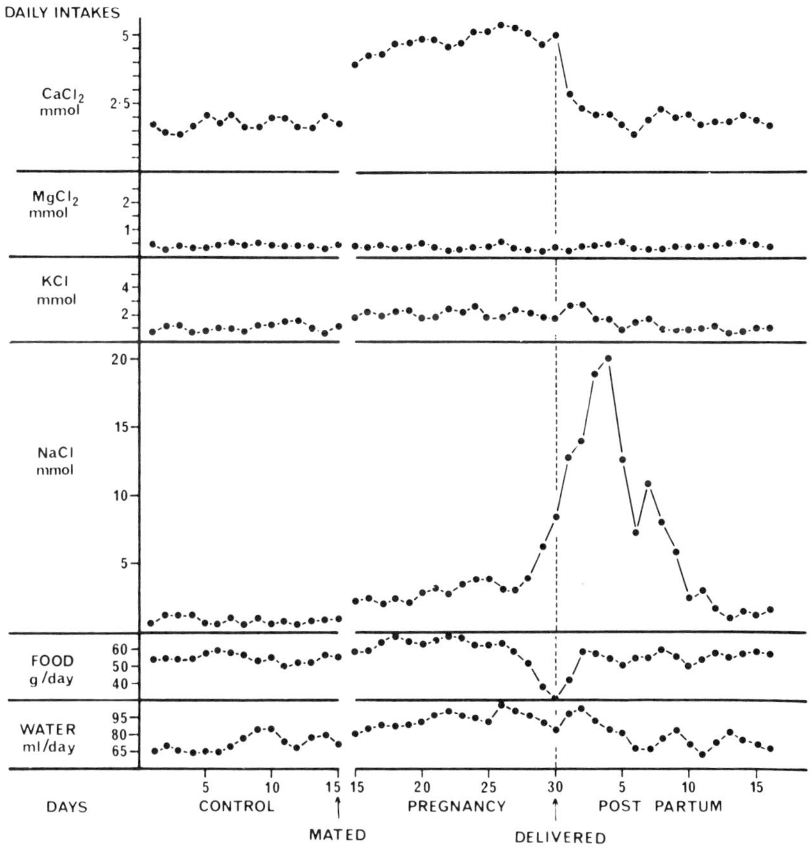

Fig. 6. Mean daily food, water, and electrolyte intakes of seven rabbits during a control period, during the second half of pregnancy, and postpartum with litter removal at birth. Reprinted from Denton and Nelson (1978) with permission.

essentially similar (Eaton and Hilliard, 1971; Bast and Melampy, 1972; Horrobin, 1973).

We therefore investigated the effects on salt appetite of physiological amounts of the hormones which are necessary for efficient lactation (Shulkes *et al.*, 1972; Blaine *et al.*, 1975). These are shown in Fig. 8. Growth hormone had no effect, oxytocin, prolactin, and ACTH produced increases of 0.8, 1.9, and 5.4 m*M*/day, respectively. When compared with the mean increase of 22 m*M*/day which occurs in lactating animals, all of these increases are small and this indicates strongly that a combination of these hormones is probably responsible for part of the increase present during lactation.

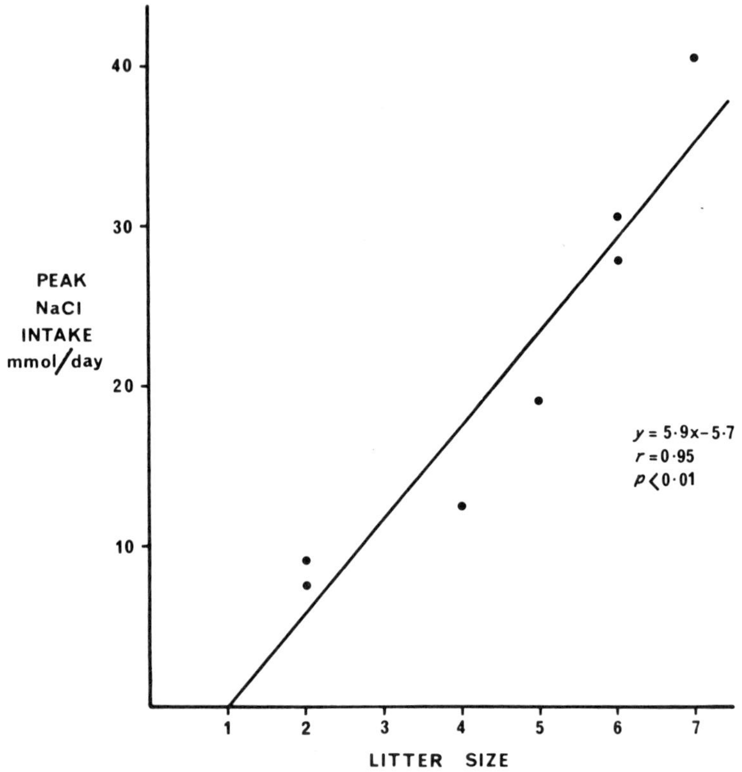

Fig. 7. Relationship between number of young in a litter and mean daily NaCl intake of the respective mothers for the first 5 days after litter removal at birth.

A study of the action mechanism of ACTH (Blaine *et al.*, 1975) revealed that its effects on salt appetite were not due solely to increased circulating glucocorticoid levels. Evidence for an extra adrenal action was obtained from findings in adrenalectomized rabbits, treated with maintenance doses of glucocorticoid and mineralocorticoid. ACTH was administered. This experiment showed that about 25% of the increase in NaCl intake produced by ACTH could be attributed to an effect elsewhere than on the adrenal. Other experiments showed that the administration of glucocorticoids in doses which produced similar blood levels to those obtained with ACTH treatment stimulated salt appetite to a lesser extent than with ACTH administration. The effect was not the result of raised aldosterone secretion with ACTH, as this hormone in relatively large doses has no effect on salt appetite in the rabbit (Denton and Nelson, 1970).

The effect of high ACTH secretion on salt appetite was well demonstrated in a study planned to administer drugs to rabbits by continuous infusion over a period

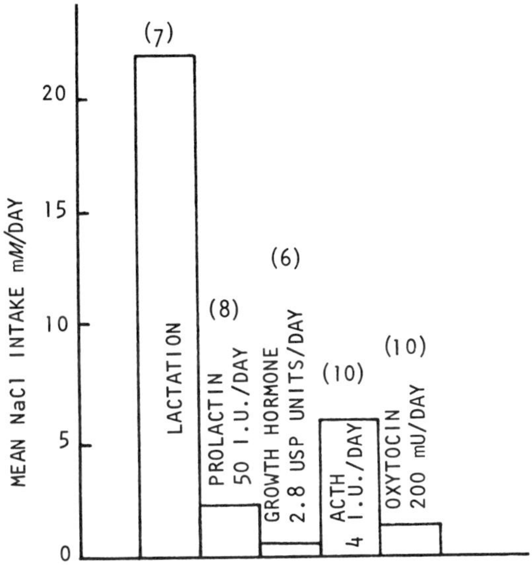

Fig. 8. Mean daily intake of NaCl during lactation, or treatment with prolactin, oxytocin, or growth hormone for 10 days or with ACTH for 7 days. The numbers in parentheses are the number of rabbits in that study.

of days. As the animals attacked the cannulae leading to perfusion pumps outside the cage, an attempt was made to carry out the procedure by means of small self-driven pumps attached to the animals' backs. These were to be protected by and carried in a jacket or backpack tied to the rabbits. The rabbits immediately tried to remove these jackets, and during the first few days they were able to remove or displace them within 8–12 hours. With modifications, jackets which would remain attached for 2–3 days, despite repeated attacks, were developed.

The investigation was ultimately abandoned because of the effect of the resultant stress on salt intake as shown in Fig. 9. During the first few days, with the less satisfactory design of jackets, the intake rose clearly but in a relatively minor fashion. Once the stress was applied more continuously a huge increase occurred with salt intake approaching that present during lactation. On removal of the jackets, salt appetite returned quickly to normal. The data seem highly relevant to the use of stressing procedures such as formalin injection to study Na appetite.

As experiments described above had shown that the individual hormones controlling lactation had relatively small effects on electrolyte intake, the influence of a series of combinations of pregnancy and lactogenic hormones was evaluated (Denton and Nelson, 1978). Elevated electrolyte intakes, similar to those produced by lactation, could only be produced by the treatment of pseudopregnant, or estrogen and progesterone-primed rabbits with a combination of

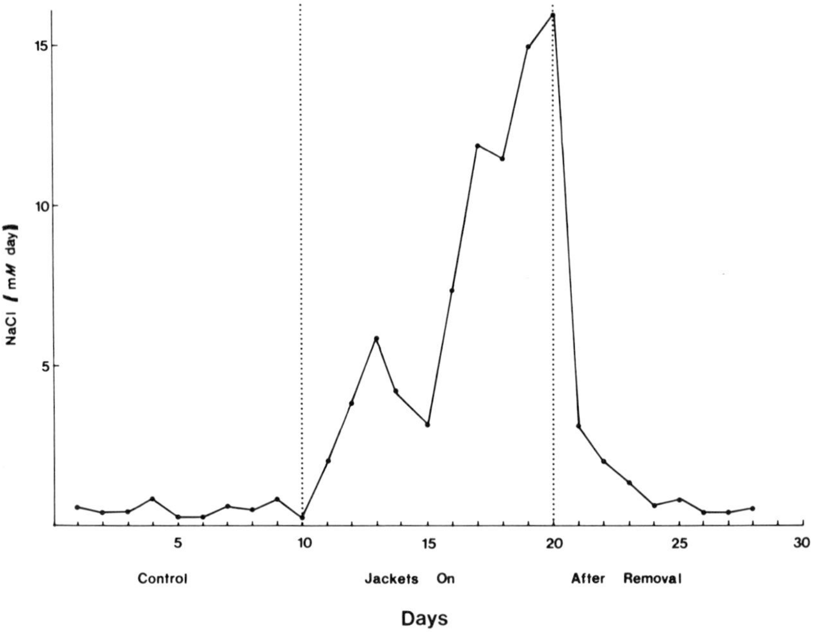

Fig. 9. Mean daily intakes of 500 m*M* NaCl by rabbits ($n = 6$) before, during, and after attachment of jackets to their backs.

ACTH, prolactin, and possibly oxytocin. The effects of one of these combinations is shown in Fig. 10. The intakes of KCl and $CaCl_2$ rose to levels approximating those in lactation and the pattern and extent of rise in water and NaCl intakes closely resembled those seen in late pregnancy and early lactation. The mean NaCl intake over the last 8 days of combined lactogenic hormone treatment was 24.5 m*M*. The results also show that, once established, the elevated water and electrolyte intakes can be maintained by ACTH alone. In other experiments which are not detailed here, it was found that prolactin and oxytocin in combination were not capable of supporting the high intakes. The fall in NaCl and KCl intakes after cessation of ACTH treatment was somewhat slower than those which follow weaning but in both cases NaCl intake remained somewhat elevated for a considerable period.

An interesting comparison can be made between the requirements for rapid development of full maternal behavior in the rat, consisting of nest building, licking and retrieving of young, and of adopting the lactating position, and those necessary for the establishment of the high electrolyte intake of lactation in the rabbit. The first requires the secretion of progesterone, estrogen, prolactin, and some other factor present in the blood for a short period before and after parturi-

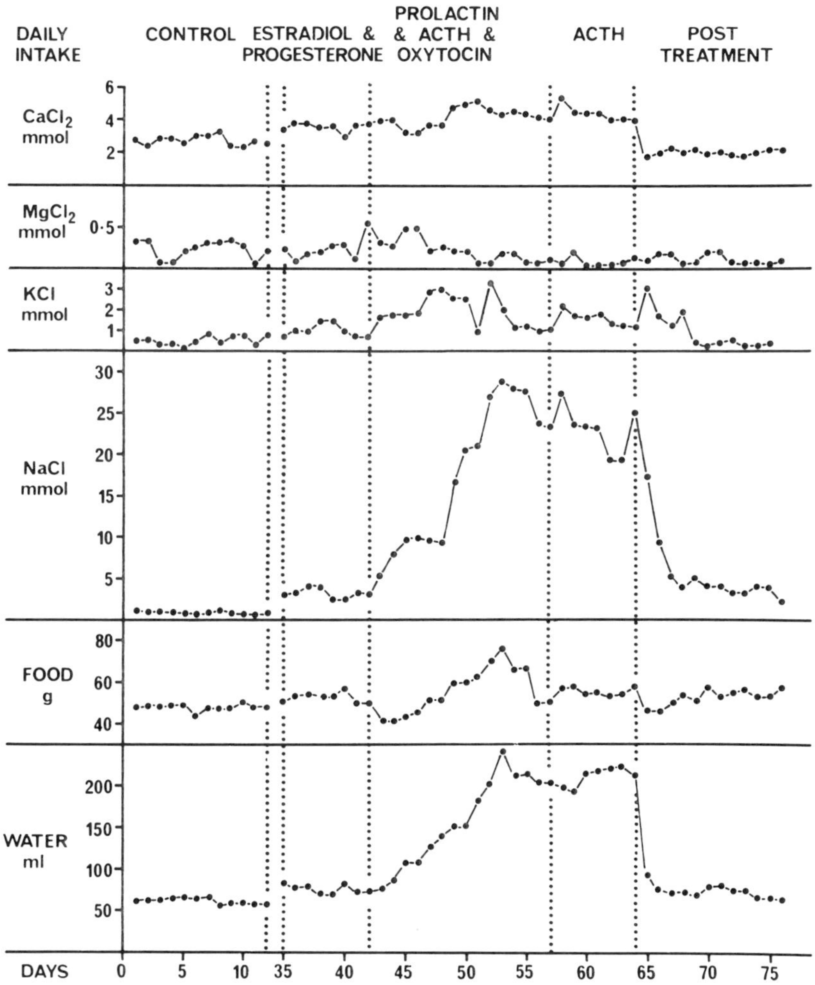

Fig. 10. Mean daily intakes of food, water, and electrolyte solutions by seven female rabbits during a control period, during the last 8 days of a 28-day treatment with 12.5 μg estradiol + 1 mg progesterone/day, during daily treatment with 50 IU prolactin + 4 IU ACTH + 200 mU oxytocin, followed by 4 IU ACTH/day and after injections ceased. Reprinted from Denton and Nelson (1978) with permission.

tion (Moltz *et al.*, 1970; Terkel and Rosenblatt, 1972). In the rat the organization of maternal behavioral responsiveness occurs during parturition (Bridges, 1975). All of these hormonal factors are required in the second and an unidentified factor, or factors, associated with parturition is involved in both situations.

Several approaches investigating the postulate that the number of young influences the subsequent salt intake of the mother are envisaged for the future. First, there is the question of whether the behavior is influenced by the number of young carried. There is evidence in mice that nest building, one of the maternal behavioral characteristics mentioned above, from the fourth day of gestation onward is determined by the number of fetuses *in utero* (Gandelman, 1975). Alternatively, is the increase influenced solely by the number of young born? This would appear to be possible from our results to date.

These two questions might be answered by (a) removal of one horn of the uterus and the associated conceptus either early or late in pregnancy, allowing the animal to give birth to the remaining young and studying salt appetite during the subsequent lactation, and (b) delivering the babies by Caesarian section at the end of the normal gestation period, and following postpartum appetite either with the young returned to the mother or permanently removed. Should either or both of these experiments provide definitive answers, it will be necessary to carry out a third study in which a number of young are removed after normal birth, and appetite investigated during the rest of lactation. In view of our finding that the increased salt appetite produced by combined hormone therapy can be maintained by ACTH alone, a further investigation in which the young are removed at birth should also be conducted, but in this case ACTH would be administered after parturition and the relationship between number of offspring and the stable salt intake determined.

The findings show that the general pattern of increased water and electrolyte intake of pregnancy and lactation may be closely replicated by the appropriate sequential administration of jointly sufficient and severally necessary physiological amounts of four or perhaps five steroid and peptide hormones which are required for maintenance of pregnancy and the establishment and continuation of normal lactation. It is proposed that the findings indicate a behavioral effect of reproductive hormones of important survival value for herbivorous and omnivorous animals in the large areas of the earth which are sodium deficient. The implications in relation to a theoretical construct of central nervous mechanisms involved in the genesis of Na appetite will be discussed.

To account for the induction of central excitation in a neuronal population specifically subserving salt appetite, the following elaboration of a hypothesis put forward in 1966 (Denton, 1966) is suggested. Any theory must account for induction of appetite by both peptide and steroid hormones in the Na-replete animal. It must also account for the classic salt hunger of Na deficiency.

Within a specific population of neurocytons, a fall of intracellular Na concentration contingent on body Na deficiency, either by direct nuclear action or a cytoplasmic effect, entrains a genetic propensity to induce specific protein synthesis. This initiates the behavioral mechanisms of appetite. By messenger RNA, there is initiated the synthesis by ribosomes of a protein which alters the ionic or membrane characteristics of the neurocytons—or their capacity to generate transmitter at the synapse (Fig. 11).

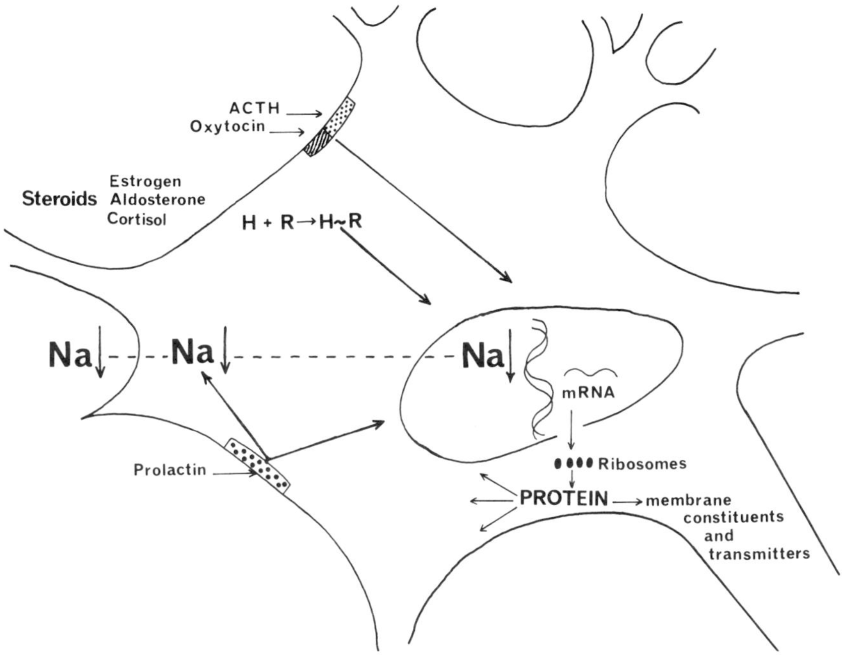

Fig. 11. Diagrammatic representation of mode of excitation of neurocytons subserving salt appetite drive.

In either way, excitation and transmission in the genetically programmed neuronal interconnections subserving salt appetite could be facilitated.

The resulting excitation in a cellular mass in the hypothalamus generates appetitive behavior and the modulation of midbrain reticular activity. Arousal and attention is biased to sensory inflow relevant to satiation of salt hunger.

We have shown experimentally that intracarotid ouabain infusion, calculated to contrive an ATPase-inhibiting concentration with resultant rise of intracellular Na concentration, abolishes salt appetite in Na deficiency. The same infusion given intravenously with a lesser degree of cerebral arterial ouabain concentration had little influence on appetite (Denton *et al.*, 1969b).

The influence of ionic changes within cells on enzymatic reactions with polyelectrolytic macromolecular cell components, including systems involved in genetic translation, has been examined by a number of workers. There is evidence that K/Na ratio and pH changes over the physiological range may play a role in regulating genomic activity (Douzou and Maurel, 1977).

Such considerations may be apposite to the postulated effect of intracellular Na concentration, in releasing structural DNA, from the inhibiting regulator influence.

In the instance of hormone action in the Na-replete animal, it is proposed, as, for example, in the case of mammary epithelium, that there are specific prolactin and also other peptide hormone receptor sites (e.g., ACTH and oxytocin) on the membranes of the salt appetite neurocytons.

The exact sequence by which perturbation in the cell membrane influences nuclear events to give messenger RNA production and, in this postulate, synthesis of excitatory protein, is not known. There is evidence that prolactin, in contrast to ACTH and some other peptides, does not activate through adenyl cyclase (Turkington, 1972). Recently, Falconer has shown that prolactin lowers the radioactive Na content of mammary cells (Falconer and Rowe, 1975). This raises the possibility of a final common pathway in the neurocyton, along with the postulated effect of Na deficiency. Ouabain abolishes this ionic effect of prolactin.

Several adrenal and sex steroid hormones are known to induce appetite. Here, entry to the cell (with or without metabolic change) and binding to specific cytosol receptors in the neurocyton would produce an activated complex. Binding of this complex to nuclear acceptor sites would trigger genetic transcription and synthesis of excitatory protein.

Now, as is basically the case with other endocrinological processes, the entire system is reversible (Mainwaring, 1975).

Our experiments with very rapid systemic infusion of sodium in the deplete animal, with "turn off" of appetite within 10–20 minutes, could be consistent with rapid intracellular influx of Na^+ in the specific neurocytons, and activation of the repressor genetic mechanism.

However, with normal physiological satiation in sheep, for example, rapid consummatory drinking of $NaHCO_3$ solution occurs over 2–5 minutes. A precipitate decline in drive follows. It is proposed that the train of a highly organized sequence of specific sensory impulses to the excitatory center via the 7th, 9th, and 10th nerves, causes a very rapid to explosive degradation of the excitatory protein. Hydén (1961) and Geiger *et al.* (1956) have considered and shown modification of brain protein by electrical impulses over, for example, 5–30 seconds—with breakage of bonds and loss of strictly ordered configuration.

Alternatively, sensory inflow may excite an inhibitory center in an excitation–inhibition type of organization of salt appetite, analogous to hunger.

In either event, inhibition of the excitatory center needs to be effective long enough for sodium drunk to be absorbed from the gut, and reverse intracellular ionic change postulated as primarily generative of excitation.

These postulates, though speculative, at least bring to focus the neurophysiological and neurochemical organization which needs experimental exploration in the face of comprehensive data which has accrued on the salt-seeking behavior of animals—and the time and quantitative characteristics of its satisfaction. Focus is immediately brought to bear on how little we know of the characteristics of the satiation process in the instance of salt hunger generated by hormones in the Na-replete animal.

Differences of salt appetite from the thirst mechanism are clear-cut in many regards. This is highlighted in one sense by the fact that when sheep are concurrently depleted of both water and sodium, they will sequentially satiate deficits when presented with $NaHCO_3$ solution and water concurrently. Satisfaction of one deficit does not modify the immediate satiation of the other—although there are sensory elements in common in the cerebri-petal inflow.

Overall, it is clear that salt, and perhaps other mineral hungers such as for phosphate, gives an easily quantifiable experimental matrix upon which to explore some of the more fundamental physiological problems of genetically programmed behaviors, and the neurochemical mechanisms which underlie them.

ACKNOWLEDGMENTS

We wish to express our thanks to the NIAMDD for the gift of the ovine prolactin used in these experiments. This work was supported by the National Health and Medical Research Council of Australia and the Robert and Helen Kleberg Foundation.

REFERENCES

Aumann, G. D., and Emlen, J. T. (1965). Relation of population density to sodium availability and sodium selection by microtine rodents. *Nature (London)* **208,** 198–199.

Bast, J. D., and Melampy, R. M. (1972). Luteinizing hormone prolactin and ovarian 20α-hydroxysteroid dehydrogenase levels during pregnancy and pseudopregnancy, in the rat. *Endocrinology* **91,** 1499-1505.

Blaine, E. H., Covelli, M. D., Denton, D. A., Nelson, J. F., and Shulkes, A. A. (1975). The role of ACTH and adrenal glucocorticoids in the salt appetite of wild rabbits [*Oryctolagus cuniculus* (L)]. *Endocrinology* **97,** 793-801.

Blair-West, J. R., Coghlan, J. P., Denton, D. A., Nelson, J. F., Orchard, E., Scoggins, B. A., Wright, R. D., Myers, K., and Junqueira, C. L. (1968). Physiological, morphological and behavioural adaptation to a sodium-deficient environment by wild native Australian and introduced species of animals. *Nature (London)* **217,** 922-928.

Bott, E., Denton, D. A., Goding, J. R., and Sabine, J. R. (1964). Sodium deficiency and corticosteroid secretion in cattle. *Nature (London)* **202,** 461-463.

Bridges, R. S. (1975). Long-term effects of pregnancy and parturition upon maternal responsiveness in the rat. *Physiol. Behav.* **14,** 245-249.

Covelli, M. D., Denton, D. A., Nelson, J. F., and Shulkes, A. A. (1973). Hormonal factors influencing salt appetite in pregnancy. *Endocrinology* **93,** 423-429.

Denton, D. A. (1966). Some theoretical considerations in relation to innate appetite for salt. *Cond. Reflex* **1,** 144-170.

Denton, D. A., and Nelson, J. F. (1970). Effect of deoxycorticosterone acetate and aldosterone on the salt appetite of wild rabbits [*Oryctolagus cuniculus* (L)]. *Endocrinology* **87,** 970-977.

Denton, D. A., and Nelson, J. F. (1971). Effects of pregnancy and lactation on the mineral appetites of wild rabbits [*Oryctolagus cuniculus* (L)]. *Endocrinology* **88,** 31-40.

Denton, D. A., and Nelson, J. F. (1978). The control of salt appetite in wild rabbits during lactation. *Endocrinology* **103,** 1880.

Denton, D. A., Orchard, E., and Weller, S. (1969a). The relationship between voluntary sodium intake and body sodium balance in normal and adrenalectomized sheep. *Commun. Behav. Biol.* **3,** 213-221.

Denton, D. A., Kraintz, F. W., and Kraintz, L. (1969b). The inhibition of salt appetite of sodium-deficient sheep by intracarotid infusion of ouabain. *Commun. Behav. Biol.* **4,** 183-186.

Douzou, P., and Maurel, P. (1977). Ionic control of biochemical reactions. *Trends Biochem. Sci.* **2,** 14-20.

Eaton, L. W., Jr., and Hilliard, J. (1971). Estradiol-17β, progesterone and 20α-hydroxypregn-4-en-3-one in rabbit ovarian venous plasma. 1. Steroid secretion from paired ovaries with and without corpora lutea, effect of LH. *Endocrinology* **89,** 105-111.

Eriksson, E. (1952). Composition of atmospheric precipitation. *Tellus* **4,** 280.

Falconer, I. R., and Rowe, J. M. (1975). Possible mechanism for action of prolactin on mammary cell sodium transport. *Nature (London)* **256,** 327-328.

Gandelman, R. (1975). Maternal nest-building performance and fetal number in Rockland-Swiss albino mice. *J. Reprod. Fertil.* **44,** 551-554.

Geiger, A., Yamasaki, A., and Lyons, R. (1956). Changes in nitrogenous components of brain produced by stimulation of short duration. *Am. J. Physiol.* **184,** 239-243.

Hammond, J., and Marshall, F. H. A. (1914). The functional correlation between the ovaries, uterus and mammary glands in the rabbit, with observations on the oestrus cycle. *Proc. R. Soc. London, Ser. B* **87,** 422-440.

Horrobin, D. F. (1973). "Prolactin: Physiology and Clinical Significance," p. 48. Med. Tech. Publ. Co., St. Leonardgate.

Hutton, J. T. (1958). The chemistry of rainwater with particular reference to conditions in southeastern Australia. *In* "Climatology and Micro-climatology," p. 285. UNESCO, Paris.

Hydén, H. (1961). *In* "The Cell" The neuron. (J. Brachet and A. Mirsky, eds.), Vol. 4, p. 306. Academic Press, New York.

Jalowiec, J. E., and Stricker, E. M. (1970). Restoration of body fluid balance following acute sodium deficiency in rats. *J. Comp. Physiol. Psychol.* **70,** 94-102.

Jalowiec, J. E., and Stricker, E. M. (1973). Sodium appetite in adrenalectomized rats following dietary sodium deprivation. *J. Comp. Physiol. Psychol.* **82,** 66-77.

Jordan, P. A., Botkin, D. B., Dominski, A. S., Lowendorf, H. S., and Belovsky, G. E. (1973). Sodium as a critical nutrient for the moose of Isle Royale. *Proc. North Am. Moose Conf. Workshop,* pp. 13-42.

Mainwaring, W. I. P. (1975). Steroid hormone receptors: A survey: *Vitam. Horm. (N.Y.)* **33,** 223-245.

Moltz, H., Lubin, M., Leon, M., and Human, W. (1970). Hormonal induction of maternal behaviour in the ovariectomized nulliparous rat. *Physiol. Behav.* **5,** 1373-1377.

Myers, K. (1967). Morphological changes in the adrenal glands of wild rabbits. *Nature (London)* **213,** 147-150.

Myers, K. (1970). The rabbit in Australia. *In* "Dynamics of Populations" (P. J. den Boer and G. R. Gradwell, eds.), pp. 478-506.

Richter, C. P., and Barelare, B., Jr. (1938). Nutritional requirements of pregnant and lactating rats studied by the self-selection method. *Am. J. Physiol.* **121,** 185-188.

Shulkes, A. A., Covelli, M. D., Denton, D. A., and Nelson, J. F. (1972). Hormonal factors influencing salt appetite in lactation. *Aust. J. Exp. Biol. Med. Sci.* **50,** 819-826.

Terkel, J., and Rosenblatt, J. S. (1972). Humoral factors underlying maternal behaviour at parturition: Cross transfusion between freely moving rats. *J. Comp. Physiol. Psychol.* **80,** 365-371.

Turkington, R. W. (1972). Molecular biological aspects of prolactin. *Lactogenic Horm., Ciba Found. Symp., 1971* pp. 111-135.

Weir, J. S. (1972). Spatial distribution of elephants in an African National Park in relation to environmental sodium. *Oikos* **23,** 1-13.

Chapter 18

Spontaneous NaCl Appetite Induced by Administration of an Oral Contraceptive and Its Components to Rats

MELVIN J. FREGLY and DEBORAH G. NEWSOME

BIOLOGICAL AND BEHAVIORAL
ASPECTS OF SALT INTAKE

ISBN 0-12-397750-9

I. INTRODUCTION

When ovariectomized rats were treated with the oral contraceptive, Enovid, at 7.5 mg/kg of food for approximately 9 months and given a choice between 0.15 *M* NaCl solution and distilled water to drink, they ingested significantly more NaCl solution and significantly less distilled water than did untreated ovariectomized control rats (Fregly, 1972). When a choice was offered between 0.25 *M* NaCl solution and distilled water, the Enovid-treated rats again ingested significantly more NaCl solution than controls. Similar NaCl appetites were induced in intact female rats administered a lower dose of Enovid (2.5 mg/kg of food) for 35 days. These rats ingested a significantly greater volume of NaCl solution (either 0.15, 0.25 or 0.35 *M*) than untreated control rats (Fregly and Newsome, 1974). Dietary administration of Enovid (7.5 mg/kg of food) to male rats was also accompanied by a significantly greater intake of 0.15 *M* NaCl solution than untreated controls when tested after 25–30 days of treatment (Fregly, 1973). Thus, an appetite for NaCl solution occurs in Enovid-treated male and female rats, both in the presence and absence of ovaries in the latter.

The objectives of the studies described below were to establish a dose–response relationship between doses of Enovid ingested with food and intake of NaCl solution, as well as to compare the preference threshold for NaCl in Enovid-treated rats with that of controls. Additional studies were designed to assess the importance of the adrenal gland in the development of the spontaneous appetite for NaCl solutions induced by oral contraceptives. A final objective was to determine the effect of the components of Enovid, i.e., norethynodrel and ethynyl estradiol, on the time course of development of the NaCl appetite and to study the effects of these components on sodium excretion after loading acutely with NaCl solutions. An additional aim of these studies was to determine whether the onset of sodium appetite correlated with an increase in sodium excretion.

II. METHODS

A. Experiment 1. Dose–Response Relationship between Intake of NaCl Solution and Dose of Administered Enovid

Twenty-eight female rats of the Long–Evans Hooded strain were kept in individual cages in a room maintained at 26 ± 1°C and illuminated from 8 AM to 6 PM. The rats were randomly divided into four equal groups. Each rat was offered a choice between distilled water and 0.15 *M* NaCl solution ad libitum for 3 days prior to beginning the experiment. Infant nursing bottles with cast aluminum fountains were used to measure fluid intakes (Lazarow, 1954). Food was finely powdered Purina Laboratory Chow and was provided ad libitum in spillproof containers (Fregly, 1960).

Group 1 served as the control group and received food without drug while groups 2, 3 and 4 received Enovid* mixed thoroughly into their food at concentrations of 1.25, 2.50, and 5.00 mg/kg, respectively. Fluid and food intakes and body weight were measured daily for 3 consecutive weeks. During the following 2 weeks the rats continued to receive Enovid and a choice between distilled water and 0.15 *M* NaCl solution to drink but intakes were not measured. During the sixth week, intakes of water, 0.15 *M* NaCl solution, and food as well as body weight were again measured daily. Intakes were not measured during the seventh week. During the eighth and ninth weeks each rat was offered a choice between distilled water and 0.25 *M* NaCl solution to drink. Fluid and food intakes and body weight were measured daily. During the next 5 weeks, intakes were not measured although the rats continued to receive Enovid and choice between distilled water and 0.25 *M* NaCl solution to drink. During the fifteenth week of the experiment, each rat was offered a choice between distilled water and 0.35 *M* NaCl solution. Food and fluid intakes and body weight were measured daily.

Statistical analysis of the data was made by means of an analysis of variance (Snedecor and Cochran, 1956). Differences between means were compared using the pooled variance and the *t* test.

B. Experiment 2. Effect of Enovid on the Preference Threshold for NaCl Solution in Rats

Twelve female rats of the Blue Spruce Farms strain, weighing 180–210 g were kept in individual cages under the same conditions, including food and fluid containers, as those described in Experiment 1. Two weeks prior to initiation of the experiment, half of the rats received food with Enovid mixed into it at a concentration of 7.5 mg/kg of finely ground Purina Laboratory Chow. During this period, each rat was allowed to choose its drinking fluid from either of two bottles, each containing distilled water. Observations of the daily fluid intake by each rat indicated that roughly half was ingested from each bottle.

At the beginning of the experiment during the first 2-day test period, each rat was allowed to choose between two bottles of distilled water. During subsequent 2-day test periods, each rat was given a choice between distilled water and the following molar NaCl solutions in chronological sequence: 0.0006, 0.001, 0.003, 0.006, 0.009, 0.012, 0.015, 0.020, 0.025, 0.030, 0.050, 0.075, 0.100, 0.150, 0.200, 0.250, and 0.00 (distilled water). Each concentration was made from a single stock solution by serial dilution, and each dilution was checked for

*Each tablet contained 15.0 mg norethynodrel and 0.075 mg mestranol.

accuracy by determination of sodium concentration by flame photometry using lithium as the internal standard. Positions of the two bottles on each cage were interchanged daily to discourage habit formation in selection of drinking fluids. Daily intakes of water and NaCl solutions were measured and expressed as ml/100 g body weight/day to relate fluid intake to a unit of body weight.

The criterion of preference threshold used was similar to that of Richter (1939), namely, the concentration of NaCl solution at and above which simultaneous mean volume taken from the bottle containing NaCl solution exceeded significantly that taken from the water bottle. Individual data for rats in each group were averaged and the means were compared statistically by a *t* test (Snedecor and Cochran, 1956).

C. Experiment 3. Effect of Chronic Administration of Norethynodrel, Ethynyl Estradiol, and Both Combined on Sodium Intake and Sodium Excretion during Acute Sodium Loading

Twenty-four male rats of the Sprague–Dawley strain weighing between 410 and 457 g were divided into four groups. The first group was implanted with a 10-mm length of Silastic tube (0.25 mm wall thickness, Silastic tubing no. 602-231) containing norethynodrel. The second group was implanted with a 10-mm length of tube containing ethynyl estradiol of the same wall thickness. The third group was implanted with a tube containing norethynodrel and another tube containing ethynyl estradiol, both of which were identical to the ones used in the first two groups. The fourth group received no treatment and served as a control group. This method of administering steroids via Silastic implants allows diffusion of crystalline steroids into various media at a constant rate over long periods of time (Dzuik and Cook, 1966; Kincl *et al.*, 1968). The amount of norethynodrel released by each tube was approximately 91 μg/kg/day while the amount of ethynyl estradiol released was approximately 41 μg/kg/day.

An experiment measuring intake of food, distilled water, and NaCl solution was conducted for 6 days during weeks 1, 3, 6, 9, and 13. The protocol for these experiments was identical to that described in Experiment 1. The concentration of the NaCl solution offered as choice with distilled water was 0.25 *M* except during week 13 when the rats were allowed to drink 0.15 *M* NaCl. On the day of each diuretic experiment, each rat was required to breathe ether for a few moments to initiate reflex emptying of the bladder. Then isotonic saline at a dose equivalent to 3% of body weight was administered ip to each rat. The saline was warmed to body temperature prior to injection. The rats were then placed in individual, stainless steel metabolic cages without food or water, and urine was collected for 5 hours. At the end of the experiment, gentle pressure was exerted on the back and lower abdomen of each rat in order to collect any urine remaining in the bladder. This urine was added to that voided during the 5-hour period and the volume was recorded. The funnel under each cage was then rinsed with 10.0 ml of distilled water. The sodium and potassium concentrations of both the urine and rinse from each rat were determined by flame photometry using a Technicon autoanalyzer.

The data were then expressed as mEq of sodium or potassium excreted per kg of body weight per 5 hours. The urinary sodium to potassium ratio and urine volume per kg body weight per 5 hours were also calculated. An analysis of variance was used to detect treatment differences, and the pooled variance and *t* test were used to detect differences between groups (Snedecor and Cochran, 1956).

An acute diuretic experiment, conducted as described above, was performed during weeks 1, 5, 11, and 14 of treatment. The concentration of the loading solution was 0.075 *M* NaCl for the experiments done during weeks 1 and 5. For those performed during weeks 11 and 14, 0.15 *M* NaCl solution was used.

After 20 weeks of treatment, each rat was anesthetized with pentobarbital (35 mg/kg) and a sample of blood was removed from the carotid artery. The blood was centrifuged at 3500 g in a refrigerated centrifuge. Serum was separated and analyzed for its sodium and potassium concentrations by flame photometry. At death, the ventricles, kidneys, testes, adrenals, and thyroid gland were removed, cleaned of extraneous tissue, and weighed on a torsion balance.

D. Experiment 4. Effect of Administration of Enovid, Norethynodrel, and Ethynyl Estradiol on the Spontaneous NaCl Intake by Adrenalectomized Rats

Three separate experiments were designed to test the effect of Enovid, norethynodrel, and ethynyl estradiol on spontaneous intakes of NaCl solution and distilled water by adrenalectomized rats. Twenty-four adrenalectomized male rats of the Sprague–Dawley strain initially weighing from 283 to 419 g were used. These rats had been adrenalectomized for 2 months. In each experiment there were three groups each containing eight rats. One group served as the control group while the other two were treated. There was an initial 5-day control period followed by a 5-day treatment period during which the drug was administered. Intakes of food, distilled water, and 0.25 *M* NaCl solution were measured during both periods in a manner already described. The drug concentrations used were: 5.0 and 7.5 mg of Enovid/kg of food; 7.5 and 15.0 mg of norethynodrel/kg of food, and 0.15 and 0.30 mg of ethynyl estradiol/kg of food. There was a 4-day rest period between experiments. Each experiment was analyzed by means of an analysis of variance. Differences between individual groups were determined by means of the pooled variance and the *t* test (Snedecor and Cochran, 1956).

E. Experiment 5. Effect of the Progestational Agent, Medroxyprogesterone, on NaCl Appetite

Twenty-four female rats of the Blue Spruce Farms (Sprague–Dawley) strain weighing initially from 169 to 207 g were divided randomly into three groups each containing eight rats. Two groups were given medroxyprogesterone (7.5 and 15.0 mg/kg of food), and the third group served as controls. Intakes of food, distilled water, and 0.25 *M* NaCl solution were measured from day 1 of drug administration until day 23. Then 0.15 *M* NaCl solution was substituted for 0.25 *M* NaCl solution, and intakes were measured again from day 24 until day 31. An analysis of variance was used to analyze the data (Snedecor and Cochran, 1956). The conditions under which this experiment was conducted and the procedures used in gathering data were identical to those already described in Experiment 1.

III. RESULTS

A. Experiment 1

Within 1 week after administration of Enovid, intake of 0.15 *M* NaCl solution by all treated groups was greater, and water intake less, than that of the control group (Table I). However, only the NaCl intake of the group given 5.00 mg of Enovid/kg of food was significantly ($p < 0.01$) greater than that of the control group. Water intakes of all treated groups were significantly ($p < 0.05$–0.01) less than that of the control group. By the criterion of NaCl intake, only the highest dose of Enovid induced an appetite for NaCl solution within the first week of drug administration.

By the end of the second week, only the group given 5.00 mg Enovid/kg of food ingested significantly ($p < 0.05$) more 0.15 *M* NaCl solution than controls (Table I). There was no significant effect of treatment on intake of NaCl solution during the third week of the experiment. However, if the criterion for development of a NaCl appetite is based on the ratio of NaCl intake to total fluid intake, it appears that all the groups receiving Enovid showed significant differences from the control group during the first and second weeks of treatment (Table I). During the third week of treatment, only the group receiving the lowest dose of Enovid failed to show a significant change in this ratio. Thus, it would appear that the ratio is a more sensitive measure of NaCl appetite than merely the volume of NaCl solution ingested.

Figure 1 illustrates the effect of administration of increasing concentrations of NaCl solution on simultaneous intakes of water and NaCl solution by each group. It is clear that in all groups, NaCl intake decreased and water intake increased as the concentration of the NaCl solutions offered increased. It is also clear that the Enovid-treated rats ingested more NaCl solution at each different concentration

TABLE I

Time Course of Development of a Salt Appetite in Rats Treated with Enovid

Experimental group	Mean body weight (g)	Intakes (ml or g/100 g body weight/day) Distilled water	0.15 *M* NaCl solution	Food	NaCl intake /Total fluid intake (%)
Week 1					
Control	190 ± 2[a]	10.1 ± 0.6	6.9 ± 1.4	9.1 ± 0.2	38.7 ± 6.1
Enovid (mg/kg food)					
1.25	187 ± 4	7.1 ± 0.9[b]	8.4 ± 0.6	7.3 ± 0.2[c]	54.8 ± 3.6[b]
2.50	181 ± 4[c]	5.2 ± 1.0[c]	10.2 ± 0.8	7.6 ± 0.4[c]	67.2 ± 5.5[c]
5.00	176 ± 3[c]	5.3 ± 0.9[c]	14.0 ± 2.1[c]	6.7 ± 0.3[c]	71.8 ± 4.4[c]
Week 2					
Control	202 ± 2	9.8 ± 0.5	9.1 ± 2.3	9.5 ± 0.2	44.2 ± 6.8
Enovid (mg/kg food)					
1.25	191 ± 4[b]	5.7 ± 0.6[c]	9.2 ± 0.9	7.7 ± 0.2[c]	61.5 ± 4.2[b]
2.50	188 ± 5[c]	4.4 ± 0.9[c]	13.8 ± 1.6	9.0 ± 0.3	75.8 ± 4.4[c]
5.00	182 ± 3[c]	5.2 ± 1.2[c]	15.5 ± 2.1[b]	8.4 ± 0.3[c]	74.6 ± 6.0[c]
Week 3					
Control	211 ± 3	9.3 ± 0.8	9.1 ± 1.9	9.1 ± 0.2	47.0 ± 5.6
Enovid (mg/kg food)					
1.25	198 ± 5[b]	5.2 ± 0.7[c]	9.7 ± 0.9	7.9 ± 0.1[c]	64.7 ± 4.7
2.50	194 ± 5[c]	4.0 ± 0.8[c]	14.2 ± 2.0	9.4 ± 0.7	76.9 ± 5.0[c]
5.00	187 ± 3[c]	5.6 ± 1.3[c]	14.0 ± 2.6	8.7 ± 0.3	68.8 ± 9.2[b]

[a] One standard error of mean.
[b] Significantly different from control ($P < 0.05$).
[c] Significantly different from control ($P < 0.01$).

offered than did controls. Enovid-treated rats actually preferred NaCl solution to water at all concentrations of NaCl solution offered. The single exception to this statement is the group given 1.25 mg Enovid/kg of food which ingested slightly less NaCl solution than water when 0.35 *M* NaCl solution was offered. In contrast, control rats rejected all concentrations of NaCl solution greater than 0.15 *M* in favor of the water offered simultaneously.

The results of this experiment suggest that a salt appetite may be induced within a week when rats are given 1.25, 2.50 or 5.00 mg of Enovid/kg of food and choice is offered between water and 0.15 *M* NaCl solution to drink. The salt appetite of Enovid-treated rats was present for hypertonic NaCl solutions that were actually aversive for control rats. This is illustrated in Fig. 2 where the ratio of [NaCl ingested/total fluid (water + NaCl solution)] × 100 is graphed against the concentration of NaCl solution offered. At all NaCl concentrations given, the percentage of the total fluid intake ingested as NaCl solution was much higher for Enovid-treated rats than for controls. There was also a dose–response relationship between dose of Enovid administered and NaCl intake ratio.

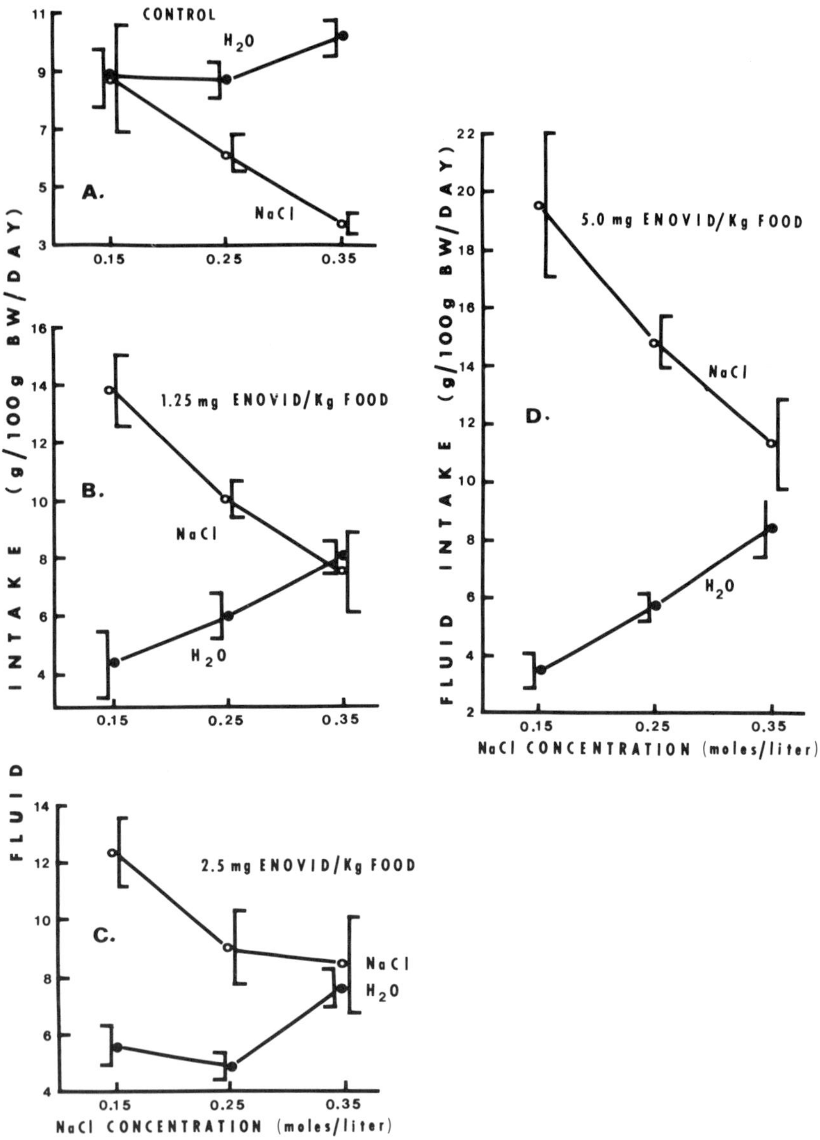

Fig. 1. Simultaneous intakes of NaCl solution and distilled water are shown at each concentration of NaCl solution offered. Intakes of the control group (A) as well as the groups given Enovid at 1.25 (B), 2.50 (C), and 5.00 (D) mg/kg of food are shown. One standard error is set off at each mean.

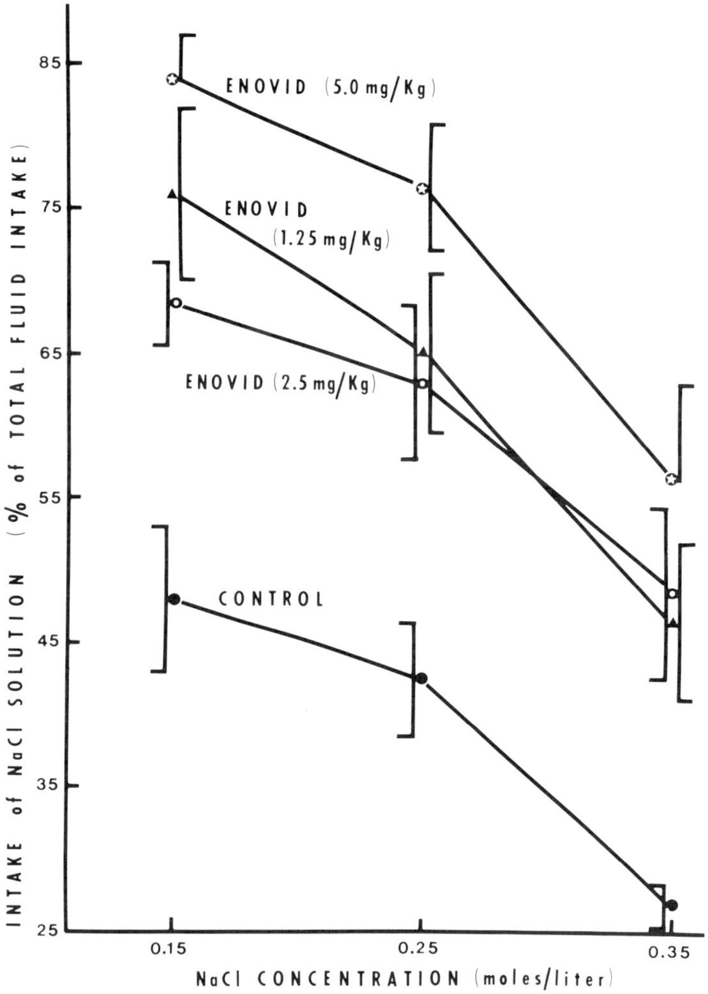

Fig. 2. The ratio of NaCl intake/total fluid intake is graphed against the concentration of NaCl solution offered simultaneously with water. The groups are designated in the figure. One standard error is set off at each mean.

Mean body weight of the four groups during the experiment is illustrated in Fig. 3. Body weight gain was reduced in proportion to the dose of Enovid administered.

B. Experiment 2

Administration of Enovid was accompanied by a significant ($p < 0.01$) reduction in preference threshold for NaCl solution (Fig. 4). The treated rats, as a

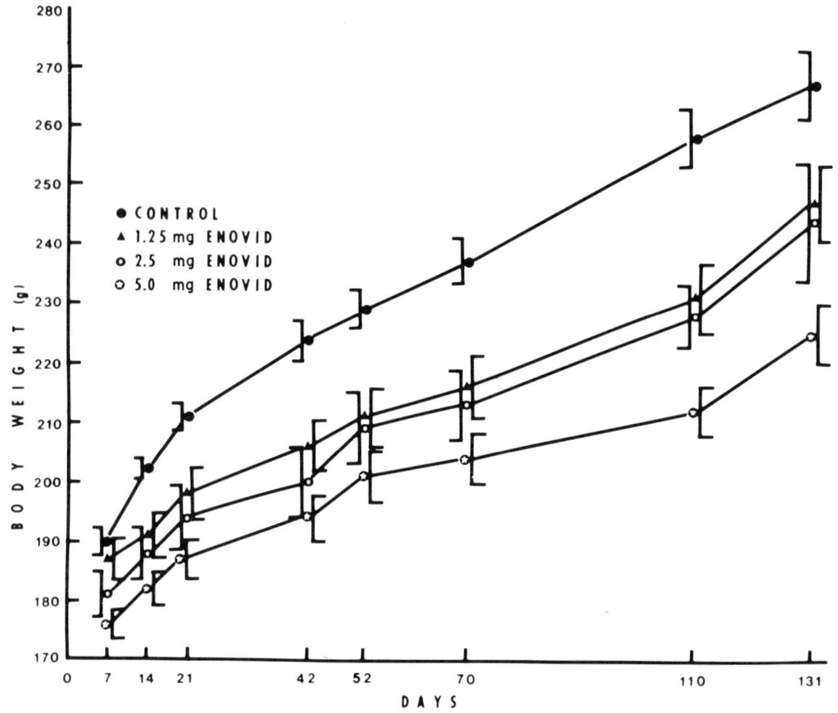

Fig. 3. Mean body weights of the four groups of rats used in Experiment 1 are shown at intervals throughout the experiment. Group designations are shown in the figure. One standard error is set off at each mean.

group, detected the difference between distilled water and NaCl solution when the concentration of the latter was 0.015 *M*, while controls detected the difference between the two bottles when the NaCl concentration was 0.030 *M*. Thus the preference threshold of the treated group lies between 0.012 and 0.015 *M* while that of the control group lies between 0.025 and 0.030 *M*.

The results indicate that Enovid-treated rats could differentiate between NaCl solution and distilled water at approximately one-third to one-half the concentration required by control rats. It should also be noted in Fig. 4 that the volume of NaCl ingested by treated rats was greater than that of control rats at all concentrations tested above threshold, including hypertonic concentrations. Mean food intake of treated rats (g/100 g body weight/day; not shown in Fig. 4) was slightly less than that of controls at all periods throughout the experiment although the difference from control value was never significant. Mean body weight of treated rats (not shown in Fig. 4) was also less than that of controls, and the difference from the control group was always significant ($p < 0.05$). Mean body weights of

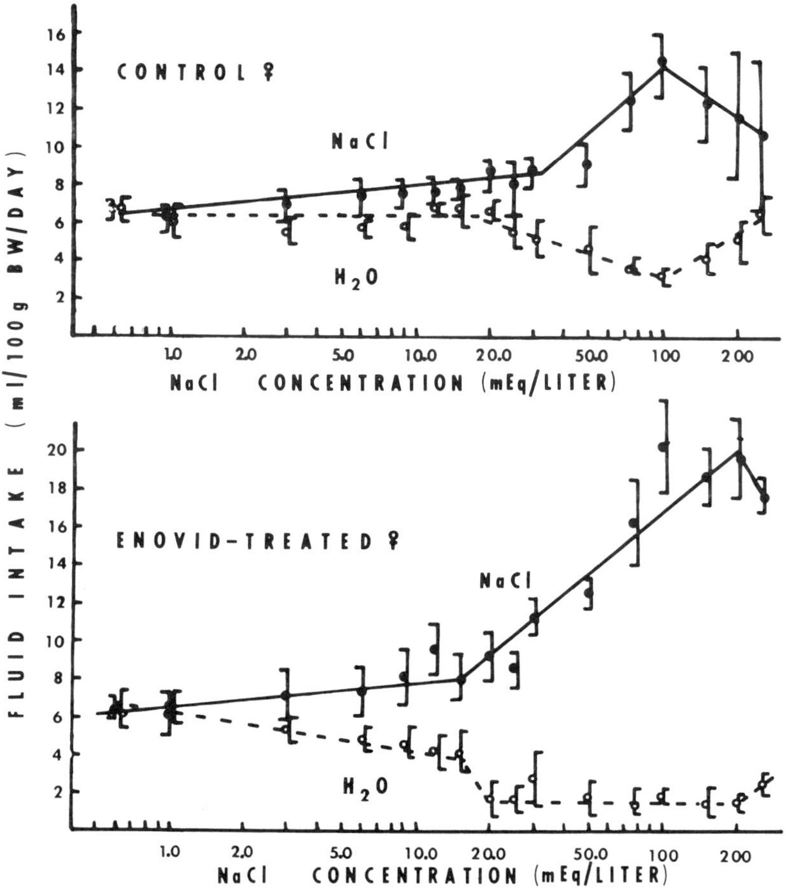

Fig. 4. Spontaneous intakes of NaCl solution (solid line) and distilled water (dashed line) are shown for control rats (upper panel) and Enovid-treated (lower panel) rats. One standard error is set off at each mean. (From Fregly, 1973; used by permission.)

the control group at the beginning and end of the experiment were 195 and 236 g, respectively, while mean body weights of the treated group were 175 and 199 g, respectively.

C. Experiment 3

The intake of 0.25 *M* NaCl solution increased for all three treated groups during the first week of steroid administration, but this increase was not significantly different from controls (Table II). The water intake of treated groups was

TABLE II

Effect of Chronic Administration of Norethynodrel, Ethynyl Estradiol, and Both Together on Spontaneous Intakes of NaCl Solution, Water, and Food

Experimental group	Number of rats	Mean body weight (g)	Intakes (ml or g/100 g body weight/day)			NaCl intake/ Total fluid intake (%)
			NaCl solution	Water	Food	
1 Week of drugs—choice between 0.25 *M* NaCl solution and distilled water						
Control	6	423 ± 16[a]	1.9 ± 0.5	8.3 ± 0.8	5.7 ± 0.2	18.6 ± 4.8
Norethynodrel[d]	6	424 ± 20	5.9 ± 1.4	6.0 ± 1.3	5.0 ± 0.2	48.5 ± 11.0[b]
Ethynyl estradiol[d]	6	370 ± 18[b]	4.7 ± 1.1	5.8 ± 1.3	3.4 ± 0.6[c]	45.0 ± 7.4[c]
Norethynodrel + ethynyl estradiol	6	366 ± 10[b]	6.1 ± 2.1	8.6 ± 1.3	3.9 ± 0.3[c]	37.7 ± 8.8[b]
3 Weeks of drugs—choice between 0.25 *M* NaCl solution and distilled water						
Control	6	443 ± 15	2.3 ± 0.6	8.2 ± 0.7	5.6 ± 0.8	21.0 ± 4.3
Norethynodrel	6	441 ± 23	6.6 ± 1.2	6.0 ± 0.9	5.2 ± 0.2	51.4 ± 8.1[b]
Ethynyl estradiol	6	370 ± 10[b]	8.9 ± 1.1[b]	8.2 ± 0.9	5.7 ± 0.2	51.9 ± 4.4[b]
Norethynodrel + ethynyl estradiol	6	373 ± 14[b]	11.1 ± 3.5[b]	11.6 ± 1.6[b]	5.8 ± 0.3	43.7 ± 9.9[b]

6 Weeks of drugs—choice between 0.25 M NaCl solution and distilled water						
Control	6	463 ± 14	2.4 ± 0.6	8.1 ± 0.7	5.2 ± 0.2	21.7 ± 4.2
Norethynodrel	6	449 ± 25	5.8 ± 1.4	6.9 ± 0.5	4.8 ± 0.1	42.8 ± 6.9[b]
Ethynyl estradiol	6	376 ± 12[c]	9.3 ± 1.3[b]	7.5 ± 0.8	4.6 ± 0.2	54.7 ± 3.7[c]
Norethynoldrel + ethynyl estradiol	6	374 ± 11[c]	11.8 ± 3.2[c]	10.9 ± 1.5	5.0 ± 0.2	47.9 ± 8.6[b]
9 Weeks of drugs—choice between 0.25 M NaCl solution and distilled water						
Control	6	468 ± 14	1.8 ± 0.3	8.5 ± 1.0	5.9 ± 0.4	17.6 ± 3.1
Norethynodrel	6	465 ± 27	4.9 ± 1.3	6.3 ± 0.7	4.2 ± 0.1[c]	41.2 ± 7.9[b]
Ethynyl estradiol	6	370 ± 11[c]	7.9 ± 1.7[b]	5.8 ± 0.6	4.1 ± 0.1[c]	50.7 ± 5.7[c]
Norethynodrel + ethynyl estradiol	6	371 ± 10[c]	12.1 ± 2.9[c]	8.7 ± 1.2	4.2 ± 0.2[c]	54.2 ± 8.6[c]
13 Weeks of drugs—choice between 0.15 M NaCl solution and distilled water						
Control	6	483 ± 13	2.5 ± 0.5	7.0 ± 0.6	5.0 ± 0.2	25.1 ± 4.3
Norethynodrel	6	476 ± 30	5.3 ± 1.2	4.3 ± 0.7	4.5 ± 0.1	53.5 ± 9.0[b]
Ethynyl estradiol	6	371 ± 12[c]	12.3 ± 1.5[c]	5.5 ± 0.3	4.9 ± 0.1	67.8 ± 3.1[c]
Norethynodrel + ethynyl estradiol	6	375 ± 9[c]	14.5 ± 3.2[c]	5.8 ± 1.3	4.9 ± 0.1	66.1 ± 10.9[c]

[a] One standard error of mean.
[b] Significantly different from control group ($p < 0.05$).
[c] Significantly different from control group ($p < 0.01$).
[d] Dose of norethynodrel was 91 μg/kg/day and dose of ethynyl estradiol was 41 μg/kg/day.

not different from the control group. When NaCl intake was expressed as a percentage of the total fluid intake, all treated groups showed a significant increase above the control group.

When the intakes of distilled water and 0.25 *M* NaCl solution were measured during the third week of treatment, the group receiving ethynyl estradiol and the one receiving norethynodrel plus ethynyl estradiol increased significantly their intake of NaCl solution (Table II). Water intakes of the groups receiving norethynodrel and ethynyl estradiol were not different from control. The group receiving both steroids had a significantly increased water intake. The ratio of NaCl to total fluid intake was increased significantly for all three treated groups.

During the sixth week of treatment, the results were essentially the same: groups receiving ethynyl estradiol and both norethynodrel and ethynyl estradiol had a significantly increased appetite for NaCl solution (Table II). There were no significant differences in water intake among groups. All groups had a significantly increased ratio of NaCl to total fluid intake.

For the ninth week of treatment, the results were the same as for the sixth week of treatment: (a) NaCl intakes of groups receiving either ethynyl estradiol or both steroids were increased significantly above that of the control group; (b) there were no differences in water intake among the groups; and (c) all treated groups ingested a significantly greater percentage of their total fluid intake as NaCl solution (Table II).

During the thirteenth week of treatment the intakes of 0.15 *M* NaCl and distilled water were measured. Most rats prefer 0.15 *M* to 0.25 *M* NaCl solution (Fig. 4), and this was reflected in the results as each group increased the volume of NaCl solution ingested during the thirteenth week compared to that ingested during the ninth week (Table II). The NaCl intake of the ethynyl estradiol-treated group and the group treated with both norethynodrel and ethynyl estradiol was increased significantly. There were no significant differences in water intake among groups. The ratio of NaCl intake to total fluid intake was increased significantly in all treated groups.

The food intake of the treated rats did not differ from that of control rats during weeks 3, 6, and 13 of treatment (Table II). During the first week of treatment, the food intakes of both the ethynyl estradiol-treated and the combined treatment groups were reduced significantly. All treated groups had a significantly reduced food intake during the ninth week. The body weights of the ethynyl estradiol-treated and combined treatment groups were reduced significantly from the controls from the first through the thirteenth weeks of treatment.

The acute diuretic experiments were performed during the first, fifth, eleventh, and fourteenth weeks of treatment (Table III). The first two studies were carried out with a loading solution of 0.075 *M* NaCl, and the second two were performed with a 0.15 *M* NaCl loading solution. The first solution is hypotonic, and resulted in roughly twice the urinary volume seen when 0.15 *M*

NaCl (isotonic) was used. Approximately the same sodium output (mEq/kg/5 hour) was seen in the control group with either concentration of loading solution.

After 1 week of treatment, there were no significant differences among groups with respect to urine output, sodium output, potassium output, or in the urinary Na/K ratio (Table III). When the same experiment was performed after the fifth week of treatment, each treated group had an increased urine output. However, this was significant only for the group given both norethynodrel and ethynyl estradiol ($p < 0.05$). Urinary sodium output was increased in all three treated groups. This increase was not significant for the group given norethynodrel only. Urinary potassium output was increased significantly in the group given both norethynodrel and ethynyl estradiol ($p < 0.01$). There was no difference in the urinary Na/K ratio among groups.

When the experiment was repeated after 11 weeks of treatment, urine output was significantly increased in both the ethynyl estradiol and the combined treatment groups ($p < 0.05$). Urine sodium output was increased significantly for each treated group ($p < 0.01$). There were no significant differences in urinary potassium output among groups. The urinary Na/K ratio increased significantly ($p < 0.01$) for all treated groups (Table III) compared to controls.

After 14 weeks of treatment, the diuretic experiment was repeated, and the results were similar to those observed after 11 weeks of treatment (Table III). Urine output increased significantly in the groups treated with ethynyl estradiol ($p < 0.05$) and both steroids ($p < 0.01$). Urinary sodium output increased significantly in all treated groups ($p < 0.01$). There were no differences among groups in urinary potassium output. The urinary Na/K ratio was increased significantly ($p < 0.01$) for the ethynyl estradiol-treated group and the group treated with both steroids.

The serum sodium and potassium concentrations of each group of rats are shown in Table IV. No differences among groups were observed in serum sodium concentration but the serum potassium concentration of the group administered both norethynodrel and ethynyl estradiol was ($p < 0.01$) reduced significantly below that of all other groups. Of the organs removed, only the weights of the testes of both groups receiving ethynyl estradiol were reduced significantly ($p < 0.01$) below those of the other two groups.

D. Experiment 4

Administration of either Enovid, norethynodrel, or ethynyl estradiol to adrenalectomized rats failed to affect significantly their intake of either distilled water or NaCl solution (Table V). In addition, the ratios of NaCl to total fluid intake were not affected significantly by administration of these steroids. When the data were expressed as mean differences between periods, there were still no significant differences among the groups with respect to intakes of distilled

TABLE III

Effects of Intraperitoneal Loads of NaCl Solution on Urinary Excretion of Sodium and Potassium in Male Rats Chronically Administered Norethynodrel, Ethynyl Estradiol, and Both

Treatment	Number of rats	Mean body weight (g)	Urine output (ml/kg BW/ 5 hours)	Sodium output (mEq/kg BW/ 5 hours)	Potassium output (mEq/kg BW/ 5 hours)	Urinary Na/K ratio
1 Week of treatment (0.075 *M* NaCl loading solution)						
Control[d]	6	427 ± 16[a]	31.2 ± 4.4	1.34 ± 0.36	1.21 ± 0.18	1.11 ± 0.16
Norethynodrel	6	435 ± 22	26.0 ± 3.9	1.26 ± 0.29	1.38 ± 0.18	0.91 ± 0.10
Ethynyl estradiol	6	429 ± 15	26.5 ± 1.7	1.03 ± 0.23	1.19 ± 0.11	0.87 ± 0.14
Norethynodrel + ethynyl estradiol	6	427 ± 16	29.1 ± 3.2	1.17 ± 0.24	1.22 ± 0.21	0.96 ± 0.14
5 Weeks of treatment (0.075 *M* NaCl loading solution)						
Control	6	465 ± 15	24.7 ± 2.3	1.81 ± 0.41	0.91 ± 0.14	2.06 ± 0.59
Norethynodrel	6	422 ± 18	33.5 ± 4.1	4.07 ± 1.45	1.43 ± 0.26	2.56 ± 0.55
Ethynyl estradiol	6	376 ± 14	33.5 ± 3.4	3.67 ± 0.57[b]	1.82 ± 0.40	2.39 ± 0.41
Norethynodrel + ethynyl estradiol	6	372 ± 9	39.9 ± 4.7[b]	5.03 ± 0.66[c]	1.94 ± 0.36[c]	2.96 ± 0.48

11 Weeks of drug treatment (0.15 *M* NaCl loading solution)						
Control	6	470 ± 2	14.1 ± 3.7	1.70 ± 0.37	1.53 ± 0.20	1.17 ± 0.24
Norethynodrel	6	475 ± 28	17.8 ± 3.0	2.49 ± 0.25[c]	1.28 ± 0.19	2.14 ± 0.38[c]
Ethynyl estradiol	6	374 ± 10[b]	29.2 ± 6.0[b]	3.99 ± 0.91[c]	1.03 ± 0.22	4.12 ± 0.55[c]
Norethynodrel + ethynyl estradiol	6	377 ± 9[b]	32.5 ± 4.2[b]	4.24 ± 0.32[c]	0.95 ± 0.14	5.40 ± 1.27[c]
14 Weeks of drug treatment (0.15 *M* NaCl loading solution)						
Control	6	477 ± 12	11.1 ± 2.4	1.75 ± 0.24	1.14 ± 0.09	1.72 ± 0.34
Norethynodrel	6	467 ± 18	15.5 ± 2.5	2.60 ± 0.16[c]	1.47 ± 0.15	1.88 ± 0.13
Ethynyl estradiol	6	385 ± 12[c]	22.2 ± 3.1[b]	3.78 ± 0.41[c]	1.07 ± 0.13	3.95 ± 0.47[c]
Norethynodrel + ethynyl estradiol	6	367 ± 7[c]	27.6 ± 2.9[c]	3.49 ± 0.51[c]	1.20 ± 0.13	3.03 ± 0.41[c]

[a] One standard error of mean.

[b] Significantly different from control ($p < 0.05$).

[c] Significantly different from control ($p < 0.01$).

[d] All rats were administered an ip load of NaCl solution (3% of body weight) and urine outputs measured during the next 5 hours. All rats had choice between 0.25 *M* NaCl solution and water as drinking fluids chronically prior to the experiments. Dose of norethynodrel was 91 μg/kg/day; dose of ethynyl estradiol was 41 μg/kg/day.

TABLE IV

Effect of Chronic Administration of Norethynodrel, Ethynyl Estradiol, and Both Combined on Organ Weight to Body Weight Ratio of Certain Organs of Male Rats

Experimental group	Number of rats	Mean body weight (g)	Organ to body weight ratio (mg/100 g body weight)					Serum Na conc. (mEq/liter)	Serum K conc. (mEq/liter)
			Ventricles	Kidneys	Testes	Adrenals	Thyroid		
Control	6	497	281.0	699.3	728.0	13.5	6.5	143.6	3.8
		±21[a]	±12.1	±37.7	±49.1	±1.0	±0.7	±4.4	±0.4
Norethynodrel	6	490	251.8	593.3	700.2	11.7	6.1	138.9	3.7
(91 μg/kg/day)		±29	± 3.5	±15.2	±31.0	±0.7	±0.9	±2.2	±0.3
Ethynyl estradiol	6	366	255.8	692.5	127.9	13.6	5.6	142.1	3.4
(41 μg/kg/day)		±12[b]	± 7.9	± 6.3	±10.2[b]	±1.9	±0.8	±3.8	±0.1
Norethynodrel +	6	371	265.4	675.6	132.1	14.6	6.6	143.3	2.6
ethynyl estradiol		±13[b]	± 5.5	±21.1	±10.1[b]	±0.9	±1.0	±1.7	±0.1[b]

[a] One standard error of mean.

[b] Significantly different from control ($p < 0.01$).

water, NaCl solution, and the ratio of NaCl to total fluid intake. Administration of either Enovid or norethynodrel decreased food intake significantly at the higher dose while administration of ethynyl estradiol was accompanied by a decrease in food intake at both doses.

E. Experiment 5

The intake of 0.25 *M* NaCl solution by the medroxyprogesterone-treated groups did not differ from that of the controls at any time (Table VI). Body weight, intake of food and distilled water, and the ratio of NaCl to total fluid intake were also not affected by administration of either concentration of medroxyprogesterone. When 0.15 *M* NaCl solution was substituted for 0.25 *M* NaCl solution at day 24, there was again no effect of treatment with medroxyprogesterone on intake of NaCl solution (Table VI). The actual amounts of medroxyprogesterone (6α-methyl-17α-hydroxyprogesterone) ingested, as calculated from the food intakes, were 1.10 and 0.56 mg/kg/day when 15.0 and 7.5 mg, respectively, were added to each kg of food.

IV. DISCUSSION

There appears to be little doubt that dietary administration of the oral contraceptive, Enovid, induces a spontaneous appetite for NaCl solution in intact as well as ovariectomized rats (Fregly, 1972, 1973; Fregly and Newsome, 1974). Hence, neither the presence nor the absence of the ovaries is requisite to the induction of a NaCl appetite. It does appear, however, that the adrenal gland may be essential (Table V).

When a choice was offered between distilled water and 0.15 *M* NaCl solution to drink, an increase in NaCl intake was induced within 1 week after initiation of treatment with 1.25, 2.50, or 5.00 mg Enovid/kg of food. The NaCl appetite of Enovid-treated rats was very strong as judged by the fact that treated rats actually preferred certain hypertonic NaCl solutions to the distilled water offered simultaneously (Fig. 1). A dose–response relationship was apparent between intake of NaCl solution and dose of Enovid administered. Intake of NaCl solution increased as a direct function of dose (Fig. 2).

The appetite for NaCl was accompanied by a reduction in the preference threshold for NaCl (Fig. 4). The preference threshold reported here for the control group is similar to values reported earlier from this laboratory (0.029 and 0.023 *M*/liter) (Fregly, 1967a, 1969; Fregly and Waters, 1965). The reduced preference threshold of Enovid-treated rats was also similar to that reported earlier to accompany administration of hydrochlorothiazide (Fregly, 1967a) and propylthiouracil (Fregly and Waters, 1965) to rats. It is also of interest that all

TABLE V

Effect of Enovid, Norethynodrel, and Ethynyl Estradiol on Body Weight, and Spontaneous Intakes of Food, Distilled Water, and 0.25 *M* NaCl Solution by Adrenalectomized Rats

		Mean body weight (g)		Spontaneous intake (ml or g/100 g BW/day) during							
				Control period				Treatment period			
Experimental group	Number of rats	Cont.	Treat.	Food	Water	NaCl solution	Ratio[d]	Food	Water	NaCl solution	Ratio[d]
A. *Experiment 1*											
Control	8	380	389	5.3	5.4	11.1	61.2	5.9	5.8	11.6	60.4
		±21[a]	±22	±0.2	±0.2	±2.6	±8.7	±0.2	±0.9	±2.9	±9.1
Enovid[e]											
5.0 mg/kg food	8	352	357	5.6	5.2	11.1	61.6	5.4	4.9	11.8	66.1
		±13	±14	±0.2	±0.2	±2.3	±8.9	±0.4	±0.7	±2.2	±8.1
7.5 mg/kg food	8	358	359	5.2	4.5	11.2	65.4	4.9[c]	3.9	12.2	69.4
		±12	±13	±0.2	±0.7	±2.3	±8.9	±0.2	±0.5	±2.3	±6.5

B. *Experiment 2*											
Control	8	349	358	6.0	5.8	10.3	57.8	6.2	5.8	10.1	56.1
		±18	±19	±0.1	±0.9	±2.4	±9.4	±0.3	±0.8	±2.6	±9.8
Norethynodrel[e]											
7.5 mg/kg food	8	354	359	6.0	5.8	11.4	60.6	5.7	4.7	12.0	64.5
		±10	±11	±0.1	±0.5	±2.4	±7.7	±0.2	±0.6	±2.2	±6.1
15.0 mg/kg food	8	340	336	5.8	5.3	11.5	62.6	4.4[c]	4.2	12.5	71.3
		±11	±17	±0.1	±0.9	±2.4	±9.6	±0.1	±0.6	±1.8	±7.2
C. *Experiment 3*											
Control	8	400	404	5.7	5.7	10.5	58.8	5.8	6.5	8.2	51.0
		±16	±15	±0.1	±0.2	±2.3	±8.7	±0.2	±0.6	±1.9	±7.2
Ethynyl estradiol[e]											
0.15 mg/kg food	8	395	394	5.7	5.7	10.8	60.2	5.1[b]	5.2	9.5	60.5
		±18	±18	±0.1	±0.1	±2.7	±8.6	±0.2	±0.4	±1.9	±5.7
0.30 mg/kg food	8	382	373	5.6	5.6	9.4	55.0	4.7[c]	5.5	9.1	53.3
		±19	±18	±0.2	±0.2	±2.5	±10.6	±0.2	±0.5	±2.6	±9.2

[a] One standard error of mean.

[b] Significantly different from control ($p < 0.05$).

[c] Significantly different from control ($p < 0.01$).

[d] Ratio of [NaCl intake to total fluid intake] × 100.

[e] Doses of Enovid were 270 and 370 μg/kg/day. Doses of norethynodrel were 430 and 660 μg/kg/day. Doses of ethynyl estradiol were 8 and 14 μg/kg/day.

TABLE VI

Effect of Dietary Administration of Medroxyprogesterone on Body Weight and Spontaneous Intakes of Distilled Water, NaCl Solution, and Food by Female Rats

Experimental group	Number of rats	Mean body weight (g)	Intakes (ml or g/100 g body wt/day): Distilled water	NaCl solution	Food	NaCl intake/ Total fluid intake %
Choice between 0.25 *M* NaCl solution and distilled water[b]						
Control	8	203 ± 5[a]	7.0 ± 0.7	8.5 ± 2.3	7.3 ± 0.2	50.7 ± 6.9
Medroxyprogesterone (7.5 mg/kg food)	8	210 ± 7	7.7 ± 0.7	8.9 ± 1.5	7.2 ± 0.1	59.7 ± 7.4
Medroxyprogesterone (15.0 mg/kg food)	8	218 ± 3	7.6 ± 0.9	8.5 ± 1.2	6.9 ± 0.1	52.8 ± 4.2
Choice between 0.15 *M* NaCl solution and distilled water[c]						
Control	8	212 ± 5	5.1 ± 0.8	13.0 ± 4.1	7.1 ± 0.1	64.1 ± 7.7
Medroxyprogesterone (7.5 mg/kg food)	8	222 ± 7	5.8 ± 0.7	10.0 ± 1.9	7.1 ± 0.1	59.7 ± 7.4
Medroxyprogesterone (15.0 mg/kg food)	8	230 ± 4	5.8 ± 0.8	10.6 ± 1.2	6.5 ± 0.3	65.4 ± 4.3

[a] One standard error of mean.
[b] Measurements made during third week of drug treatment.
[c] Measurements made during fourth week of drug treatment.

experimental procedures thus far tested inducing a chronic appetite for NaCl solution (viz. adrenalectomy, hypothyroidism, and administration of deoxycorticosterone acetate, propylthiouracil, Enovid, or hydrochlorothiazide) are also accompanied by a reduced preference threshold for NaCl solution (Fregly, 1967a, 1969; Fregly and Waters, 1965; Herxheimer and Woodbury, 1960; Richter, 1939).

The apparent relationship between reduced preference threshold for NaCl solution and NaCl appetite in rats has not been explained satisfactorily, although a number of possibilities exist and have been presented (Fregly, 1967b). For example, it has been suggested that these two phenomena may be related directly to the sodium concentration of saliva bathing taste receptors and indirectly to blood concentration of aldosterone which appears to control salivary electrolyte concentration (Fregly, 1967b; Blair-West *et al.*, 1963; Frawley and Thorn, 1951). Blood levels of aldosterone are most likely increased by administration of oral contraceptives. Thus, increases in plasma renin activity and plasma levels of renin substrate, as well as an increased rate of excretion of aldosterone, are reported for women ingesting oral contraceptives (Crane and Harris, 1969a,b, 1974; Saruta *et al.*, 1970; Weinberger *et al.*, 1969) and rats administered estradiol (Llaurado *et al.*, 1962) or diethystilbesterol (Menard *et al.*, 1970). It is also possible that the salt appetite and reduced preference threshold are induced by central nervous mechanisms responding to either altered aldosterone or electrolyte concentrations of blood or to altered extracellular fluid volume. Changes in body sodium content resulting from increased renal sodium loss induced by both ethynyl estradiol and norethynodrel may also play a role in the rat (Table III).

The results of Experiment 4 favor a role for the adrenal gland in oral contraceptive-induced NaCl appetite. Adrenalectomized rats failed to increase their intake of NaCl solution when administered Enovid, and its components, norethynodrel and ethynyl estradiol (Table V).

Since administration of estrogenic steroids can induce fluid retention, at least in the dog, by acting on the renal tubule at a site different from that of the mineralocorticoids (Johnson *et al.*, 1970), an additional objective of Experiment 4 was to determine whether fluid retention, as assessed by increases in body weight, could be observed in the estrogen-treated, adrenalectomized rats. Increases in body weight did not occur (Table V). However, since estrogen-treated rats seldom grow at a normal rate, it is difficult to assess by body weight gain whether fluid retention contributes significantly to the induction of the NaCl appetite (Fig. 3).

The results of Experiment 3 indicate that chronic administration of ethynyl estradiol is accompanied by an increased rate of excretion of a sodium load (Table III). The first significant increase was measured during the fifth week of treatment but could have occurred sometime between the first and fifth weeks of treatment. Since the NaCl appetite occurred during the first week of drug treatment, the results suggest, but do not prove, that the appetite for NaCl occurs prior to the occurrence of increased loss of sodium into urine. However, the possibility that the increased urinary sodium loss accompanying chronic administration of ethynyl estradiol supports the NaCl appetite of these rats seems a likely one. The latter results are of particular interest in view of the reported effect of estrogen on sodium exchange in dogs (Johnson *et al.*, 1970, 1977; Davis *et al.*, 1974). Whether the increase in sodium excretion requires an initial extracellular volume expansion in rats is not known at present but is currently under study in this laboratory.

When the components of Enovid, i.e., ethynyl estradiol and norethynodrel, were administered alone, both appeared to increase spontaneous intake of NaCl solution although the increase was considerably more variable for norethynodrel and never reached a level of statistical significance (Table II). However, treatment with norethynodrel was accompanied by a significantly increased urinary sodium loss during e diuretic studies conducted in Experiment 3 (Table III). These results with norethynodrel, a synthetic testosterone derivative and progestational agent, are of interest because progesterone, the naturally occurring progestational agent, is known to inhibit the renal effects of aldosterone (Landau and

Lugibihl, 1958) as well as other renal tubular mechanisms concerned with sodium reabsorption (Oparil *et al.*, 1974). Medroxyprogesterone is a synthetic progestational agent and derivative of progesterone that is reported to have no effect on either renin substrate concentration of plasma or on urinary aldosterone excretion in women (Crane and Harris, 1969a, 1974). In a delay of menses test, which measures progestational activity in women, norethynodrel was approximately three times more potent than medroxyprogesterone acetate (Goodman and Gilman, 1970). Although the progestational activity of a contraceptive steroid in women is not necessarily related to its activity in rats, the dose of medroxyprogesterone used in Experiment 5 was chosen to be approximately ten times larger than the daily amount of norethynodrel ingested with the minimally effective dose of Enovid (1.25 mg/kg of food). The doses of medroxyprogesterone used failed to affect intake of NaCl solution despite the fact that they were large enough to account for a possible difference in potency between norethynodrel and medroxyprogesterone (Table VI). However, they were not high enough to induce adrenal atrophy and block release of ACTH (Givner and Rocheford, 1972). Doses 30 to 80 times higher than those used here would be required for this to occur. These results, while not conclusive of themselves, also support a role for the adrenal gland in the increased NaCl intake induced by the progestational agent, norethynodrel.

Thus, of the possible mechanisms by which an increase in the spontaneous NaCl intake can be induced by oral contraceptive treatment of rats, the results of the studies reported here favor an effect mediated, at least initially, by the adrenal cortex. However, the participation of changes in extracellular volume and of increased urinary sodium loss as a result of treatment cannot be ruled out by present data and remain for additional study. The possibility that the proximate physiological change responsible for induction of an appetite for NaCl solution is a change in salivary sodium concentration remains attractive but will require additional experimental support (Thrasher and Fregly, this volume).

V. SUMMARY

Dietary administration of the oral contraceptive, Enovid, at 1.25, 2.50, and 5.00 mg/kg of food to female rats induced a spontaneous appetite for NaCl solution within 1 week of drug administration. The appetite was present for isotonic as well as hypertonic NaCl solutions. Administration of Enovid (7.5 mg/kg of food) was also accompanied by a reduction in the preference threshold for NaCl. Treated rats could distinguish between distilled water and a NaCl solution when the latter was 0.015 moles/liter compared with 0.030 moles/liter for control rats.

The adrenal gland may play a role in the increased NaCl intake of oral contraceptive-treated rats since chronic administration of norethynodrel and ethynyl estradiol, the components of Enovid, failed to affect NaCl intake of adrenalectomized rats.

Other studies in intact rats suggest that both norethynodrel and ethynyl estradiol induce an increase in spontaneous NaCl intake. Both also increase sodium loss following acute ip loading with NaCl solutions. The results suggest that the increased NaCl intake may precede the increased sodium loss.

Although the progestational agent, norethynodrel, appeared to increase NaCl intake, administration of medroxyprogesterone failed to do so. Thus, progestational agents differ with respect to their effect on spontaneous NaCl intake in the rat. The differences may be related to their respective effects on the adrenal cortex. Progesterone and norethynodrel are known to increase adrenal cortical secretion of aldosterone while medroxyprogesterone, in the doses used here, does not. These results suggest a role for the adrenal cortex in initiating the increase in intake of NaCl solution.

ACKNOWLEDGMENT

Supported by Grant HL 14526-07 from the National Heart, Lung and Blood Institute.

REFERENCES

Blair-West, J. R., Coghlan, J. P., Denton, D. A., Goding, J. R., and Wright, R. D. (1963). The effect of aldosterone, cortisol and corticosterone upon the sodium and potassium content of sheep's parotid saliva. *J. Clin. Invest.* **42,** 484–495.

Crane, M. G., and Harris, J. J. (1969a). Plasma renin activity and aldosterone excretion rate in normal subjects. I. Effect of ethynyl estradiol and medroxyprogesterone acetate. *J. Clin. Endocrinol. Metab.* **29,** 550–557.

Crane, M. G., and Harris, J. J. (1969b). Plasma renin activity and aldosterone excretion rate in normal subjects. II. Effect of oral contraceptive agents. *J. Clin. Endocrinol. Metab.* **29,** 558–562.

Crane, M. G., and Harris, J. J. (1974). Effect of estrogens and gestagens on the renin–aldosterone system. *In* "Oral Contraceptives and High Blood Pressure" (M. J. Fregly and M. S. Fregly, eds.), pp. 100–117. Dolphin Press, Gainesville, Florida.

Davis, J. O., Johnson, J. A., and Taylor, A. A. (1974). Mechanisms of salt and water retention during pregnancy in the dog. *In* "Oral Contraceptives and High Blood Pressure" (M. J. Fregly and M. S. Fregly, eds.), pp. 247–257. Dolphin Press, Gainesville, Florida.

Dzuik, P. J., and Cook, B. (1966). Passage of steroids through silicone rubber. *Endocrinology* **78,** 208–211.

Frawley, P. F., and Thorn, G. W. (1951). The relation of the salivary Na/K ratio to adrenal cortical activity. *Proc. Clin. ACTH Conf., 2nd, 1950* Vol. 1, pp. 115–122.

Fregly, M. J. (1960). A simple and accurate feeding device for rats. *J. Appl. Physiol.* **15,** 539.

Fregly, M. J. (1967a). Effect of hydrochlorothiazide on preference threshold of rats for NaCl solutions. *Proc. Soc. Exp. Biol. Med.* **125,** 1079–1084.

Fregly, M. J. (1967b). The role of hormones in regulation of salt intake by rats. *In* "The Chemical Senses and Nutrition" (M. R. Kare and O. Maller, eds.), pp. 115-138. Johns Hopkins Univ. Press, Baltimore, Maryland.

Fregly, M. J. (1969). Preference threshold and appetite for NaCl solution as affected by propylthiouracil and deoxycorticosterine acetate in rats. *Olfaction Taste, Proc. Int. Symp., 3rd, 1968* pp. 554-561.

Fregly, M. J. (1972). Effect of an oral contraceptive on spontaneous running activity, salt appetite and blood pressure of ovariectomized rats. *J. Pharmacol. Exp. Ther.* **182,** 335-343.

Fregly, M. J. (1973). Effect of an oral contraceptive on NaCl appetite and preference threshold in rats. *Pharmacol., Biochem. Behav.* **1,** 61-65.

Fregly, M. J., and Newsome, D. G. (1974). Oral contraceptive-induced salt-appetite in rats. *In* "Oral Contraceptives and High Blood Pressure" (M. J. Fregly and M. S. Fregly, eds.), pp. 141-158. Dolphin Press, Gainesville, Florida.

Fregly, M. J., and Waters, I. W. (1965). Effect of propylthiouracil on preference threshold of rats for NaCl solutions. *Proc. Soc. Exp. Biol. Med.* **120,** 637-640.

Givner, M. L., and Rocheford, J. G. (1972). Effect of synthetic progesterones and estradiol 17β on adrenal function in the rat. *Endocrinology* **90,** 1238-1244.

Goodman, L. S., and Gilman, A., eds. (1970). "The Pharmacological Basis of Therapeutics," 4th ed., p. 1555. MacMillan, New York.

Herxheimer, A., and Woodbury, D. M. (1960). The effect of deoxycorticosterone on salt and sucrose preference thresholds and drinking behaviour in rats. *J. Physiol. (London)* **151,** 253-260.

Johnson, J. A., Davis, J. O., Baumber, J. S., and Schneider, G. (1970). Effects of estrogen and progesterone on electrolyte balance in normal dogs. *Am. J. Physiol.* **210,** 1691-1697.

Johnson, J. A., Davis, J. O., Hanson, R. C., Stubbs, D. H., and Keitzer, W. F. (1977). Acute sodium-retaining effects of estrogens in dogs. *Proc. Soc. Exp. Biol. Med.* **156,** 241-246.

Kincl, F. A., Benagiano, G., and Angee, I. (1968). Sustained release preparations. 1. Diffusion of various steroids through polymer membranes. *Steroids* **11,** 673-680.

Landau, R. L., and Lugibihl, K. (1958). Inhibition of the sodium-retaining influence of aldosterone by progesterone. *J. Clin. Endocrinol. Metab.* **18,** 1237-1245.

Lazarow, A. (1954). Methods for quantitative measurement of water intake. *Methods Med. Res.* **6,** 225-229.

Llaurado, J. G., Claus, J. L., and Trunnell, J. B. (1962). Aldosterone excretion in feces of rats treated with estradiol. *Endocrinology* **71,** 598-604.

Menard, J., Malmejac, A., and Milliez, P. (1970). Influence of diethylstilbesterol on the renin-angiotensin system of male rats. *Endocrinology* **86,** 774-780.

Oparil, S., Ehrlich, E. N., and Lindheimer, M. D. (1974). Effects of progesterone on volume-homeostasis in man: Alterations in intrarenal sodium reabsorption, aldosterone excretion, and renin activity. *In* "Oral Contraceptives and High Blood Pressure" (M. J. Fregly and M. S. Fregly, eds.), pp. 170-183. Dolphin Press, Gainesville, Florida.

Richter, C. P. (1939). Salt taste threshold of normal and adrenalectomized rats. *Endocrinology* **24,** 367-371.

Saruta, T., Saade, G. A., and Kaplan, N. M. (1970). A possible mechanism for hypertension induced by oral contraceptives; diminished feedback suppression of renin release. *Arch. Intern. Med.* **126,** 621-626.

Snedecor, G. W., and Cochran, W. G. (1956). "Statistical Methods," p. 333. Iowa State University Press, Ames.

Weinberger, M. H., Collins, R. D., Dowdy, A. J., Nokes, G. W., and Luetscher, J. A. (1969). Hypertension induced by oral contraceptives containing estrogen and gestagen. *Ann. Intern. Med.* **71,** 891-901.

PART IV
NEUROLOGICAL ASPECTS OF SALT INTAKE

Chapter 19

Membrane Transitions in Taste Receptor Cell Activation by Sodium Salts

GREGORY MOOSER

I. INTRODUCTION

A number of models have been proposed to account for the initial events in salt activation of taste receptor cells (Price and DeSimone, 1977). Evidence presented in this chapter does not refute the major hypotheses supporting most of the models, but it does implicate the involvement of a membrane transition in salt stimulation. More specifically, the transition is based on an equilibrium between an active and an inactive state of the membrane. Differences between the two states can involve alterations in ion affinity for fixed sites on the membrane as well as alterations in ion permeation properties. For convenience, the model is discussed in the context of ion interaction with fixed sites (Beidler, 1954), although the concept and data do not exclude other mechanisms of

BIOLOGICAL AND BEHAVIORAL
ASPECTS OF SALT INTAKE

ISBN 0-12-397750-9

stimulus-dependent cell depolarization (Eyzaguirre *et al.*, 1972; Kamo *et al.*, 1974; DeSimone and Price, 1976). Since stimulus interaction with fixed sites is coupled to functional events, the sites will be considered, in the broadest sense, as receptors.

One of the earliest models with experimental support was proposed by Beidler (1954) who found, using summated chorda tympani activity in rats, that the form of salt concentration–response profiles was consistent with a Langmuir isotherm and, therefore, could be explained on the basis of formation of a simple salt–receptor complex as the initial event in receptor activation. The publication of this model in the early 1950's was not only pertinent to taste perception, but has since proved to be valid, with some modification, for a large number of membrane receptor systems (Kahn, 1976).

This chapter describes an allosteric mechanism as a model for activation of taste receptors. It is a site occupation model which can be considered as a modification of the Beidler model based on relatively recent concepts in membrane receptor activation. A reevaluation of summated chorda tympani activity similar to the measurements made by Beidler is warranted for several reasons. First, concentration–response profiles deviate slightly from a simple Langmuir adsorption isotherm. Some of the data cannot be adequately fit to the equations for a single site model; reciprocal plots, used as a linear transformation of the equations, do not give a data distribution pattern which is linear throughout the concentration range. Second, certain characteristics of sodium salt activation, such as reversible anion inhibition and irreversible inhibition by certain protein modification reagents (Mooser and Lambuth, 1977), can be explained more conveniently on the basis of a multiple state allosteric mechanism as opposed to a single state mechanism. In addition, since two important events (stimulus binding and a conformational transition) are implicit in all allosteric mechanisms, they have understandably been proposed to account for the initial activation of several membrane receptor systems (Edelstein, 1972; Limbird and Lefkowitz, 1976; DeMeyts, 1976).

II. THEORY

Of the several published allosteric models, that found to be most applicable to taste receptor activation is the concerted transition model of Monod, Wyman, and Changeux (1965; Rubin and Changeux, 1966). It involves an equilibrium between an active (R) and an inactive (T) state of the receptor. The position of the equilibrium in the absence of stimulus is defined solely by an equilibrium or allosteric constant (L) as indicated in Eq. (1).

$$L = T/R = \text{inactive state/active state} \tag{1}$$

For the system to be functional, the allosteric constant must be high enough for the major portion of receptors to be in the inactive state when no stimuli are present. The equilibrium, however, can be easily displaced toward the active state by addition of a stimulus which has a higher affinity for the active state compared to the inactive state. The model is shown schematically in Fig. 1. It is important to note that the degree of activation is determined by the total number of receptors in the R state. All R state receptors have identical activity whether they contain no or multiple equivalents of bound stimulus. Therefore, the level of activity at any stimulus concentration, S, is related to the proportion of receptors in the R state, $\bar{R}$, and is a function of the equilibrium parameters as defined in Eq. (2),

$$\bar{R} = \frac{(1+\alpha)^n}{(1+\alpha)^n + L(1+c\alpha)^n} \quad (2)$$

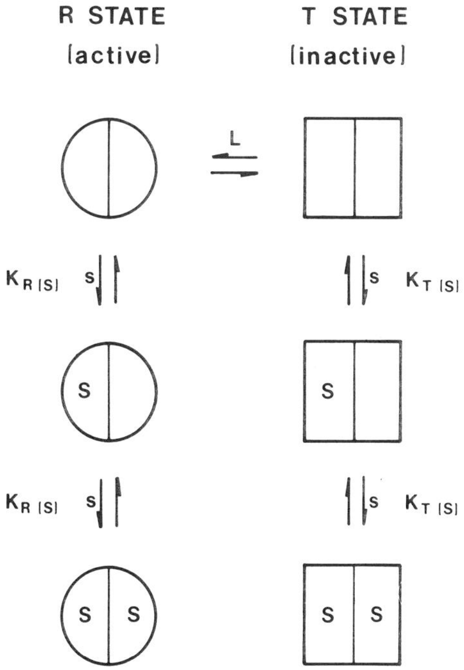

Fig. 1. A schematic representation of the equilibrium between the active state, R, and inactive state, T, in the allosteric model of Monod, Wyman and Changeux. Two equivalent binding sites per receptor unit are shown. The equilibrium in the absence of stimulus favors the inactive state. Addition of stimulus with a higher affinity for the active compared to the inactive state results in displacement of the equilibrium in favor of the active state. All R state receptors, with or without bound stimulus, are equally active.

where α is the normalized stimulus concentration $(S/K_{S(R)})$*, c is the nonexclusive binding coefficient or ratio or R state to T state dissociation constant $[K_{S(R)}/K_{S(T)}]$, and n is the number of equivalent binding sites per receptor (e.g., $n = 2$ in Fig. 1).

III. APPLICATION TO TASTE RECEPTOR CELL ACTIVATION BY SODIUM SALTS

While the proportion of R state receptors in the absence of stimulus is dependent solely on the value of L, a finite number of receptors is always in the activated state as shown in Eq. (3).

$$\bar{R} = \frac{1}{1+L} \text{ at } S = 0 \tag{3}$$

Generally, L is high enough for a very large majority of receptors to be in the inactive state at zero stimulus concentration, but this does not appear to be the case in the taste receptor system where the calculated value for L was found to be 8.8, resulting in about 10% of the receptors in the R state at $S = 0$. Thus, when measuring receptor activity relative to a baseline in the absence of stimulus, the observed fraction of R state receptors, $\bar{R}_{obs}$ is:

$$\bar{R}_{obs} = \frac{(1+\alpha)^n}{(1+\alpha)^n + L(1+c\alpha)^n} - \frac{1}{1+L} \tag{4}$$

In addition to being a required part of the equation, this may account for the relatively high spontaneous activity observed in whole nerve chorda tympani recordings as well as the potential to decrease activity below baseline with certain potassium salts (Beidler, 1962).

Both reversible inhibition of the sodium response by organic anions (acetate and propionate) and irreversible inhibition by protein modification reagents, such as dimethyl(2-hydroxy-5-nitrobenzyl)sulfonium bromide (HNB-dmS), can be theoretically accounted for by the allosteric model.

The basis of the model is best established if the receptor unit is conceptualized to include a multimolecular section or the entire receptor cell membrane where

*The dissociation constants are identified with a subscript indicating either stimulus, S, or inhibitor, I, binding to either the R or T state of the receptor, e.g., $K_{S(R)}$ for stimulus binding to the R state of the receptor, and $K_{I(T)}$ for inhibitor binding to the T state of the receptor.

†The ratio of dissociation constants (nonexclusive binding coefficient) is as important as the absolute values of the constants since the degree and direction of displacement of the equilibrium is a function of the ratio. Ligands with a nonexclusive binding coefficient less than 1 are receptor activators, and those with coefficients greater than 1 are receptor inhibitors. If the value is equal to 1, no displacement of the equilibrium results. Equation 2 reduces to $1/(1+L)$ when either $c = 1$ or $S = 0$. This is a consideration in chloride binding as discussed in the text.

the transition between the active and inactive states involves an active and inactive form of the membrane. In this context, sodium activation would result if sodium affinity is higher when the membrane is in the active state compared to the inactive state. By an analogous mechanism, organic anions can counteract sodium activation if they bind at a site independent of sodium but with a higher affinity for the inactive state compared to the active state. Receptor activators simply displace the equilibrium toward the active state by virtue of a higher affinity for the active state, and receptor inhibitors displace the equilibrium toward the inactive state by virtue of a higher affinity for the inactive state. The algebraic expression that relates the observed activity to the equilibrium parameters when an independently acting receptor inhibitor is included is given in Eq. (5),

$$\bar{R}_{\text{obs}} = \frac{(1+\alpha)^n\,(1+\beta)^m}{(1+\alpha)^n\,(1+\beta)^m + L(1+c\alpha)^n\,(1+d\beta)^n} - \frac{1}{1+L} \quad (5)$$

where β is the normalized inhibitor concentration $[I/K_{I(R)}]$, d is the nonexclusive binding coefficient for the inhibitor $[K_{I(R)}/K_{I(T)}]$, and m is the number of equivalent sites that bind inhibitor. Frequently, m is equal to n; however, in taste receptor cells where membrane transitions can involve nonreceptor macromolecules which are integrally related to transformations of the receptor itself, an inhibitor may bind at a site remote from the receptor which places constraints on receptor transformation. In this case, an equivalence of n and m would only be fortuitous. Neither n nor m represent the total number of ion binding sites on a cell membrane. Rather, they refer to the smallest common denominator of the system. In the analyses presented here, the value of n which provided the best fit to the data was 2, and the value of m was 1, although 2 also gave a reasonable approximation. In all the analyses, $n = 2$ and $m = 1$ were used.

Irreversible inhibition by HNB-dmS can also be accounted for by this mechanism. HNB-dmS reacts with taste receptor cells by a simple bimolecular reaction with the receptor cell membrane. In general, a finite but reduced ($24 \pm 3\%$ at 0.3 M NaCl) response to sodium stimulation remains after HNB-dmS treatment, even though inhibition is irreversible (Mooser and Lambuth, 1977). The inhibition and residual activity may be a consequence of stabilization of the inactive state which would be mathematically manifest as an increase in the value of the allosteric constant. Sodium and organic anion interaction with the cell membrane need not be altered by HNB-dmS; treatment only has to increase the energy (or concentration of ions) required for transition to the activated state.

The validity of the allosteric model as an explanation of sodium salt stimulation in rats is evaluated here by analysis of the summated chorda tympani nerve response to salt stimulation. Concentration–response profiles of NaCl and Na propionate, before and after treatment with HNB-dmS, are examined for consistency with the appropriate allosteric equations.

IV. MATERIALS AND METHODS

All measurements are steady-state summated chorda tympani recordings using male Holtzman strain white rats. The recording procedures have been described previously (Mooser, 1976). The magnitude of the steady-state activity remained essentially constant for 120 seconds or longer and was generally measured a few minutes after a constant stimulus application. All measurements were linearly reduced to values relative to 100 for 0.3 *M* NaCl. Preparations were discarded after any significant change in the response to the standard. Salt stimuli were reagent grade and prepared in distilled water without further purification. All solutions were adjusted to pH 7.0 prior to use. HNB-dmS was obtained from Pierce Chemical Company. Inhibition was performed in 35 m*M* HNB-dmS as previously described (Mooser and Lambuth, 1977). Data reduction was performed by computer-assisted nonlinear least squares regression.

V. RESULTS

Figure 2 shows concentration-response profiles for NaCl and sodium propionate (NaPr) in both untreated and HNB-dmS treated preparations. In the untreated

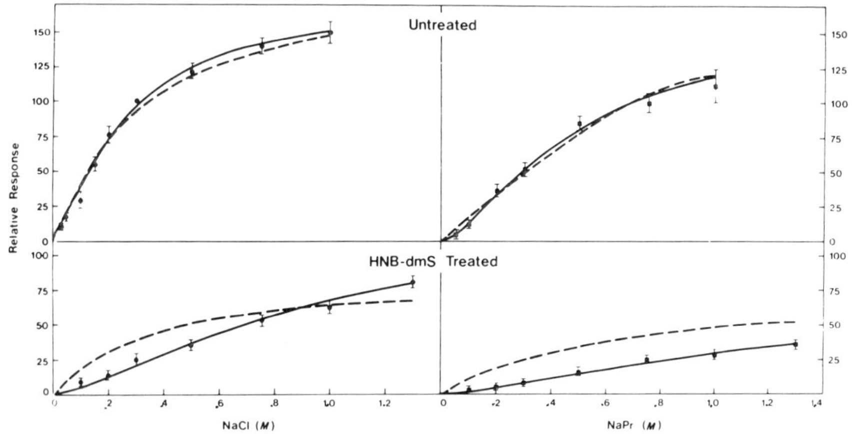

Fig. 2. Concentration–response profiles of the summated chorda tympani activity after taste receptor stimulation by NaCl (circles) and sodium propionate (squares). The data were generated from twelve preparations of untreated animals and eight treated animals. Data from all animals are normalized to a value of 100 for the response to 0.3 *M* NaCl in the untreated preparation. The inhibited preparations (bottom) were treated with 35 m*M* HNB-dmS at pH 4.0 for 20 minutes followed by a 10-minute water rinse prior to stimulation. The data points are shown with ± standard error of the mean. *Solid lines:* regressions based on the allosteric mechanism [Eqs. (4) and (5)]; *Dashed lines:* regressions based on a single state mechanism [Eq. (6)].

preparations, the data are well resolved by the regressions on the allosteric equations indicated by the solid curve. Equation (4) was used for the NaCl profile, and Eq. (5) was used for the sodium propionate profile with the organic anion treated as an allosteric inhibitor. In the latter case, the allosteric constant and the sodium ion dependent parameters [$K_{S(R)}$ and c] were maintained within ±15% of the values determined for NaCl by Eq. (4).

Analysis of the NaCl data by the single state mechanism was based on a Langmuir isotherm given in Eq. (6) as proposed by Beidler (1954),

$$R_{obs} = \frac{R_{max} S}{K_R + S} \tag{6}$$

where R_{obs} is the observed response, R_{max} is the maximum response, and K_R is the receptor–sodium salt dissociation constant. The equation, as was shown over 20 years ago (Beidler, 1954), adequately approximates the data in the untreated preparations, but not quite as well as the allosteric equations. When plotted as a linear transformation of Eq. (6) (Beidler, 1954), the data points were slightly curved.

Regressions were then used to examine the concentration–response profiles after treatment with HNB-dmS. The regression analyses using allosteric Eqs. 4 and 5 are shown in the lower half of Fig. 2 and use all of the parameter values (±15%) determined in the uninhibited preparations except the allosteric constant, L, which is increased about tenfold.

When the single state equation was used for the inhibited profiles, a reasonable approximation to the data was not possible. In this analysis, salt ion affinities, but not R_{max}, were maintained within ±15% of the values obtained in the uninhibited preparation. The alternative situation in which R_{max} is maintained constant and the values for the ion affinities are permitted to vary, also did not provide an acceptable fit. This possibility, however, is less likely. It has been shown that NaCl does not affect the rate of HNB-dmS inhibition, indicating no significant relationship exists between stimulus affinity and inhibition (Mooser and Lambuth, 1977). For the same reason, a partial competitive mechanism is not consistent with available data.

If the sodium salt response from taste receptors is consistent with an allosteric mechanism, it should be possible to predict the pattern of the response from a mixed stimulus solution. The experiment designed to test this involved stimulation with a series of solutions which contained a constant concentration of sodium ions, but variable concentrations of chloride and propionate ions. The results of the experiment are shown in Fig. 3 with sodium constant at 0.75 *M*, chloride varying from 0.75 to 0.0 *M*, and propionate equal to 0.75 *M* − {*chloride*}.

An initial regression analysis based on the parameter values determined from Fig. 3 did not provide an acceptable fit to the data as shown by the dashed curve.

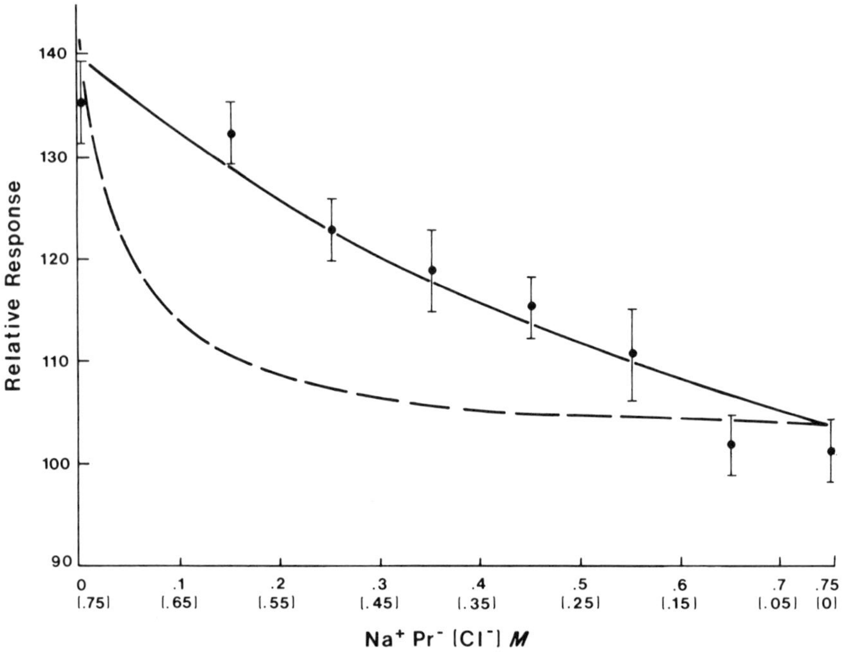

Fig. 3. Response profile of steady-state summated chorda tympani activity after stimulation with NaCl–NaPr mixtures. The data were generated from five rat preparations. Sodium ion and chloride plus propionate ions were constant at 0.75 *M*. The vertical lines are ± standard error of the mean. *Dashed line:* nonlinear regression based on the allosteric equation without consideration of chloride binding; *Solid line:* nonlinear regression based on the allosteric equation modified to incorporate chloride binding with a dissociation constant of 0.074 *M* for both states.

The allosteric mechanism has an interesting characteristic which can account for this discrepancy. This relates to the fact that any ligand that binds with equal affinity to the active and inactive states of the membrane does not affect the level of activation [see footnote (indicated by dagger)]. A high concentration of a ligand may bind to all available sites but will cause neither activation nor inhibition unless there is a different affinity for the two states. In the analysis of the NaCl data in Fig. 2, chloride ion was not considered because the data were easily resolved without this parameter. However, it is impossible to distinguish the absence of chloride binding from binding with equal affinity to both states. This is best demonstrated by noting that Eq. (5) reduces to Eq. (4) when $d = 1$. While the data in Fig. 2 do not permit a distinction between the absence of binding and equivalent binding to the two states, there would be a significant effect on the mixed stimulus experiment due to competition between the two anions if they bind to the same site. This possibility was tested by nonlinear regression on the data in Fig. 3 using the sodium and propionate binding parameters calculated

TABLE I

Equilibrium Parameters for NaCl and NaPr Binding before and after Treatment with HNB-dmS[a]

	Sodium parameters		Propionate parameters		
Stimulus	$K_{S(R)}$	c	$K_{I(R)}$	d	L^b
Untreated					
NaCl	0.098	0.060			8.8
NaPr	0.099	0.057	0.057	2.6	8.8
HNB-dmS treated					
NaCl	0.097	0.061			91.2
NaPr	0.102	0.067	0.054	2.5	91.2
NaCl–NaPr mixture	0.099	0.057	0.057	2.6	8.8

[a] $K_{S(R)}$ and $K_{I(R)}$ are in molar units; c, d, and L have no units. The NaCl parameter values are derived from Eq. (4) and the NaPr parameters from Eq. (5) based on the data in Figs. 2 and 3. In the NaCl–NaPr mixture regression, chloride ion binding with a dissociation constant of 0.074 *M* for both states was included.

[b] The value of the allosteric constant was not permitted to vary in the regression except after HNB-dmS treatment.

from Fig. 2 with the assumption that chloride binds to the propionate site but with equal affinity for both states. The data are reasonably well resolved by this regression as shown by the solid curve. Thus, the magnitude of the response from a mixture of NaCl and NaPr is consistent with that predicated from the response from each stimulus alone.

The consistency of the data with the allosteric mechanism is demonstrated in Table I where the values of the experimental parameters from the nonlinear regressions of the data in Figs. 2 and 3 are given. Note that the values of the sodium binding parameters [$K_{S(R)}$ and c] are independent of the anion (chloride and propionate), and both the sodium binding parameters and the propionate parameters [$K_{I(R)}$ and d] are independent of HNB-dmS treatment. The large decrease in activity after HMB-dmS treatment is resolved by an approximately tenfold increase in the value of the allosteric constant (L). The value of the nonexclusive binding coefficient for sodium (c) is less than 1 as expected for a receptor activator; a value greater than 1 for the analogous propionate parameter (d) is consistent with a receptor inhibitor.

VI. DISCUSSION

The validity of an allosteric mechanism as a model for sodium salt activation of taste receptor cells is enhanced by the use of three experimental approaches which have overlapping characteristics. First, NaCl and NaPr stimulation vary in anion effects, yet, because of the common cation, possess equivalent sodium activation parameters. As noted in Table I, the reversible decrease in activity caused by propionate can be resolved easily by incorporation of an independent anion site with an affinity for propionate which is somewhat higher (about 2.5-fold) in the inactive state. Distinct anion and cation binding sites have been previously proposed (Beidler, 1967) with the former serving an inhibitory role. Since the inhibitory effect increases as the anion becomes more hydrophobic (Beidler, 1954), it is reasonable to suggest that the membrane around the anion site is slightly more hydrophobic in the inactive than the active state. Second, irreversible inhibition by HNB-dmS can be accounted for without proposing any alterations in ion affinities. This is expected since HNB-dmS inhibition is independent of salt stimulus parameters. The observation that the concentration of stimulus has no effect on the rate of HNB-dmS inhibition demonstrates that there is no interaction between the site of HNB-dmS reaction and the site of sodium stimulation (Mooser and Lambuth, 1977). The range of activity in HNB-dmS-treated preparations is severely limited because of the magnitude of inhibition. Nevertheless, the reduced activity can be readily resolved by a tenfold increase in the allosteric constant without invoking any significant changes in salt binding constants. Finally, the magnitude of activity of mixed stimulus solutions which contain a constant concentration of sodium ions and a variable ratio of chloride to propionate ions is consistent with all equilibrium parameters calculated from the previous experiments. The one modification required to resolve the data involves a weak, but significant, chloride ion interaction at the propionate site with equal chloride affinity for both states. This further supports the importance of the hydrophobic portion of the anion in inhibition. Chloride can bind to the propionate site, but a lack of hydrophobic interaction eliminates any potential inhibition.

One difficulty in establishing a quantitative mechanism for taste receptor activation is that all available methods for monitoring salt occupancy are indirect. No isolated salt receptor preparations exist, and the apparent dissociation constant for sodium binding ($\sim$0.2 *M*) is too high to design a feasible approach. Beidler's original mechanism and the allosteric mechanism presented here are based on the assumption of a linear relationship between receptor occupancy and summated chorda tympani activity. In other systems, such as the eel electroplax, apparent dissociation constants based on *in situ* measurements of receptor potentials can be compared to dissociation constants determined from direct ligand binding measurements (Popot *et al.*, 1976). While direct salt binding measurements are not yet possible with taste receptor cells, a relationship between receptor potential and steady-state chorda tympani activity has been demonstrated (Kimura and Beidler, 1961; Sato, 1976). The possibility that this relationship is linear is supported by inhibition studies with irreversible inhibitors which act directly on receptor cells (Mooser, 1976; Mooser and Lambuth, 1977). Inhibition follows classical pseudo first order kinetics, suggesting summated neural activity is a direct function of events which occur at the receptor cell.

Only measurements which were clearly in the steady-state portion of the response gave results which were consistent with an allosteric mechanism. Analysis of independently measured NaCl responses, kindly provided by Dr. David V. Smith, was consistent with the model using measurements made 120 seconds after stimulus application. Measurements from the transient portion of the response did not adequately fit the model.

It is important to emphasize that this type of model analysis can only establish a consistency with the experimental data and provide a basis to analyze results obtained from different experimental approaches. While only one out of twenty-two allosteric type models considered in the course of this study adequately fit all of the data, many more are possible. For example, anion inhibition resulting from binding of neutral ion pairs in a low dielectric region (DeSimone and Price, 1976), as opposed to absorption to an inactive state of the membrane, cannot be excluded. An appropriate assignment of parameter values in the allosteric equations which are modified to include anion–cation association may prove to resolve the data adequately.

However, the unique aspect of this mechanism which has not been considered to date is the requirement for an *equilibrium* between distinct active and inactive states of the membrane. The model does not exclude the possibility that ion interaction leads to depolarization through effects on surface charge and/or ion permeability (Eyzaguirre *et al.*, 1972; Kamo *et al.*, 1974; DeSimone and Price, 1976), as long as the events involve a conformational transition between two membrane states. In particular, HNB-dmS inhibition results are most readily explained on this basis. The reagent, under the conditions of inhibition, is selective for tryptophan and cysteine residues in proteins (Horton and Tucker, 1970), does not react with phospholipids, and does not form charged modification products (Horton and Koshland, 1972; Heinrich *et al.*, 1973). While HNB-dmS would not be expected to alter membrane potential through a direct modification of surface charge, it could cause inhibition through incorporation of a reaction product in the membrane which alters the energy required for transition to the active state as suggested here. It is the transition itself which is responsible for a change in membrane properties and cell depolarization.

Through the use of an analogous approach, allosteric events have been implicated in the activation of the Na^+ ionophore in neuroblastoma cells (Catterall, 1977). Alkaloid neurotoxins activate the ionophore through preferential binding to the active state of the membrane, and scorpion toxin enhances activation by altering the allosteric constant. The former effect involves a mechanism comparable to the proposed events which cause anion inhibition, and the latter effect is similar to that proposed for HNB-dmS inhibition. Related arguments support an allosteric mechanism for acetylcholine receptor activation in cholinergic membranes (Edelstein, 1972).

The scope of this report is limited to taste receptor cell activation by sodium salts. Stimulation by potassium salts at low concentration has an interesting characteristic that can be considered in the context of the allosteric mechanism. Potassium salts of hydrophobic anions, such as potassium benzoate, decrease the magnitude of summated activity below the level of a water rinse response (Beidler, 1962). This could result as a consequence of the observation that the calculated value of the allosteric constant is 8.8 (Table I) which results in about 10% of the receptors in the active state in the absence of stimulus (Eq. 3). At low concentrations, a stimulus could decrease the proportion of active receptors if the nonexclusive binding coefficient is slightly less than that calculated for sodium. This possibility is under consideration as part of an analysis of the response from various potassium salts and will be treated in a subsequent report.

ACKNOWLEDGMENT

This work was supported in part by grant number DE 03739 from the National Institutes of Health, National Institute of Dental Research.

REFERENCES

Beidler, L. M. (1954). A theory of taste stimulation. *J. Gen. Physiol.* **34,** 133–139.

Beidler, L. M. (1962). Taste receptor stimulation. *Prog. Biophys. Biophys. Chem.* **12,** 107–151.

Beidler, L. M. (1967). Anion influences on taste receptor responses. *Wenner-Gren Cent. Int. Symp. Ser.* **8,** 509–534.

Catterall, W. A. (1977). Activation of the action potential Na^+ ionophore by neurotoxins: An allosteric model. *J. Biol. Chem.* **252,** 8669–8676.

DeMeyts, P. (1976). Cooperative properties of hormone receptors in cell membranes. *J. Supramol. Struct.* **4,** 241–258.

DeSimone, J. A., and Price, S. (1976). A model for the stimulation of taste receptor cells by salt. *Biophys. J.* **16,** 869–881.

Edelstein, S. J. (1972). An allosteric mechanism for the acetylcholine receptor. *Biochem. Biophys. Res. Commun.* **48,** 1160–1165.

Eyzaguirre, C., Fidone, S., and Zapata, P. (1972). Membrane potentials recorded from the mucosa of the toad's tongue during chemical stimulation. *J. Physiol. (London)* 515–532.

Heinrich, C. P., Adam, S., and Arnold, W. (1973). The reaction of dimethyl(2-hydroxy-5-nitrobenzyl)sulfonium bromide with *N*-acetyl-L-tryptophan amide. *FEBS Lett.* **33,** 181–183.

Horton, H. R., and Koshland, D. E., Jr. (1972). Modification of proteins with active benzyl halides. *In* "Methods in Enzymology" (C. H. W. hirc and S. N. Timasheff, eds.), Vol. 25, pp. 468–482. Academic Press, New York.

Horton, R. H., and Tucker, W. P. (1970). Dimethyl(2-hydroxy-5-nitrobenzyl) sulfonium salts: Water soluble environmentally sensitive reagents. *J. Biol. Chem.* **425,** 3397–3401.

Kahn, C. R. (1976). Membrane receptors for hormones and neurotransmitters. *J. Cell Biol.* **20,** 261–286.

Kamo, N., Miyade, M., Kurihara, K., and Kobatake, Y. (1974). Physicochemical studies of taste reception. I. Model membrane stimulating taste receptor potential in response to stimuli of salts, acids, and distilled water. *Biochim. Biophys. Acta* **367,** 1–10.

Kimura, K., and Beidler, L. M. (1961). Microelectrode study of taste receptors of rat and hampster. *J. Cell. Comp. Physiol.* **58,** 131–139.

Limbird, L. E., and Lefkowitz, R. J. (1976). Negative cooperativity among β-adrenergic receptors in frog erythrocytes. *J. Biol. Chem.* **251,** 5007–5014.

Monod, J., Wyman, J., and Changeux, J.-P. (1965). On the nature of allosteric transitions: A plausible model. *J. Mol. Biol.* **12,** 88–118.

Mooser, G. (1976). *N*-substituted maleimide inactivation of the response to taste cell stimulation. *J. Neurobiol.* **7,** 457–468.

Mooser, G., and Lambuth, N. (1977). Inactivation of taste receptor cell function by two cationic protein modification reagents. *J. Neurobiol.* **8,** 193–206.

Popot, J.-L., Sugiyama, H., and Changeux, J.-P. (1976). Studies on the electrogenic action of acetylcholine with *Torpedo marmorata* electric organ. II. The permeability response of the receptor-rich membrane fragments to cholinergic agonists in vivo. *J. Mol. Biol.* **106,** 469–483.

Price, S., and DeSimone, J. A. (1977). Models of taste receptor cell stimulation. *Chem. Senses Flavor* **2,** 427–456.

Rubin, M. M., and Changeux, J.-P. (1966). On the nature of allosteric transitions: Implications of nonexclusive ligand binding. *J. Mol. Biol.* **21,** 265–274.

Sato, T. (1976). Does an initial phasic response exist in the receptor potential of taste cells. *Experientia* **32,** 1426–1428.

Chapter 20

Peripheral Mechanisms in Salty Taste Reception

JOSEPH G. BRAND and DOUGLAS L. BAYLEY

I. INTRODUCTION

The taste receptor theory proposed by Beidler (1954, 1962, 1971) is predicated on the observation that the integrated neural response in the rat chorda tympani nerve can be related to stimulus concentration by a simple Langmuir adsorption isotherm. The theory assumes that salt adsorbing to the taste cell surface generates a proportional response in the innervating nerve. Beidler also pointed out the possibility of anion inhibition, since salts possessing the same cation but different anions are not equally effective in eliciting a neural response. This theory is still widely employed to explain many results in taste physiology and remains a reasonable working hypothesis for taste receptor stimulation. Recent results from Mooser's laboratory have forced us to reexamine the implications of this simple theory (Mooser, 1976, also this volume; Mooser and Lambuth, 1977).

When attempting to conceptualize the actual physical processes which occur on the taste cell membrane during salt stimulation, one can begin with a model of salt taste reception proposed by Gross and elaborated in a review by Beidler and Gross (1971). This model considers the possibility that macromolecules in the

BIOLOGICAL AND BEHAVIORAL
ASPECTS OF SALT INTAKE

ISBN 0-12-397750-9

taste cell plasma membrane undergo conformational changes with the addition of stimulus molecules. Such mechanochemical interactions are well known in chemical polymers where, for example, ionic strength of the bulk medium can markedly affect the size of several types of polymers. The model also assumes that the taste cell receptor is composed of a matrix of lipid and protein, with the protein being capable of reacting in a mechanochemical manner to changes in salt concentration. Changing salt concentration in the surrounding medium will immediately lead to changes in the electrostatic field of the macromolecule causing it, in their theory, to decrease ("shrink") its effective molecular volume. In this essentially nonstoichiometric process, the simple one-to-one correspondence often assumed between receptor and stimulus need not hold. In addition, various types of conformationally deformable macromolecules can be interlaced within the membrane which can then respond optimally to various types of stimuli. This concept leads to tremendous flexibility of response as well as to considerable complexity in interpretation—two facts we know from experience to be both relevant and frustrating.

In addition to reception, their theory also treats taste cell response. When macromolecules at one part shrink, others at other membrane regions should expand. They consider these expanding macromolecules to be effectors—molecules below the level of the tight junctions which expand and thereby affect the permeability of the membrane leading to the generation of the receptor potential. What may be of peripheral interest in this theory is that it does not exclude the possibility of "dirty" receptors; that is, receptors which may display only partial stimulus specificity. For example, simple sugars may, to a degree, excite salt receptors. This may be a microscopic conception for the macroscopic observations of von Békésy (1964).

Recent work from Kurihara's laboratory has suggested that the receptor macromolecules postulated in Gross's theory need not be proteins at all, but rather, can be simple lipids. Kamo *et al.* (1974b) recorded zeta potentials of liposomes upon the addition of salts to the medium. Interesting parallels were observed between their results and known results of taste responses observed neurophysiologically. For example, the 1:1 salts, NaCl and KCl, gave identical functions of concentration versus ζ-potential while the 2:1 salts, $CaCl_2$ and $MgCl_2$, gave functions different from the 1:1 salts. In addition, the 1:1 salts never gave positive potentials with increasing concentration, while the 2:1 salts eventually did. Even though these functions followed the same form as the Beidler taste equation (Beidler, 1954), strict binding of cations to the presumed anionic phosphate surface was not sufficient to explain the result. The surface density of negative charge at the liposome surface actually increased with rising ζ-potential and increasing Na^+ concentration. So strict adsorption of cations is not alone responsible for these results. Using 2:1 salts, however, negative charge density did decrease, suggesting direct adsorption of the divalent cation to phospholipid. The observation of sign reversal on Na^+ addition to a membrane coated with Fe^{3+} or cocaine was also reproduced in this simple model.

In these experiments (Kamo *et al.*, 1974b) the liposomes were made of an extract from bovine tongue (presumably, nontaste) epithelium. No direct Na^+ binding to these vesicles was observed. Until recently, it was assumed that monovalent cations did not bind to the lipid bilayer. Consequently, all effects observed with increasing monovalent cation concentration were thought to be due to screening. Whether actual binding of Na^+ to the receptor surface occurs is not in practice relevant to the use of the Langmuir adsorption isotherm as proposed by Beidler's early work (1954). However, the fact of Na^+ (or any other monovalent cation) binding to the receptor surface could lend a degree of specificity to the receptor response that is conceptually more difficult to envision in the case of simple electrostatic screening. To this end, a recent report of Puskin (1977) is relevant. He found that Mn^{2+} binding to phosphatidylserine liposomes is altered by the presence of monovalent cations. Strength of alteration generally followed the lyotropic series. What is of relevance, however, is that the results cannot be completely explained by screening effects based on the Gouy–Chapman diffuse double layer theory (see Puskin, 1977). Rather this work suggests that the discrepancy between theory and experiment may be due to some specific monovalent cation–phospholipid binding or to penetration of the cations between the head group spaces of the lipid sheet. In either case, a suggestion for specificity via direct cation binding is made. Recent work (Nir *et al.*, 1978; McLaughlin and Eisenberg, 1979) demonstrates not only direct binding of monovalent cations to phosphatidylserine vesicles but also yields differential binding for these cations. The binding affinity for Na^+ to these vesicles is estimated to be near 0.6 liters/mole, a value not unreasonable if it were to be responsible for the initiation of salty taste.

In a recent theoretical paper, DeSimone and Price (1976) further compact the model for salt stimulation by introducing the concept that fixed anionic surface charges can interact with both mobile cations and mobile ion pairs. Interaction with mobile ion pairs makes it possible at least to theoretically model the observation of anion inhibition. A phospholipid layer at an aqueous interface is essentially a sheet of negative charge. It should attract cations and repel anions. DeSimone and Price argue that the interaction of salt with the taste cells involves an initial change in surface potential due to ion binding (or electrostatic screening), but that neutral ion pairs may compete for the fixed anion sites on the membrane without, of course, significantly altering the charge density. This model thus eliminates the unsettling necessity of having to bring an anion in contact with a sheet to which it should normally be electrostatically excluded. Their model also accounts for the effect of Fe^{3+} and pH on salt taste as well as the generation of the water taste. Their model predicts a decrease in the fraction of surface charge for both an increase in salt concentration of the bulk solution or a dilution of the bulk concentration.

After investigating the effect of water (or dilution) on phase boundary potential it was suggested (Kamo *et al.*, 1974a) that the so-called water taste of sour-after-salty was due to a diffusion potential caused by ion flow from the membrane surface back to the bulk solution. However, recent work reported by DeSimone *et al.* (1979a,b) has suggested a simpler mechanism. They show that the surface pressure of charged phospholipid monolayers is a nonmonotonic function of the ionic strength of the solution subphase. Hydrogen ions as well as other cations may determine the surface charge density. Since H^+ is titrating the membrane surface almost exclusively, the effect of Na^+ is predominantly nonstoichiometric, serving to screen the surface charge. Since surface pressure is low for very dilute as well as very concentrated salt subphases but high at intermediate ranges (DeSimone *et al.*, 1979a,b) the model resembles the characteristics observed off of "water-sensitive" nerve fibers. The water-after-salt response can thus be simply modeled as a decrease in surface pressure at the receptor cell surface induced by a decrease in local pH. The hypertonic salt response can also be explained if one assumes that a lowered surface pressure represents a stimulation. This theory, unlike that proposed by Kamo *et al.* (1974a) predicts a water response to KCl adaptation. Such a response has been observed both in the cat (Bartoshuk, 1965) and the frog (Coté, 1976).

These studies have collectively led to the hypothesis that the membrane is a patchwork or mosaic of lipid domains, each domain being more responsive to one type of salt than another. This is not an idea far removed from that of Beidler and Gross, except that the fundamental nature of the receptor macromolecule has changed from a conformationally deformable protein to a conformationally cooperative structure—the lipid bilayer. Whether the membrane can undergo structural changes with salt addition as proposed in the thesis outlined by Beidler and Gross is a question which may be approached using liposomes impregnated with appropriate fluorescent dyes.

These observations all would predict that there is very little specificity at the receptor level for salty taste. Yet what, for example, gives us the ability to distinguish NaCl from KCl? Both of these 1:1 salts interact practically identically with the liposomes used by Kamo *et al.* (1974b) and probably would behave similarly in phospholipid monolayers. Direct binding of Na^+ and K^+ to phosphatidylserine liposomes suggests a mechanism for discrimination in taste, but qualitative differences have yet to be demonstrated among the ions in these simple systems. Obviously, the taste cell is not a simple bilayer so that the considerable complexity of the plasma membrane may aid in this specificity determination. Different salts would, additionally, be expected to interact differently with other types of receptor cells. Thus the taste of KCl is often termed bitter–salty. Also participating in specificity could be any intracellular events which may be activated as a result of salty stimuli.

We have found recently, for example, that the addition of salty stimuli to taste receptor tissue causes changes in reduced pyridine nucleotide fluorescence (Brand and Bayley, 1978). We record reduced pyridine nucleotide fluorescence via a front-surface technique in which we illuminate the receptor sheet with appropriate excitation energy and read fluorescent light at right angles to the incident beam. The taste receptor tissue is continuously bathed in a cuvette with either an adapting medium or a stimulation medium. Media can be exchanged by a simple continuous-exchange procedure.

II. POSSIBLE INVOLVEMENT OF REDUCED PYRIDINE NUCLEOTIDE IN SALTY RECEPTION

For these experiments, we employed a simple flow design using a normal quartz fluorescence cuvette. A hollow needle was set down the center of the cuvette. Two small holes were milled near the bottom of the needle. Solution could thus be introduced through this needle and be mixed with the contents already in the cuvette. Exchange was effected and cuvette volume was kept constant by a tube at the meniscus to which a vacuum was applied. Preliminary experiments indicated that complete exchange could be achieved within 1 minute.

Circumvallate papillae from steer tongue are impaled on the hollow needle so that their taste bud-rich epithelial surface is facing the cuvette sides and thus the light source. Five to six papillae are normally stacked one on top of the other so that the excitation source and emission analyzer see a continuous receptor sheet. The excitation source (Xenon) is followed by a monochromator set at 350 nm, then by an interference filter (Corion #3478-132) so that excitation energy reaching the sample is very sharp. No stray light from the Xenon source can be detected from 370 to 700 nm. A nominal short wavelength filter with cutoff at 390 nm is placed between the sample and the analyzer. The instrument used is a Perkin–Elmer MPF-2A Fluorescence Spectrophotometer.

Excitation of the tissue with 350 nm light leads to an emission spectrum indicative of the presence in the tissue of reduced pyridine nucleotide (Fig. 1). The emission maximum (447 nm) of this intrinsic reduced nucleotide is consistent with that of other published spectra of cell-associated NADH. The excitation spectrum of the tissue (filters removed) displays a maximum at 344 nm, also consistent with other published excitation spectra of tissue-associated NADH (see, for example, Davis and Canessa-Fischer, 1965). The slight shoulder at 295 nm probably reflects a tryptophan excitation.

If the emission maximum is now continuously monitored during the addition of stimuli, we find a characteristic change in emission intensity with change in

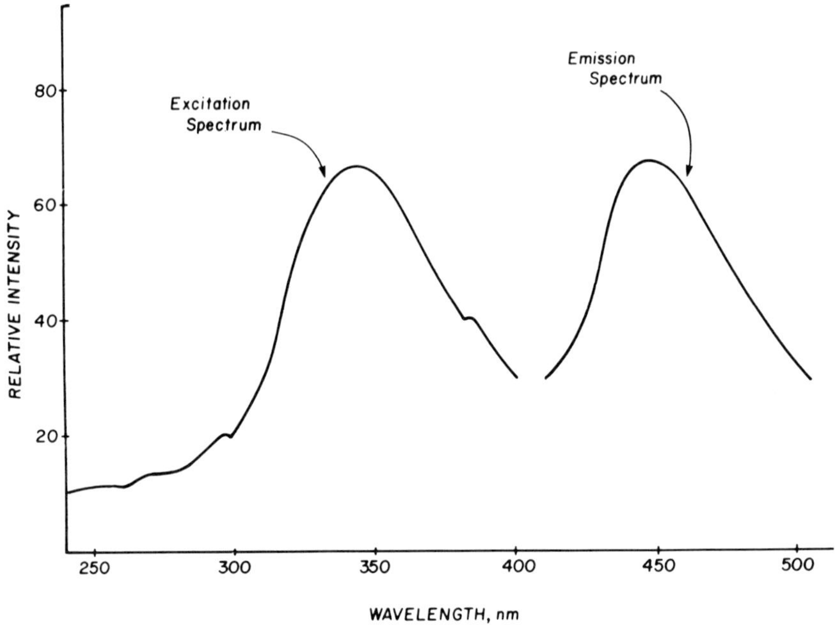

Fig. 1. The excitation and emission spectra of presumed reduced pyridine nucleotides from taste papillae. The excitation spectrum was obtained by setting the emission monochromator to 450 nm. The emission spectrum was obtained by setting the excitation monochromator to 350 nm with an interference filter between the monochromator and the papillae.

salt concentration. Figure 2 shows the character of this change during a typical run. The peak (monitored at 450 nm) decreases in intensity after the introduction of NaCl until a steady state is reached. This steady state is maintained even though salt is being continuously flowed through the apparatus. Upon replacement of the salt solution by the original (''adapting'') medium (6 m*M* $CaCl_2$ in 0.05 *M* NaCl), the emission intensity at 450 nm begins to return toward its original position, but never reaches the initial level. The longer the period of flow of the stimulating NaCl solution, the smaller this return. Also, alternating between adapting medium and stimulating medium eventually leads to the inability of the tissue to respond to either the addition of NaCl or its removal.

Figure 2 also shows results of an experiment where nitrogen was bubbled through both the adapting medium and a 1 *M* NaCl stimulating medium. Prior to any addition of NaCl, the level of emission at 450 nm increases upon changing from adapting medium with normal atmosphere to adapting medium containing all N_2 (less than 2% 0_2 could be detected in this N_2 saturated solution by a Clark oxygen electrode). The rise in emission intensity reflects the fact that anerobic conditions drive most of the oxidized pyridine nucleotide to the reduced (fluores-

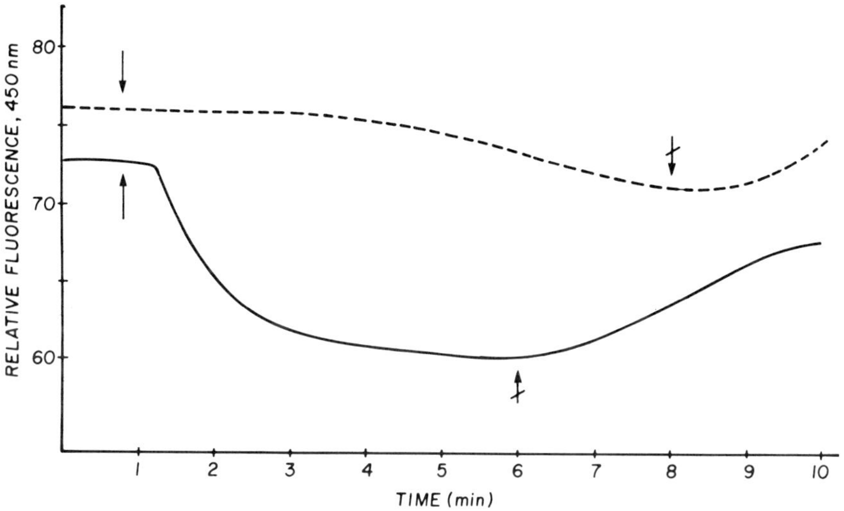

Fig. 2. Change in relative fluorescence intensity at 450 nm versus time upon the addition of 1 *M* NaCl under conditions of normal (oxygenated) atmosphere and deaerated (nitrogen) atmosphere. The addition of 1 *M* NaCl (at ↑) causes a decrease in the signal observed at 450 nm (———). The change is sustained for the length of the stimulation and partially recovers after exchange of the 1 *M* NaCl for the original "adapting" medium (at ↟). Introduction of an adapting medium which has been deaerated by bubbling nitrogen through it for 4 hours prior to the experiment leads to an increase in the signal at 450 nm over that normally observed with aerated medium. Subsequent introduction of 1 *M* NaCl also deaerated with N_2 (at ↓) leads to a very slight reduction in the signal and then only after several minutes (-------). Exchange of this stimulating medium with the deaerated adapting medium (at ↡) reverses the change. In this case, reversal is complete. Adapting medium is 0.05 *M* NaCl, 6 m*M* $CaCl_2$. Stimulating medium is 1 *M* NaCl, 6 m*M* $CaCl_2$.

cent) form. The addition of deoxygenated 1 *M* NaCl (Fig. 2) to this tissue leads to only a slight decrease in the 450 nm signal and then only after 5–6 minutes of flow of this stimulating salt solution. The exchange of the stimulating NaCl medium with the deoxygenated adapting medium brings the emission intensity back to the original baseline. This is in contrast to experiments performed in oxygenated media where there is no return to initial emission levels (compare bottom and top traces of Fig. 2).

These observed changes in the level of intrinsic tissue emission at 450 nm are quite general for all compounds which have some salty taste character. For example, the general phenomenon can be observed using not only NaCl, but also KCl, LiCl, NH_4Cl, $MgCl_2$, Na_2SO_4, and K_2SO_4. However, the bitter salt, $MgSO_4$, even at 1 *M*, produces no change in intensity at 450 nm. Likewise other bitter stimuli, sucrose octaacetate and Bitrex, and the sugars, sucrose and glucose, are without effect.

Under what conditions is this effect inhibited? If the tissue fails to respire, the intensity changes are no longer observable. For example, freeze–thawing, heating, or treatment with strong acid (pH 1–2) destroys the effect. Exposure of the tissue to ouabain (10 m*M*) for 5 min does not inhibit the effect but exposure to the sulfhydryl complexers (maleimides) employed by Mooser in his study (Mooser, 1976) did abolish these salt-induced changes.

The lowest level of NaCl that can initiate this effect (using an adaptation medium consisting of only 6 m*M* $CaCl_2$) is about 0.025 *M*. Interestingly, Goatcher and Church (1970) demonstrated a discrimination threshold for NaCl in the calf near 0.02 *M*.

The response of cells to sodium stimulation has been studied neurophysiologically. Most cutaneous cells respond to salt stimulation, be they either specialized taste cells or simple undifferentiated epithelial cells (Eyzaguirre *et al.*, 1972; Teeter, 1974). This suggests the possibility that taste cells may make use of intracellular metabolic processes extant in all cells to transduce salty information. It has been demonstrated (Lehninger *et al.*, 1978) that oxidation of reduced pyridine nucleotide is accompanied by Ca^{2+} release from mitochondria. Perhaps a similar release of Ca^{2+} accompanies the changes in nucleotide fluorescence observed here, and these changes in Ca^{2+} levels may initiate membrane changes necessary to induce the receptor potential (see Brand, 1978, for review). However, the experiments reported here could not distinguish between NADH responding in taste cells as opposed to epithelial cells. We are currently attempting to use microfluorescence techniques to monitor only taste bud cells or only surrounding epithelial cells. Results of these experiments may aid in determining whether cellular specificity exists for salt taste.

III. SUMMARY

Classical taste receptor theories assume that salty taste is initiated by the adsorption of the salt ions to the taste cell receptor plasma membrane. However, recent experiments using charged liposomes as models for the taste receptor have demonstrated that alterations in apparent surface charge density and surface pressure can be caused by electrostatic screening by monovalent cations. These experiments would seem to eliminate the necessity for direct binding of monovalent cations to the receptor surface. While the binding of monovalent cations to charged phospholipid surfaces may be weak, such binding, nevertheless, has been demonstrated for high cation concentrations. The combination of electrostatic screening by and weak binding of monovalent ions to the receptor surface may lend a degree of specificity to the generation of the salty taste, providing us with the ability to distinguish among several types of salts.

Ions which have a salty character also change the levels of reduced pyridine nucleotides within the tissue of the taste papilla. Upon introduction of salty stimuli, the fluorescence due to reduced pyridine nucleotide decreases, suggesting a shift from the reduced nucleotide state to the oxidized state. The level is partially restored following removal of the stimuli. It is suggested that the change in the level of reduced nucleotides may be reflecting a transductive process in the taste cell.

ACKNOWLEDGMENTS

The suggestions of and helpful discussions with Drs. J. A. DeSimone, G. L. Heck and J. S. Puskin are gratefully acknowledged.

REFERENCES

Bartoshuk, L. M. (1965). Effects of adaptation of responses to water in cat and rat. Ph.D. Thesis, Brown University, Providence, Rhode Island.

Beidler, L. M. (1954). A theory of taste stimulation. *J. Gen. Physiol.* **38,** 133–139.

Beidler, L. M. (1962). Taste receptor stimulation. *Prog. Biophys. Biophys. Chem.* **12,** 107–151.

Beidler, L. M. (1971). Taste receptor stimulation with salts and acids. *In* "Handbook of Sensory Physiology" (L. M. Beidler, ed.), Vol. 4, Part 2, pp. 220–220. Springer-Verlag, Berlin and New York.

Beidler, L. M., and Gross, G. W. (1971). The nature of taste receptor sites. *In* "Contributions to Sensory Physiology" (W. D. Neff, ed.), Vol. 5, pp. 97–127. Academic Press, New York.

Brand, J. G. (1978). Biophysics of taste receptors. *In* "Sweeteners and Dental Caries" (J. H. Shaw and G. G. Roussos, eds.), pp. 13–32. Information Retrieval, Inc., Washington, D.C.

Brand, J. G., and Bayley, D. L. (1978). Monitoring fluorescence from intact taste papillae. Applications to the biophysics of taste reception. *Biophys. J.* **21,** 136a.

Coté, J. A. (1976). Investigation into the mechanism of the frog's water response. Ph.D. Thesis, Temple University, Philadelphia, Pennsylvania.

Davis, R. P., and Canessa-Fischer, M. (1965). Spectrofluoremetric identification of reduced pyridine nucleotide in the intact isolated urinary bladder of the toad. *Anal. Biochem.* **10,** 325–343.

DeSimone, J. A., and Price, S. (1976). A model for the stimulation of taste receptor cells by salt. *Biophys. J.* **16,** 869–881.

DeSimone, J. A., Heck, G. L., and DeSimone, S. K. (1979a). A surface chemical model of salt, acid and "water" taste. *In* "Bioelectrochemistry: Ions, Surfaces, Membranes" (M. Blank, ed.), ACS Symp. Ser. Am. Chem. Soc., Washington, D.C. (in press).

DeSimone, J. A., Heck, G. L., and DeSimone, S. K. (1979b). The antagonistic effects of sodium and calcium on the surface pressure of phosphatidic acid monolayers. *Biophys. J.* **25,** 177a.

Eyzaguirre, C., Fidone, S., and Zapata, P. (1972). Membrane potentials recorded from the mucosa of the toad's tongue during chemical stimulation. *J. Physiol. (London)* **221,** 515–532.

Goatcher, W. D., and Church, D. C. (1970). Taste responses in ruminants. III. Reactions of pygmy goats, normal goats, sheep, and cattle to sucrose and sodium chloride. *J. Anim. Sci.* **31,** 364–372.

Kamo, N., Miyake, M., Kurihara, K., and Kobatake, Y. (1974a). Physicochemical studies of taste reception. I. Model membrane simulating taste receptor potential in response to stimuli of salts, acids and distilled water. *Biochim. Biophys. Acta* **367,** 1–10.

Kamo, N., Miyake, M., Kurihara, K., and Kobatake, Y. (1974b). Physicochemical studies of taste reception. II. Possible mechanisms of generation of taste receptor potential induced by salt stimuli. *Biochim. Biophys. Acta* **367,** 11-23.

Lehninger, A. L., Vercesi, A., and Bababunmi, E. A. (1978). Regulation of Ca^{2+} released from mitochondria by the oxidation-reduction state of pyridine nucleotides. *Proc. Natl. Acad. Sci. U.S.A.* **75,** 1690-1694.

McLaughlin, S., and Eisenberg, M. (1979). The adsorption of alkali metal cations to bilayer membranes containing phosphatidyl serine. *Biophys. J.* **25,** 262a.

Mooser, G. (1976). N-Substituted maleimide inactivation of the response to taste cell stimulation. *J. Neurobiol.* **7,** 457-468.

Mooser, G., and Lambuth, N. (1977). Inactivation of taste receptor cell function by two cationic protein modification reagents. *J. Neurobiol.* **8,** 193-206.

Nir, S., Newton, C., and Papahdjopoulos, D. (1978). Binding of cations to phosphatidylserine vesicles. *Bioelectrochem. Bioenerg.* **5,** 116-133.

Puskin, J. S. (1977). Divalent cation binding to phospholipids: An EPR study. *J. Membr. Biol.* **35,** 39-55.

Teeter, J. H. (1974). Electrical properties of taste bud cells and surrounding epithelial cells in catfish and mudpuppies. Ph.D. Thesis, University of Pennsylvania, Philadelphia., Pennsylvania.

von Békésy, G. (1964). Sweetness produced electrically on the tongue and its relation to taste theories. *J. Appl. Physiol.* **19,** 1105-1113.

Chapter 21

Peripheral Neural Changes Associated with Sodium Deprivation

ROBERT J. CONTRERAS

In deficit conditions, many mammals show an overwhelming craving for sodium salts. This behavior has been observed in wild herbivores (rabbits, kangaroos, deer) suffering varying degrees of sodium deprivation (Blair-West *et al.*, 1968), in laboratory rats maintained on sodium-free diets (Nachman, 1962; Contreras, 1975), and in calves with parotid fistulae (Bell and Sly, 1977). Salt appetite also occurs in humans who have experienced salt loss induced by sweating and consuming a low salt diet (McCance, 1936) or who have a pathological adrenal cortex (Wilkins and Richter, 1940). More recently, Schechter *et al.* (1974) reported that hypertensive individuals consumed more than four times as much saline as did normotensive controls. Langford *et al.* (1977) reported that human patients treated for hypertension with diuretics had an increased salt appetite and sodium intake that may have counteracted the therapeutic efforts of the physician. The immediate intake of sodium salts over other nonsodium salts

BIOLOGICAL AND BEHAVIORAL
ASPECTS OF SALT INTAKE

ISBN 0-12-397750-9

in these situations implies that animals recognize, by taste, the appropriate stimulus. In so doing, this unleashes the aggressive consumption of salt.

I. SODIUM INTAKE, A MANIFESTATION OF HOMEOSTASIS

In mammals, sodium is such an important constituent of the extracellular fluid that disruptions in sodium balance produce profound effects upon cellular metabolism, affecting most bodily functions. To cite some examples, sodium is important for maintaining blood volume, pressure, and osmolarity, is involved in carbohydrate, protein, and amino acid metabolism, and is important in the production of electrical signals by the nervous system (Meneely and Battarbee, 1976). From a homeostatic viewpoint, it is generally assumed that there are two primary mechanisms which have evolved to protect an animal against sodium imbalance (Denton, 1965). Sodium regulation depends upon a dynamic balance between aldosterone secretion controlling sodium loss and sodium appetite controlling sodium intake. Sodium deprivation results in an activation of the renin-angiotensin system which induces an increased secretion of sodium-retaining aldosterone (Spielman and Davis, 1974; Douglas *et al.*, 1978) which acts to reduce sodium levels in urine, perspiration, and saliva (Ganong, 1971). In addition, sodium deprivation, in many terrestrial species, stimulates the specific hunger for sodium known as sodium appetite. According to a homeostatic view, cessation of salt intake is associated with a return to sodium balance and a brake on endocrine systems responsible for controlling sodium excretion.

II. ROLE OF GUSTATION IN CONTROL OF SALT INTAKE

Curt Richter, a pioneer in the investigation of self-regulatory behaviors, and others have provided substantial evidence that the gustatory sense is important both for the initiation and satiation of the salt intake behavior of a sodium-deficient rat (Denton, 1965; Nachman and Cole, 1971). Richter studied the behavior of the adrenalectomized rat, which because of its condition loses considerable amounts of salt, but compensates for this loss by ingesting large quantities of NaCl solution. Using the relative intake method, where water and NaCl solutions were simultaneously presented to the animal, Richter found that adrenalectomized rats immediately consumed moderate or strong saline usually rejected by normal rats (Richter, 1936) and would drink NaCl solution at low concentrations to which intact controls were indifferent (Richter, 1939). Gustatory sensibility seemed to be crucial for the expression of salt appetite; after surgical denervation of the taste receptors on the tongue, several adrenalectomized rats lost the ability to increase their intake of salt and consequently died (Richter, 1956).

Subsequent research has demonstrated that the sensory signal from the taste receptors elicited by a sodium salt is a factor, to some degree, in determining the amount of salt ingested. Ingestion accompanied by NaCl stimulation of the taste receptors leads to a rapid (Denton, 1965), short-term satiation (Nachman and Valentino, 1966; DiCara and Wilson, 1974) which does not occur without taste receptor stimulation (e.g., when solutions are introduced into the stomach via an esophageal fistula). If cessation of salt intake were simply under the control of postingestional effects, peripheral stimulation would not have this effect (Morrison and Young, 1972). The fact that adrenalectomized (Jalowiec and Stricker, 1973) and sodium-deprived rats (Contreras and Hatton, 1975) continued to ingest NaCl solution after sodium repletion might suggest that there is a learned preference for salt due to positive postingestional consequences (Pfaffmann, 1963). Garcia *et al.* (1974) reported that negative and positive shifts in taste preference occur due to an association between the taste of a substance and the physiological consequences of illness or recuperation from illness, respectively. Cabanac (1971) claims that a given taste stimulus can be pleasant or unpleasant depending upon the physiological state of the organism.

Rats will consume sodium salts when sodium replete (Richter, 1936; Bare, 1949). This is consistent with Richter's notion that gustatory stimulation by salt is instinctively (genetic) rewarding at moderate concentrations, and this confers survival advantage. When gustatory sensibility is reduced by sectioning the taste nerves (Pfaffmann, 1952) or by thalamic lesions (Oakley and Pfaffmann, 1962), salt preferences are reduced. Salt receptors and fibers have been found in a wide variety of organisms. Denton (1967) believes that these receptors were adapted specifically to protect an animal against sodium deficiency. Dethier (1977) suggests that these receptors did not evolve as part of a mechanism responsive to sodium need but in warning against a hypersaline environment. This does not preclude the possibility, however, that salt receptors are utilized by some animals for sodium preference. Salt preferences exhibited by need-free rats may also be attributable to experiential as well as genetic factors. Theios *et al.* (1962) reported that the saline intake of rats was modified by experience with particular salt concentrations.

III. BEHAVIORAL AND PHYSIOLOGICAL EFFECTS OF SODIUM DEPRIVATION

Since sodium deprivation more closely approximates that which occurs in nature and has more limited physiological consequences, under most circumstances, it has been my method for inducing sodium appetite. In all of my experiments, animals were fed a powdered, sodium-free diet for at least 9–10 days before testing; control animals were fed the same diet to which 1 g of NaCl crystals was added to each 99 g of powder.

Ten days of sodium deprivation in the intact rat results in sodium appetite and increased NaCl intake, as presented in Fig. 1. These animals were given two-bottle preference tests between distilled water and 0.4 *M* NaCl solution for 1 hour. Two tests were administered. The first test was given to animals that had free access to water and food; the second was given to the same animals adapted to a 23-hour schedule of water deprivation. In both tests, sodium-deprived rats

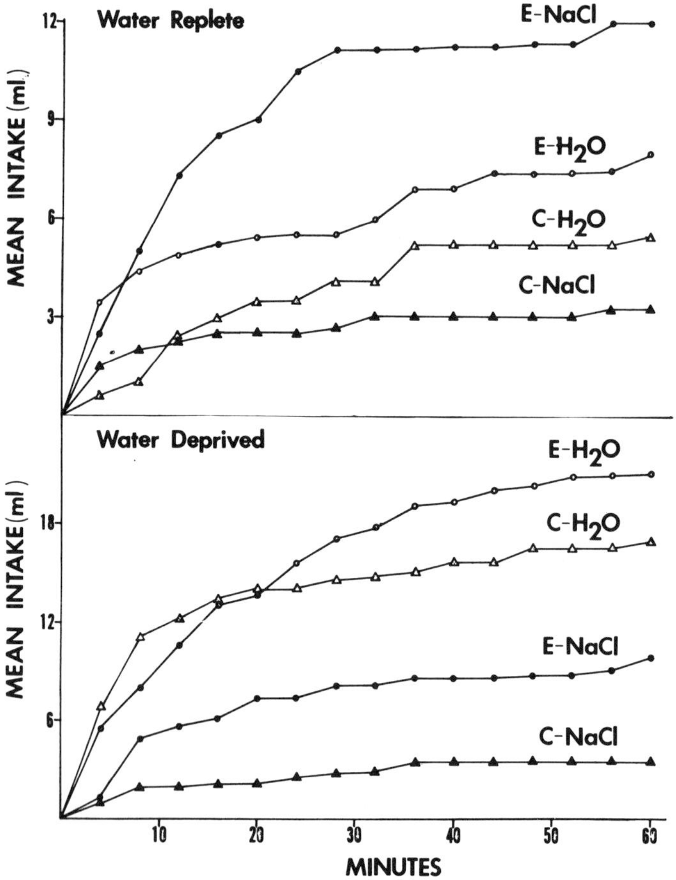

Fig. 1. The average cumulative intakes of distilled water and 0.4 *M* NaCl as a function of time are plotted for sodium-deprived (E-NaCl, E-H_2O) and control, sodium-replete (C-NaCl, C-H_2O) rats. The top graph represents data collected from rats that were water replete and the bottom graph from rats that were water deprived. Reprinted from Contreras and Hatton (1975) with permission.

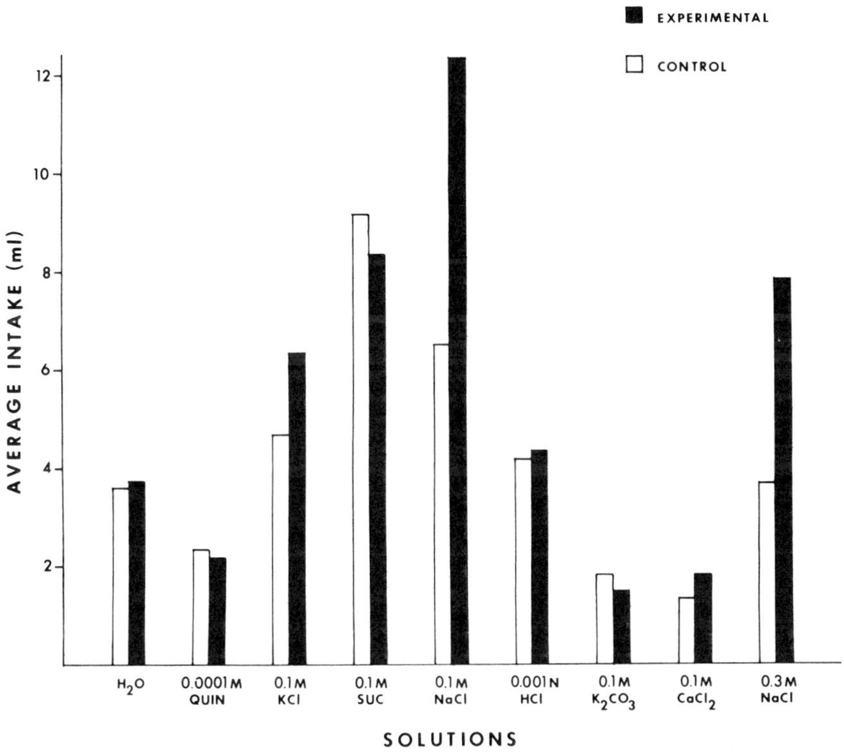

Fig. 2. The average intakes of NaCl solutions (0.1 *M* and 0.3 *M*), water, nonsodium salts, and other gustatory stimuli in sodium-deprived and control animals. The animals were given one-bottle tests for 10 minutes. Sodium-deprived rats differed from controls only in their intakes of NaCl, consuming significantly larger quantities.

showed significantly greater intakes of saline than control sodium-replete rats. In another set of animals, sodium deprivation resulted in a specific increase in intake of NaCl solution (0.1 *M* NaCl and 0.3 *M* NaCl) but not for nonsodium salts or other gustatory stimuli (Fig. 2). The animals of this experiment were given one-bottle tests for 10 minutes on successive days. The rats had been adapted to a 23-hour schedule of water deprivation. After the animals received their daily ration of water for 1 hour, all food and water were removed from each animal's cage for another hour. Following this, either a sapid solution or distilled water was presented to each animal to drink and the total intake of that solution was recorded over the ensuing 10-minute period.

The effects of sodium deprivation on electrolyte concentration in urine and saliva, and on blood chemistry, have been determined (Contreras and Hatton, 1975; R. J. Contreras and F. A. Catalanotto, unpublished observations). Var-

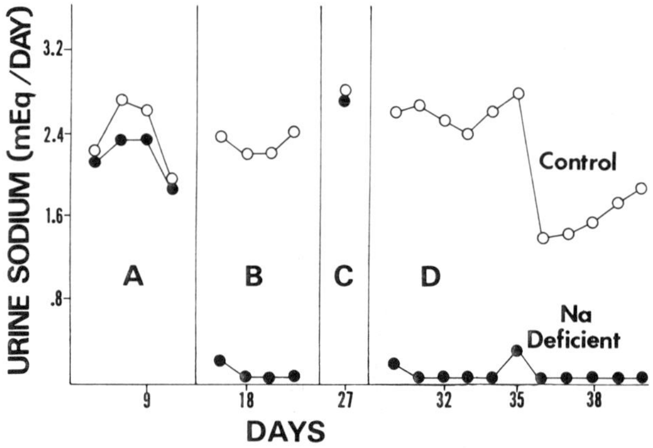

Fig. 3. Average amounts of sodium excretion in sodium-deprived and control rats across days and under conditions of being fed: (A) normal, sodium-replete diet, (B) sodium-free diet, (C) normal diet, (D) sodium-free diet, and beginning on day 35, a 23-hour schedule of water deprivation was introduced. Reprinted from Contreras and Hatton (1975) with permission.

iations in the amount of sodium excreted per day as a consequence of sodium deprivation are shown in Fig. 3. The amount of sodium eliminated in urine dropped dramatically when sodium was no longer added to the animals' diet. Sodium loss was kept to a minimum for the duration of the sodium deprivation period. Sodium deprivation of normal intact rats was associated with urinary sodium losses averaging 0.37 mEq in 10 days, which compares with 23.0 mEq in the same period for sodium-replete rats (Contreras and Hatton, 1975). R. J. Contreras and F. A. Catalanotto (unpublished observations) have reported that rats deprived of sodium for 10 days also show a decrease in sodium, but not potassium, concentration of whole saliva. Samples from whole saliva were collected from animals anesthetized with sodium pentobarbital and injected with pilocarpine (Table I). These changes in urinary and salivary sodium presumably

TABLE I

Sodium and Potassium Concentration of Saliva in Sodium-Deprived and Control Animals

	Sodium-deprived	Control
Salivary sodium (mEq/liter)	23.1 ± 5.8[a]	43.8 ± 10.98
Salivary potassium	52.8 ± 9.6	55.3 ± 11.5

[a] $p < 0.01$, *t* test, two-tailed. From R. J. Contreras and F. A. Catalanotto, unpublished observations.

TABLE II

Sodium, Potassium, and Protein Concentrate in Plasma of Sodium-Deprived and Control Animals[a]

	10 day	20 day
Experimental group		
Plasma Na (mEq/liter)	143.00 ± 1.417	148.20 ± 4.771
Plasma K[b] (mEq/liter)	4.46 ± 0.074	5.33 ± 0.285
Plasma protein (g/100 ml)	6.53 ± 0.120	6.35 ± 0.051
Control group		
Plasma Na (mEq/liter)	142.90 ± 0.945	146.40 ± 2.616
Plasma K (mEq/liter)	4.53 ± 0.056	4.45 ± 0.146
Plasma protein (g/100 ml)	6.58 ± 0.109	6.38 ± 0.108

[a] Two plasma samples were taken: one after 10 and a second after 20 days of sodium deprivation. Reprinted with permission from Contreras and Hatton (Copyright 1975, Pergamon Press and Brain Research Publication.)

[b] $p < 0.05$.

reflect the operation of an efficient salt-retaining mechanism in the intact deprived organism. The effects of sodium deprivation on 3 plasma parameters are presented in Table II. When rats were deprived of dietary sodium continuously for 10 or 20 days, the concentrations of sodium and protein (an indirect measure of blood volume) were not altered, most likely because the adrenal gland and kidney responded quickly and efficiently to minimize sodium loss. Bone contains appreciable amounts of sodium, almost as much as the body fluids, which can be mobilized to counteract obligatory losses due to sodium deprivation (Michell, 1976). An increase in plasma potassium was detected, however, when deprivation was extended to 20 days. It appears that plasma potassium is a more sensitive barometer to changes in sodium status than plasma sodium. This is one of the reasons that Michell (1978) suggested that sodium appetite and increased NaCl intake is a response to both potassium and sodium metabolism.

IV. SODIUM DEPRIVATION ALTERS PERIPHERAL NEURAL RESPONSES TO GUSTATORY STIMULI

With some knowledge of the behavioral and physiological effects of sodium deprivation, a number of studies were conducted (Contreras, 1977; Contreras and Frank, 1979) to examine peripheral neural mechanisms of gustation potentially involved in controlling the short-term intake of salt in a sodium-deprived rat. Several years ago, in order to explain the role gustatory sensibility plays in the salt intake of the adrenalectomized rat, Richter (1939) suggested that sodium deficiency might make the taste receptors more sensitive to NaCl stimulation. Changed sensitivity of the peripheral receptors was apparently ruled out when Pfaffmann and Bare (1950) reported that the concentration of NaCl necessary to evoke a reliable discharge of the taste nerve (chorda tympani) greater than that evoked by water was the same in intact and adrenalectomized rats. Subsequently, Nachman and Pfaffmann (1963) measured the activity of the total chorda tympani nerve to threshold and suprathreshold concentrations of NaCl solution and several other stimuli. They found that responses to these stimuli, measured relative to the activity evoked by 0.01 *M* NaCl, were the same in normal and sodium-deprived rats.

More than a decade later, however, work based on a technique for recording from single afferent taste fibers revealed a peripheral effect of sodium deprivation (Contreras, 1975, 1977) that was not evident in previous whole nerve preparations. Contreras showed that there was a specific decrease in the discharge frequency of taste units most reactive to 0.1 *M* NaCl solution, primarily NaCl-best units (Fig. 4). Frank (1973) divided chorda tympani units into four groups according to which of the four basic tastes elicits the largest response, naming them sucrose-best, NaCl-best, HCl-best, and quinine-best units. Responses to 0.5 *M* sucrose, 0.01 *N* HCl, or 0.02 *M* quinine in units from sodium-deprived and control, sodium-replete animals did not differ.

That sodium deprivation desensitizes the taste receptors was surprising in view of Richter's suggestion that the taste receptors might become more sensitive to NaCl stimulation in sodium-deficient rats. In Contreras' study, however, only the responses to a single suprathreshold concentration of each of the four basic tastes were studied. Nevertheless, the notion was entertained that this reduced signal to a suprathreshold sodium stimulus might account, in part, for the observation that sodium-deprived rats accept salt solutions at concentrations that would be rejected by sodium-replete rats.

Contreras and Frank (1979) recently determined the effects of sodium deprivation on the responses of single chorda tympani neurons in rat to the four standard taste solutions across a wide range of concentrations. It was also determined whether recently discovered reductions in single fiber activity to NaCl (Contreras, 1975, 1977) could be detected in whole nerve recordings. To ensure against experimenter bias, both whole nerve and single fiber recordings were obtained and analyzed without knowledge of the animal's deprivation condition.

Experimental animals were fed a sodium-free diet for a 9- or 10-day period before being used for chorda tympani recording. Control animals were fed the same diet except that 1 g of NaCl crystals were added to each 99 g of powdered food. Since sodium-deprived rats excrete less sodium (Contreras and Hatton, 1975), analysis of urinary sodium was used to verify diet conditions. All animals were anesthetized with urethane, the chorda tympani was surgically isolated, and its responses to chemical stimulation of the tongue were studied by standard

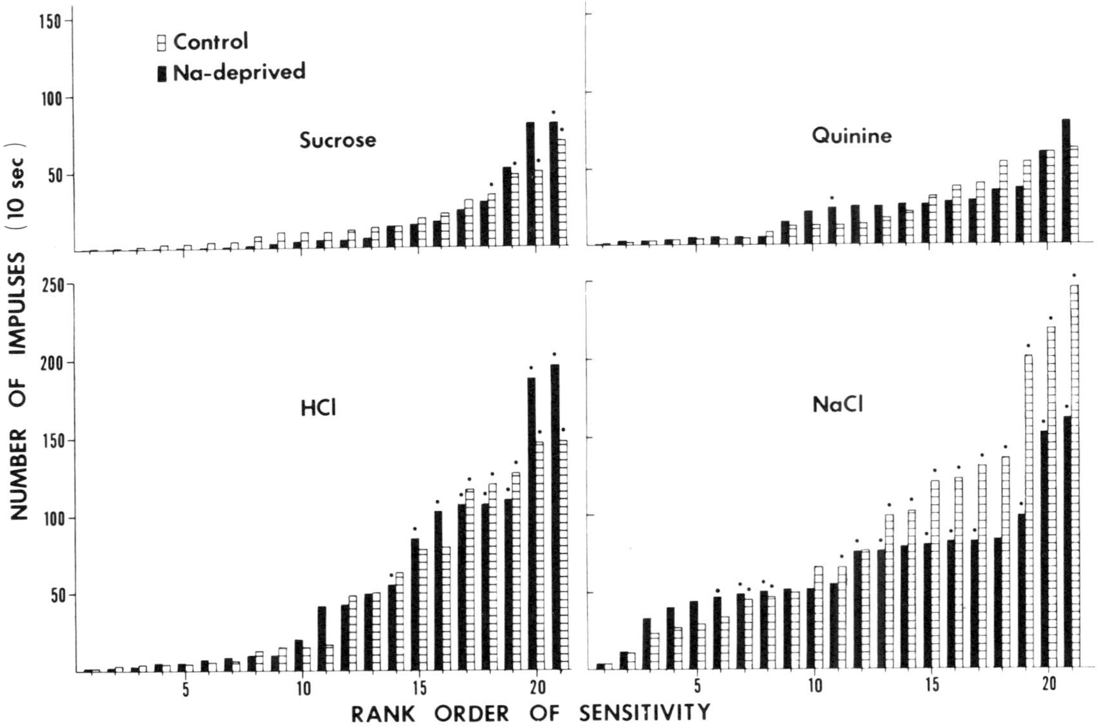

Fig. 4. The distribution of responses of 21 fibers from sodium-deprived rats and 21 fibers from controls to 0.5 *M* sucrose, 0.02 *M* quinine, 0.01 *N* HCl, and 0.1 *M* NaCl. These fibers are ranked ordered (from low to high) four different times according to response frequency (number of impulses elicited in 10 seconds of stimulation). A dot above a bar indicates whether a particular fiber is a sucrose-best (top left), a quinine-best (top right), and HCl-best (bottom left), or a NaCl-best (bottom right) fiber. The chief difference between fibers from sodium-deprived and control animals is in responses to NaCl, where fibers that are more reactive to NaCl (75 or more impulses) were smaller in deprived animals' nerves. Reprinted from Contreras (1977) with permission.

electrophysiological procedures. Test solutions flowed over the animals' tongues for at least 10 seconds and were separated by a distilled water rinse.

The whole nerve responses of 10 sodium-deprived and 10 control animals are shown in Fig. 5. Two measures of whole nerve activity during stimulation were taken: one was the maximal response that usually appeared immediately after stimulus onset, the second was the response approximately 10 seconds after the beginning of the response. The first is a measure of the initial peak neural discharge and the second a measure of the later tonic neural discharge. The functions in this figure show that the size of the chorda tympani response, either earlier peak (A) or later tonic (B) increases with concentration. In deprived rats whole nerve recordings show a decrease in median response to NaCl for both peak and tonic measures. Threshold concentrations of NaCl (0.001 *M* for peak and 0.01 *M* for tonic response) do not change but the slopes and maximal responses to NaCl solutions (0.03 *M* to 3.0 *M*) are lower after sodium deprivation for both peak and tonic responses (chi-square, $p < 0.05$). The response functions for sucrose, HCl, or quinine generated from the sodium-deprived and control animals' nerves do not differ in threshold, slope, or maximal response magnitude. The median absolute responses to water, the measure to which all plotted responses were made relative, were the same for the two groups.

The responses of a total of 100 units were studied; the responses from 42 units

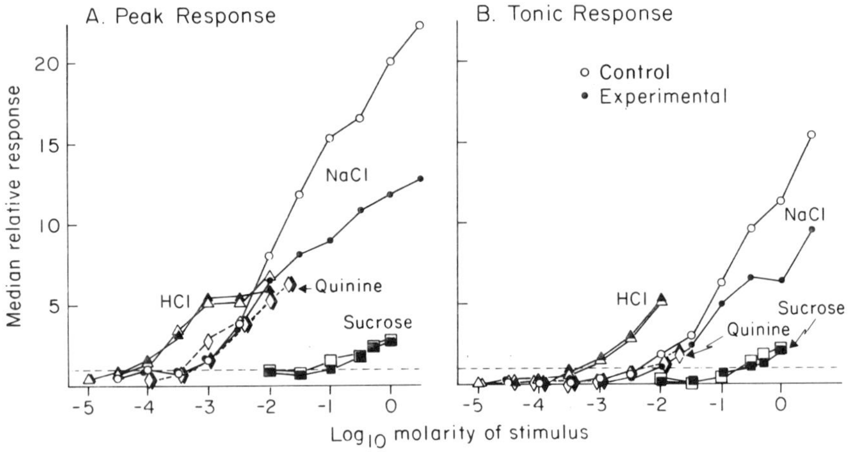

Fig. 5. The median responses of 10 whole nerves of sodium-deprived (filled symbols) and 10 whole nerves of control (open symbols) rats to a range of concentrations of NaCl, HCl, sucrose, and quinine. Two measures of the summed evoked activity of the nerve were taken: one (A) a measure of the peak discharge, the other (B), a measure of the tonic discharge. The numbers plotted are ratios of evoked responses to a reference level of activity during continuous water flow. A dashed line marks the reference level. Both peak and tonic responses to NaCl (0.03–3.0 *M*) are smaller after deprivation. Reprinted from Contreras and Frank (1979) with permission.

(21 in each group) have been previously reported (Contreras, 1977). Of the 100 units, 45 were from sodium-deprived and 55 from control rats' nerves. In Fig. 6, the responses of these single fibers are rank ordered (from low to high) 5 different times. They are ordered according to the frequency (number of impulses in 10 sec) of responses to each standard solution and water. Fibers from sodium-deprived rats differ from fibers from sodium-replete rats in their responses to 0.1 *M* NaCl; the average response ($p < 0.05$) and response variance ($p < 0.001$) are smaller in deprived animals' nerves. Comparable differences in the response distributions to 0.5 *M* sucrose, 0.01 *N* HCl, 0.02 *M* quinine, or water from the two groups of fibers were not found. It is especially noteworthy that there are no differences in the response distributions to 0.01 *N* HCl since this HCl solution and 0.1 *M* NaCl have similar response distributions.

The difference between NaCl response distributions stems primarily from the more responsive fibers, the responses of which occur at the top half of each distribution. Most of these are NaCl-best fibers, those that respond more to NaCl than the other taste stimuli. Of the 45 fibers in the sodium-deprived group, 22 responded best to NaCl, 21 best to HCl, 2 best to sucrose, and 0 best to quinine. Of the 55 fibers in the control group, the numbers are 27, 22, 5, and 1, respectively. It was determined that NaCl-best fibers from experimental animals generated a smaller response mean to NaCl ($p < 0.05$) than corresponding fibers from control animals. Sucrose-best fibers from the experimental group, however, generated larger responses to sucrose than corresponding fibers from control animals.

For some of the units, response functions were obtained. Figure 7 is divided into separate graphs showing the average response functions for (A) NaCl-best fibers, (B) HCL-best fibers, and (C) all fibers, regardless of classification, which includes only the NaCl-best and HCl-best since no complete response functions were obtained from sucrose-best units. There appear to be two prominent groups of fibers in the rat chorda tympani. One group of fibers, the NaCl-best fibers, respond strongly to NaCl and very little, if at all, to the other stimuli. A second group, the HCl-best fibers, responds strongly to both HCl and NaCl. After sodium deprivation, the NaCl-best units show, on the average, a decreased reactivity to suprathreshold NaCl solutions between 0.1 *M* to 3.0 *M* ($p < 0.05$). Anomalously, HCl-best fibers from sodium-deprived rats responded more to 3.0 *M* NaCl than comparable fibers from control rats. Nevertheless, the combined effects of NaCl-best and HCl-best fibers (C) approximate the response of the whole nerve (see Fig. 5). The measure used for the responses of single fibers (number of impulses in 10 seconds of stimulation), however, is a more integral measure over the entire stimulation period than either of the two measures of whole nerve activity.

These results reaffirm and extend Contreras' original observation that the chorda tympani nerves of sodium-deprived rats are less reactive to solutions of

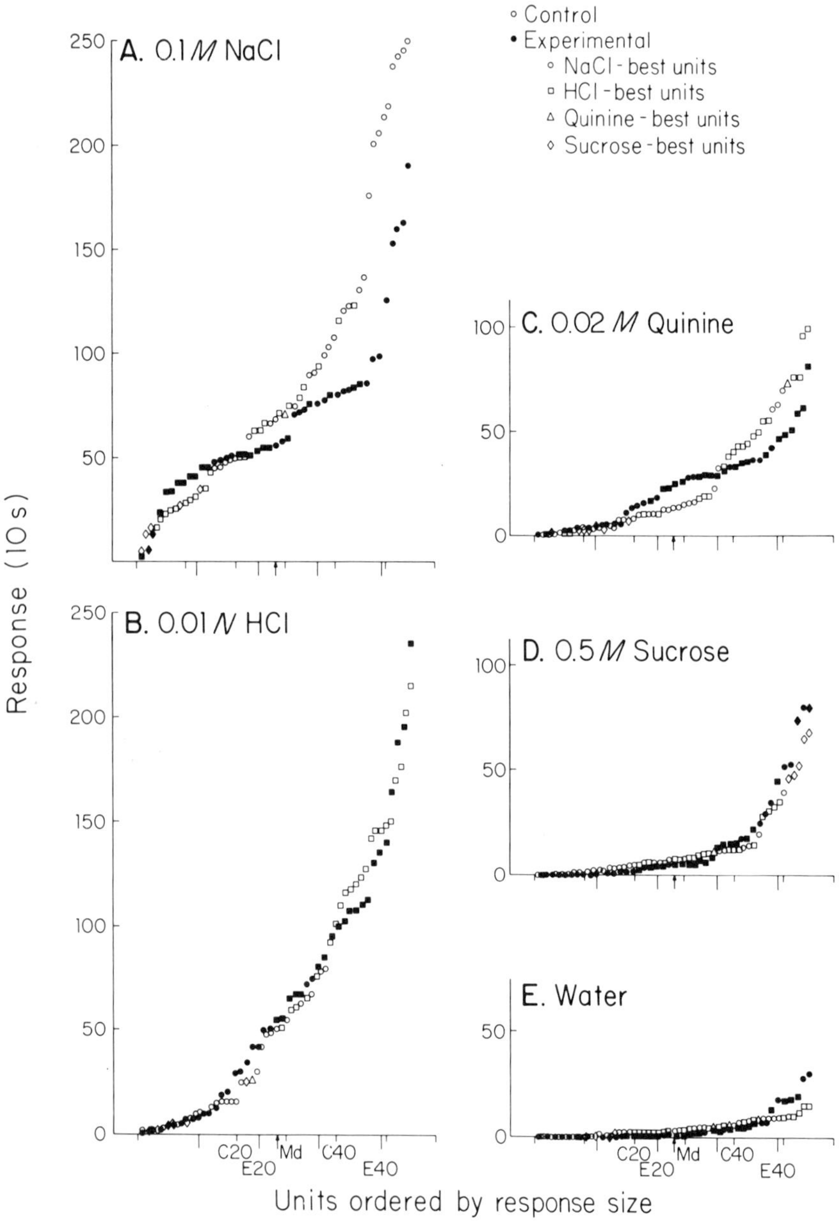

Fig. 6. Responses of 45 chorda tympani units (*E*'s) from sodium-deprived (experimental) and 55 units (*C*'s) from control rats rank ordered from low to high according to their response frequencies (number of impulses elicited in 10 seconds) to each standard solution (0.1 *M* NaCl, 0.01 *N* HCl, 0.02 *M* quinine, 0.5 *M* sucrose) and water; position of medians along abscissa is marked *Md*. The relative positions of the twentieth and fortieth units along the abscissa are marked *C20* and *C40* for the control group and *E20* and *E40* for the experimental group. The major difference between the fibers sampled from experimental and control rats is in their responses to NaCl, with NaCl-best units from sodium-deprived animals showing lower response frequencies to NaCl than corresponding fibers from controls. Reprinted from Contreras and Frank (1979) with permission.

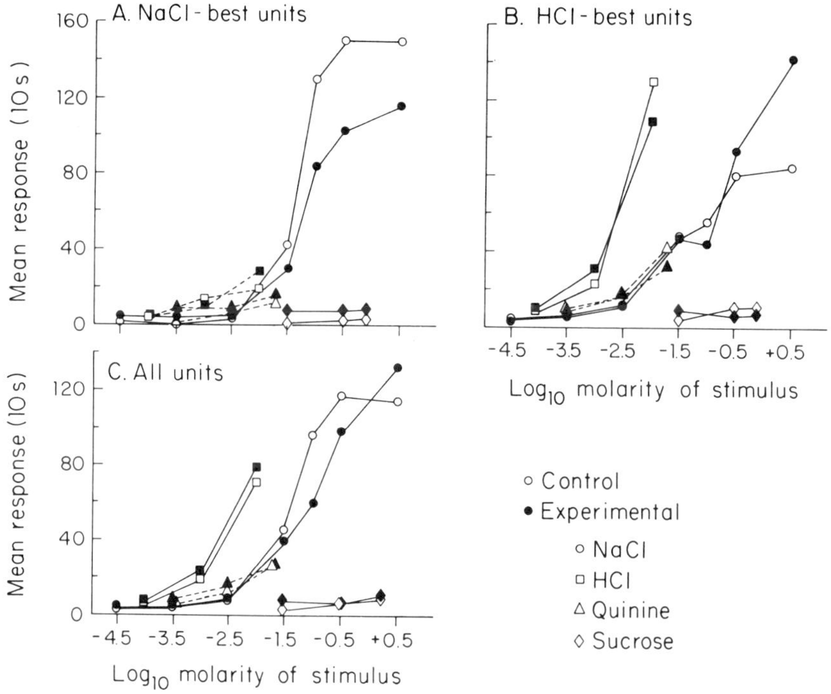

Fig. 7. Average responses of single fibers of the chorda tympani nerve of sodium-deprived (experimental) or control rats as a function of the logarithm of stimulus molarity. Response (number of impulses elicited in 10 seconds of stimulation) functions for NaCl-best (A), HCl-best (B), and all fibers, regardless of classification (C), were averaged separately. The points plotted are means of responses of from 10 to 15 control, or 7 to 8 experimental NaCl-best units; from 13 control, or 9 to 13 experimental HCl-best units; or from a total of 23 to 28 control or 16 to 21 experimental units. The mean response to water, presented as a stimulus, was similar for all the control (4.8 impulses/10 seconds) and all the experimental (6.0 impulses/10 seconds) units. Smaller responses to NaCl (0.03–3.0 *M*) in the NaCl-best fibers but a larger response to 3.0 *M* NaCl in the HCl-best fibers resulted from sodium deprivation. Reprinted from Contreras and Frank (1979) with permission.

NaCl (0.03–3.0 *M*) than the nerves from control (sodium-replete) rats. An analysis of single fiber responses shows the NaCl-best fibers are most affected. No differences in response to sucrose, HCl, quinine, or water were found. The possibility exists that this specific reduction in peripheral nerve responsivity may be related to the increased salt intake of sodium-deprived rats. It is not known, however, whether this same decrease in responsivity would occur in adrenalectomized rats (or any other animal model) that also show increased salt appetite and salt intake.

V. ADRENALECTOMY VERSUS SODIUM DEPRIVATION

Nevertheless, it might be particularly instructive to compare the sodium-deprived rat as a model for the study of salt appetite to the more classical model, the adrenalectomized rat, on several physiological variables. This comparison is summarized in Fig. 8, which indicates whether a particular variable is affected and the direction and relative amount of the effect. Adrenalectomized rats, without sodium-retaining aldosterone, rapidly lose sodium in urine and saliva (Catalanotto and Sweeney, 1979) and have reduced levels of plasma sodium, reduced blood volume, and elevated levels of plasma potassium (Jalowiec and Stricker, 1973). Sodium-deprived rats, with an intact sodium-retaining mechanism, do not lose enough sodium to alter the sodium concentration of plasma or plasma volume.

Sodium-deprived and adrenalectomized rats differ in their sodium concentration of saliva, the former having reduced levels, the latter having elevated levels. It is known that the salt content of saliva influences the sensitivity of the taste receptors through the process of adaptation. To humans, a solution of NaCl is recognized as salty if the concentration is more intense than the adapting NaCl solution, and taste intensity increases as the test concentration increases from the adapting concentration (McBurney and Pfaffmann, 1963; Bartoshuk, 1974). If these same principles apply to rats, then the effect of adrenalectomy, with its accompanying increase in salivary sodium, could not increase the sensitivity of the taste receptors to NaCl, it could only decrease it. With consideration to the possible role salivary sodium might play in salt preference, it is not known how adrenalectomized rats are able to make the discrimination between very weak NaCl solutions and water, although Bartoshuk (1974) has offered some suggestions. The fact that sodium-deprived animals have lower salivary sodium levels

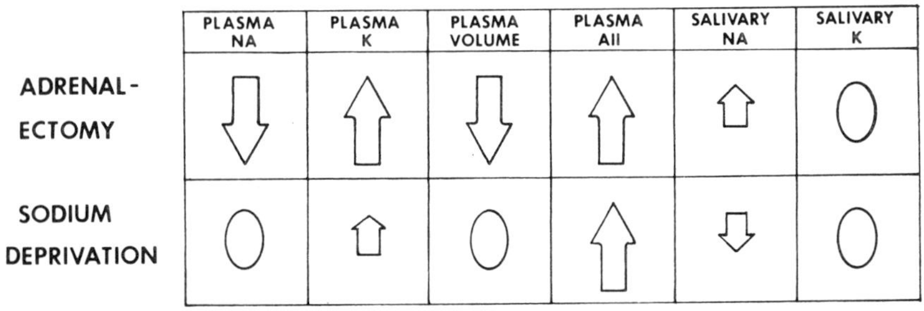

Fig. 8. The effects of adrenalectomy versus sodium deprivation in rat are compared across six physiological variables. This figure indicates whether a particular variable is affected and the direction and relative amount of the effect. Adrenalectomy and sodium deprivation both alter potassium and angiotensin II concentrations in plasma in similar ways.

would suggest that their receptors are more sensitive to low concentrations of stimulating salt solutions. In the neural studies of Contreras and Frank (1979), a water rinse always preceded test stimulus presentation, eliminating the role of saliva in affecting NaCl thresholds.

In sodium-deprived rats, interest is focused on the behavior of an intact organism responding to a nutritional deficiency; in adrenalectomized rats, interest is focused on an organism with a major component of its reactive system missing. Mechanisms underlying salt appetite in these two preparations may be different. Alternatively, both sodium-deprived (Douglas and Catt, 1976) and adrenalectomized rats have elevated levels of angiotensin II in plasma. Recent evidence suggests that intraventricular infusion of angiotensin II in the brains of rats induces an increase in consumption of NaCl solution (Fischer and Buggy, 1975; Chiaraviglio, 1976; Avrith and Fitzsimons, 1978; Bryant *et al.*, 1979). Since angiotensin II is involved in sodium regulation by stimulating aldosterone secretion, it might also be involved in stimulating sodium appetite.

Adrenalectomy (Jalowiec and Stricker, 1973) and sodium deprivation (Contreras and Hatton, 1975) in rats both result in an increase in potassium concentration of plasma. Michell (1978) has recently argued that there is enough evidence to entertain the notion that there is significant relationship between salt appetite and extracellular potassium. He proposes that sodium appetite is a response to both potassium and sodium metabolism and that sodium appetite might be triggered by a mechanism in the brain that monitors the transport of sodium and potassium across a particular site.

VI. SUMMARY

The physiological mechanisms which may be crucial in mediating an animal's behavior to search and ingest salt in deficit conditions are presumably triggered through some innate and centrally organized processes. The sensory signal from the taste receptors, however, plays a role both in the initial detection of the appropriate stimulus, a sodium salt, and in determining, to some extent, the amount ultimately ingested. It is not known how sodium deprivation leads to a vigorous response to the taste of salt. Nevertheless, the possibility exists that the reduced signal from the taste receptors to salt stimulation may be related to the sensory control of a concomitant increase in NaCl intake displayed by sodium-deprived rats. There are several possibilities for mechanisms affecting the sensory change after sodium deprivation (Contreras and Frank, 1979). Regardless of what the mechanisms may turn out to be, physiological changes due to sodium deprivation alter the information that is transmitted from the gustatory receptors to the brain. These sensory changes might allow a sodium-deprived animal to accept salt solutions that are usually rejected by normal animals.

ACKNOWLEDGMENTS

Original data reported in this paper were collected with support from an NIH Biomedical Research Support Grant 5-507-RR-07015. I thank L. K. Contreras for editing and typing.

REFERENCES

Avrith, D., and Fitzsimons, J. T. (1978). Intracranial angiotensin II stimulates sodium appetite in the rat. *J. Physiol. (London)* **282,** 40P.

Bare, J. K. (1949). The specific hunger for sodium chloride in normal and adrenalectomized white rats. *J. Comp. Physiol. Psychol.* **42,** 242–253.

Bartoshuk, L. M. (1974). NaCl thresholds in man: Thresholds for water taste or NaCl taste? *J. Comp. Physiol. Psychol.* **87,** 310–325.

Bell, F. R., and Sly, J. (1977). Correlation of behavioral activity and biochemical status of sodium-deficient calves assessed by operant conditioning. *Olfaction Taste, Proc. Int. Symp., 6th, 1977* p. 274.

Blair-West, J. R., Coghlan, J. P., Denton, D. A., Nelson, J. F., Orchard, E., Scoggins, B. A., Wright, R. D., Myers, K., and Junqueira, C. L. (1968). Physiological, morphological and behavioral adaptation to a sodium-deficient environment by wild native Australian and introduced species of animals. *Nature (London)* **217,** 922–928.

Bryant, R. W., Epstein, A. N., and Fluharty, S. J. (1979). A possible role for angiotensin II in the elicitation of salt appetite. *Int. Symp. Biol. Behav. Aspects Salt Intake, 1979* p. 000.

Cabanac, M. (1971). Physiological role of pleasure. *Science* **173,** 1103–1107.

Catalanotto, F. A., and Sweeney, E. A. (1978). Salivary sodium and potassium concentrations in adrenalectomized rats. *Behav. Biol.* **24,** 467–473.

Chiaraviglio, E. (1976). Effect of renin–angiotensin system on sodium intake. *J. Physiol. (London)* **255,** 57–66.

Contreras, R. J. (1975). Changes in gustatory nerve discharges with sodium deficiency: A single unit analysis. Doctoral Dissertation, Michigan State University, East Lansing.

Contreras, R. J. (1977). Changes in gustatory nerve discharges with sodium deficiency: A single unit analysis. *Brain Res.* **121,** 373–378.

Contreras, R. J., and Frank, M. (1979). Sodium deprivation alters neural responses to gustatory stimuli. *J. Gen. Physiol.* **73,** 569–594.

Contreras, R. J., and Hatton, G. I. (1975). Gustatory adaptation as an explanation for dietary-induced sodium appetite. *Physiol. Behav.* **15,** 569–576.

Denton, D. A. (1965). Evolutionary aspects of the emergence of aldosterone secretion and salt appetite. *Physiol. Rev.* **45,** 245–295.

Denton, D. A. (1967). Salt appetite. *In* "Handbook of Physiology" (C. F. Code, ed.), Sect. 6, Vol. 1, pp. 453–459. Am. Physiol. Soc., Washington, D.C.

Dethier, V. G. (1977). The taste of salt. *Am. Sci.* **65,** 744–751.

DiCara, L. V., and Wilson, L. M. (1974). Role of gustation in sodium appetite. *Physiol. Psychol.* **2,** 43–44.

Douglas, J., and Catt, K. J. (1976). Regulation of angiotensin II receptors in the rat adrenal cortex by dietary electrolytes. *J. Clin. Invest.* **58,** 834–843.

Douglas, J., Hansen, J., and Catt, K. J. (1978). Relationships between plasma renin activity and plasma aldosterone in the rat after dietary electrolyte changes. *Endocrinology* **103,** 60–65.

Fischer, A. E., and Buggy, J. (1975). Central mediation of water and sodium intake: A dual role for angiotensin? *In* "Control Mechanisms of Drinking" (G. Peters, J. T. Fitzsimons, and L. Peters-Haefeli, eds.), pp. 139–147. Springer-Verlag, Berlin and New York.

Frank, M. (1973). An analysis of hamster afferent taste nerve response functions. *J. Gen. Physiol.* **61,** 588–618.

Ganong, W. F. (1971). "Review of Medical Physiology," pp. 264-287. Lange Med. Publ., Los Altos, California.

Garcia, J., Hankins, W. G., and Rusiniak, K. W. (1974). Behavioral regulation of the milieu interne in man and rat. *Science* **185,** 824-831.

Jalowiec, J. E., and Stricker, E. M. (1973). Sodium appetite in adrenalectomized rats following dietary sodium deprivation. *J. Comp. Physiol. Psychol.* **83,** 63-77.

Langford, H. G., Watson, R. L., and Thomas, J. G. (1977). Salt intake and the treatment of hypertension. *Am. Heart J.* **93,** 531-532.

McBurney, D. H., and Pfaffmann, C. (1963). Gustatory adaptation to saliva and sodium chloride. *J. Exp. Psychol.* **65,** 523-529.

McCance, R. A. (1936). Experimental sodium chloride deficiency in man. *Proc. R. Soc. London, Ser. B* **119,** 245-268.

Meneely, G. R., and Battarbee, H. D. (1976). Sodium and potassium. *Nutr. Rev.* **34,** 225-235.

Michell, A. R. (1976). Skeletal sodium: A missing element in hypertension and salt excretion. *Perspect. Biol. Med.* **20,** 34-43.

Michell, A. R. (1978). Salt appetite, salt intake, and hypertension: A deviation of perspective. *Perspect. Biol. Med.* **21,** 335-347.

Morrison, G. R., and Young, J. C. (1972). Taste control over sodium intake in sodium deficient rats. *Physiol. Behav.* **8,** 29-32.

Nachman, M. (1962). Taste preferences for sodium salts by adrenalectomized rats. *J. Comp. Physiol. Psychol.* **55,** 1124-1129.

Nachman, M., and Cole, L. P. (1971). Role of taste in specific hungers. *In* "Handbook of Sensory Physiology" (L. Beidler, ed.), Vol. 4, Part 2, pp. 337-362. Springer-Verlag, Berlin and New York.

Nachman, M., and Pfaffmann, C. (1963). Gustatory nerve discharges in normal and sodium-deficient rats. *J. Comp. Physiol. Psychol.* **56,** 1007-1011.

Nachman, M., and Valentino, D. A. (1966). Roles of taste and postingestional factors in the satiation of sodium appetite in rats. *J. Comp. Physiol. Psychol.* **62,** 280-283.

Oakley, B., and Pfaffmann, C. (1962). Electrophysiologically monitored lesions in the gustatory thalamic relay in the albino rat. *J. Comp. Physiol. Psychol.* **55,** 155-160.

Pfaffmann, C. (1952). Taste preference and aversion following lingual denervation. *J. Comp. Physiol. Psychol.* **45,** 393-400.

Pfaffmann, C. (1963). Taste stimulation and preference behavior. *Wenner-Gren Cent. Int. Symp. Ser.* **1,** 257-273.

Pfaffmann, C., and Bare, J. K. (1950). Gustatory nerve discharges in normal and adrenalectomized rats. *J. Comp. Physiol. Psychol.* **43,** 320-324.

Richter, C. P. (1936). Increased salt appetite in adrenalectomized rats. *Am. J. Physiol.* **115,** 155-161.

Richter, C. P. (1939). Salt taste thresholds of normal and adrenalectomized rats. *Endocrinology* **24,** 367-371.

Richter, C. P. (1956). Salt appetite in mammals: Its dependence on instinct and metabolism. *In* "L'instinct dans le comportement des animaux et de l'homme," p. 577. Masson, Paris.

Schechter, P. J., Horwitz, D., and Henkin, R. I. (1974). Salt preference in patients with untreated and treated essential hypertension. *Am. J. Med. Sci.* **267,** 321-326.

Spielman, W. S., and Davis, J. O. (1974). The renin-angiotensin system and aldosterone secretion during sodium depletion in the rat. *Circ. Res.* **35,** 615-624.

Theios, J., DeRivera, J., and Aronson, E. (1962). Modification of the rat's saline intake gradient by experience with specific concentrations. *Psychol. Rep.* **10,** 487-490.

Wilkins, L., and Richter, C. P. (1940). A great craving for salt by a child with corticoadrenal insufficiency. *J. Am. Med. Assoc.* **114,** 866-868.

PART V
PHYSIOLOGICAL AND PATHOLOGICAL ASPECTS OF SALT INTAKE

Chapter 22

Glycinamide Hydrochloride, a Compound with Common Salt Flavor

M. STERNBERG, D. A. CORNELIUS, N. J. EBERTS,
F. J. SCHWENDE, and J. P. C. CHIANG

I. INTRODUCTION

Salt has been valued for a long time as a flavoring agent of foods. Pliny the Elder, the Roman author of *Natural History*, commented on this subject in the year A.D. 77.

> The higher enjoyments of life could not exist without the use of salt. So necessary is this substance to mankind that even the pleasures of the mind can be expressed by no better term than the word salt.

Salt is mentioned in the Odyssey and in the Bible (Leviticus II 13, Numbers XVIII 19, Ezra IV 14). Yet not every historical civilization had salt available or used it. In some parts of America and even in India salt was first introduced by Europeans (Encyclopaedia Britannica, 1941). The *Odyssey* speaks of inlanders who did not know the sea and used no salt with their food (Encyclopaedia Britannica, 1941). Early man probably required little salt so long as raw animal flesh

ISBN 0-12-397750-9

was available. As communities became pastoral and began to rely more on farinaceous foods, the need for salt increased (Thorpe and Whiteley, 1941).

From the turn of the century evidence started to accumulate suggesting that patients with either cardiac failure or hypertension might benefit by a reduction in the daily intake of sodium chloride (Talbott, 1950; Weinsier, 1976; Fries, 1976). Salt substitutes were developed both to satisfy the salt appetite and to decrease the actual intake of the sodium ion. The substitutes most frequently encountered are based on KCl, NH_4, Ca, and Mg salts, as well as organic acids and their salts of K, Ca, or NH_4. None succeeded in duplicating perfectly the flavor of real salt. The one which came closest to sodium chloride was lithium chloride. This was put on the market around 1949 and seemed to have a flavor very close to sodium chloride; however, it had to be withdrawn after serious signs of intoxication and alleged death (Talbott, 1950).

Currently there are a number of salt substitutes available in grocery and drug stores. They all contain as the principal ingredient, potassium chloride (Table I).

Potassium, however, has important physiological effects (Meneely and Battarbee, 1976). In a recent study, Yap *et al.* (1976) reported "serious cardiac arrhythmias" developed after excessive use of potassium-containing salt substitutes. The same authors qualify hyperkalemia as one of the most serious electrolyte disturbances because of "its profound effect on the cardiac conduction and impulse formation."

We searched for a substitute for salt flavor which did not contain potassium

TABLE I

Commercial Salt Substitutes

Name	Manufacturer	Ingredients
1. Salt Substitute	The Kroger Company	KCl, glutamic acid, KH glutamate, $Ca_3(PO_4)_2$, KI
2. Adolph's	Adolph's Ltd.	KCl, glutamic acid, KH glutamate, SiO_2, tartaric acid, KI
3. CO-Salt	USV Pharmaceutical Corporation	KCl, NH_4Cl, choline bitartrate, silica, lactose
4. Nu-Salt	Cumberland Packing Corporation	KCl, dextrose, cream of tartar
5. Morton Salt Substitute	Morton Salt Company	KCl, fumaric acid, $Ca_3(PO_4)_2$, $CaHPO_4$
6. DIASAL	E. Fougera and Co.	KCl, glutamic acid
7. Featherweight	Chicago Dietic Supply Inc.	KCl, glutamic acid, K glutamate, $Ca_3(PO_4)_2$
8. Neocurtasal	Winthrop Laboratories	KCl, glutamic acid, K glutamate, $CaSiO_3$, $Ca_3(PO_4)_2$, KI
9. Lite Salt	Morton Salt Company	KCl, NaCl

$$\underset{\text{glycinamide hydrochloride}}{H_2NCH_2CONH_2 \cdot HCL} + H_2O \rightarrow \underset{\text{glycine}}{H_2NCH_2COOH \cdot HCL} + \underset{\text{ammonia}}{NH_3}$$

Fig. 1. Hydrolysis of glycinamide hydrochloride into glycine hydrochloride.

chloride or other inorganic cations and found glycinamide hydrochloride. This compound imparts an acceptable salty flavor to foods. It is structurally related to the amino acid glycine, and is not likely to be more toxic than glycine (Fig. 1).

II. SYNTHESIS OF GLYCINAMIDE HYDROCHLORIDE

Glycinamide hydrochloride is commercially available from several sources, yet we felt that the only way to control the chemical purity of the compound was to prepare it ourselves. The synthetic route we chose (Bergell and von Wülfing, 1910) was to condense chloroacetamide with ammonia. The product was thoroughly purified by multiple crystallization and ion exchange chromatography. The synthesis is convenient from a preparative standpoint, although more expensive than other reported methods. This, however, was not considered important at this stage of assessing the value of glycinamide as a salt flavor substitute. The advanced purification which we used, including crystallization and ion exchange chromatography, was meant to ensure removal of impurities such as chlorinated organic compounds and peralkylation compounds of ammonia.

The purified glycinamide hydrochloride was characterized by the following analytical results (Table II).

III. TOXICITY STUDIES

To be assured that the ingestion of glycinamide·HCl by taste panelists was a safe practice, an oral LD_{50} determination in mice by Miles Laboratories toxicol-

TABLE II

Analytical Characterization of Synthetic Glycinamide Hydrochloride

N (Dumas) found	25.2% (Theory 25.2%)
Cl found	31.73% (Theory 32.0%)
Organic Cl found	Less than 4 ppm
Glycinamide · HCl found	102%
Iminodiacetamide (Durrum)	1.036%
Glycine (Durrum)	0.61%

ogy services and a subchronic 90-day toxicity study in rats by the Central Institute of Nutrition and Food Research TNO in the Netherlands, were done.

The acute oral toxicity of glycinamide hydrochloride, expressed as LD_{50}, was 6000 mg/kg with a 95% confidence limit. The subacute feeding study was conducted on 90 female and male weanling albino rats to compare the toxicity of glycinamide HCl with that of glycine. The conclusion of the study, based on 5 and 10% of the active compound present in the diet, was that glycinamide HCl is not more toxic than glycine (Till *et al.*, 1976).

IV. ORGANOLEPTIC EVALUATIONS: FLAVOR PROFILE AND FLAVOR THRESHOLD

The salty flavor of glycinamide · HCl is evident when present in a food such as hamburgers. In contrast, water solutions of glycinamide·HCl have a bitter component. We found that addition of 15–25% sodium glutamate to the glycinamide·HCl either in a food system or in solution decreases some of this bitterness, making the salty taste more evident.

In later practice we found that a mixture of 85:15 w/w glycinamide·HCl–monosodium glutamate had optimal salting properties. The amount of sodium in the mixture corresponds to 1.8% while an equal quantity of sodium chloride contains 39.36% sodium. Although addition of 15–25% w/w monosodium glutamate gave the most acceptable flavor, it could be replaced with potassium glutamate, glutamic acid, or glutamic acid hydrochloride if a Na-free substitute was desired. A slightly bitter taste was evident in hamburger patties containing potassium glutamate, whereas a slight acid taste was noted with glutamic acid or glutamic acid hydrochloride.

Salts of glycinamide combined with food-approved acidulants were prepared and evaluated to determine the role of the anion in the salty flavor. The salts were added to hamburger patties mixed with monosodium glutamate in a 75:25 w/w ratio, at a total level of 1.0% versus uncooked patty weight. The patties were fried and evaluated for flavor by a group of 6 trained tasters (Table III).

Salts having the most acceptable flavors in hamburgers were evaluated in egg salad at a level of 0.7%. Monosodium glutamate was not added because it was felt that its flavor did not blend well with that of eggs (Table IV).

In both systems, the hydrochloride salt of glycinamide had the most acceptable salty flavor.

A search of other amino acid amide hydrochlorides did not reveal salty taste superior to that of glycinamide hydrochloride. Tasting was first performed in distilled water with solutions containing 0.028 g amino acid amide and 0.0094 g monosodium glutamate per 100 ml. This gave a final concentration of 0.0375 g

TABLE III

Flavor of Salts of Glycinamide Tested in Hamburgers

Anion	Flavor description
Adipic (monobasic)	Sour, slightly salty
Adipic (dibasic)	Bland, little salty flavor
Tartaric (monobasic)	Sour
Tartaric (dibasic)	Slightly salty, bland
Fumaric (monobasic)	Slightly sour, slightly salty
Fumaric (dibasic)	Slightly salty, bland
Malic (dibasic)	Slight to moderate saltiness
Succinic (monobasic)	Very sour
Succinic (dibasic)	Bitter
Citric (monobasic)	Sour
Citric (dibasic)	Sour
Citric (tribasic)	Slightly salty, slightly sour
Glutamic (monobasic)	Slight to moderate saltiness
Hydrochloric	Moderately salty, slightly bitter

per 100 ml which is the concentration at which sodium chloride was perceived as having a salty taste (Table V).

This experiment failed to show that any of the tested amino acid amide hydrochlorides had a stronger salty taste than sodium chloride. Some compounds including glycinamide hydrochloride were not perceived at all at the threshold concentration of sodium chloride. Further evaluation was conducted in hamburger patties where each compound was mixed in at 0.525 g/100 g ground beef. Also, except for the control of sodium chloride, all samples contained 0.175 g of monosodium glutamate per 100 g ground beef (Table VI).

In this experiment glycinamide hydrochloride mixed with monosodium glutamate in a 75:25 w/w ratio had the best salty taste compared to sodium chloride.

TABLE IV

Flavor of Salts of Glycinamide Tested in Egg Salad

Anion	Flavor description
Fumaric (dibasic)	Bland, off flavor
Tartaric (dibasic)	Bland
Adipic (dibasic)	Slightly salty
Malic (dibasic)	Slightly salty, bland
Citric (tribasic)	Slightly salty, off flavor
Glutamic (monobasic)	Slightly salty, MSG off flavor
Hydrochloride	Slight to moderate saltiness

TABLE V

Taste of Amino Acid Amide Solutions in Water

Component	Taste evaluation
Sodium chloride	Saline
L-Valine amide · HCl + MSG[a]	Slightly bitter, slightly saline
L-Isoleucine amide · HCl + MSG	Bitter, chemical taste
L-Phenylalanine amide · HCl + MSG	Very bitter
L-Histidine amide · HCl + MSG	Not distinguishable
L-Proline amide · HCl + MSG	Not distinguishable
L-Alanine amide · HCl + MSG	Not distinguishable
Glycylglycine amide · HCl + MSG	Not distinguishable
L-Tryptophan amide · HCl + MSG	Moderately bitter
L-Leucine amide · HCl + MSG	Not distinguishable
L-Glycinamide · HCl + MSG	Not distinguishable

[a] MSG, Monosodium glutamate.

The value of glycinamide hydrochloride as a salt substitute in a variety of foods was assessed by a 24-member taste panel. All panelists were healthy individuals on a normal salt diet. They were asked to evaluate on a nine-point hedonic scale, foods unsalted and salted with a mixture of glycinamide hydrochloride and monosodium glutamate 85:15 w/w or a mixture of glycinamide hydrochloride-monopotassium glutamate-glutamic acid 92:5:3. The results (Table VII), statistically analyzed by the two-way analysis of variance, indicate that foods seasoned with the mixtures based on glycinamide hydrochloride compared favorably with unseasoned ones.

Most of the meats seasoned with glycinamide hydrochloride-monosodium glutamate were significantly preferred over those with no seasoning. This was

TABLE VI

Taste of Amino Acid Amides in Ground Beef Patties [0.525 g Compound and 0.175 g Monosodium Glutamate (MSG) Where Indicated]

Compound	Taste evaluation
Sodium chloride	Good salty flavor
L-Glycinamide · HCl + MSG	Less salty flavor than sodium chloride but flavor good
L-Valine amide · HCl + MSG	Slightly bitter, chemical taste
L-Leucine amide · HCl + MSG	Very bitter
L-Isoleucine amide · HCl + MSG	Very bitter
L-Alanine amide · HCl + MSG	Slightly bitter, chemical taste
L-Proline · HCl + MSG	Slightly bitter, chemical taste

TABLE VII

Preference Test of Glycinamide Hydrochloride in Various Foods

Product evaluated	Salt substitute level (%)	Group means[a]	Level of significance[b]
Beef broth	0.5	1. 5.12	1 different from 3 ($p < 0.05$)
		2. 4.50	
		3. 4.00	
Tomato sauce	0.6	1. 6.26	NS
		2. 5.66	
		3. 5.54	
Vegetable soup	0.3	1. 5.29	1, 2 different from 3 ($p < 0.05$)
		2. 5.20	
		3. 4.45	
Popcorn	0.7	1. 4.91	NS
		2. 4.70	
		3. 5.25	
French fries	0.7	1. 5.58	NS
		2. 5.08	
		3. 6.00	
Frozen corn	0.5	1. 5.50	NS
		2. 5.33	
		3. 6.12	
Mashed potatoes	0.7	1. 5.62	NS
		2. 5.08	
		3. 4.95	
Broiled steak	1.0	1. 7.00	NS
		2. 6.44	
		3. 6.33	
Fried hamburgers	1.0	1. 6.20	1 different from 3 ($p < 0.05$)
		2. 5.58	
		3. 5.38	
Baked halibut	1.0	1. 6.54	1 different from 2, 3 ($p < 0.05$)
		2. 5.25	
		3. 5.75	
Baked turkey	1.0	1. 6.58	1 different from 3 ($p < 0.05$)
		2. 5.95	
		3. 5.54	
Scrambled eggs	0.5	1. 6.70	1, 2 different from 3 ($p < 0.05$)
		2. 6.41	
		3. 5.70	
French salad dressing	2.0	1. 5.41	NS
		2. 5.41	
		3. 5.66	

(continued)

TABLE VII (*continued*)

Product evaluated	Salt substitute level (%)	Group means[a]	Level of significance[b]
Frozen green beans	0.7	1. 4.79	1, 3 different from 2 ($p < 0.05$)
		2. 3.70	
		3. 5.54	
Yeast bread	1.1	1. 5.20	3 different from 2 ($p < 0.5$)
		2. 5.00	
		3. 5.58	
Spice cake	0.7	1. 7.16	NS
		2. 7.08	
		3. 7.16	

[a] 1. Glycinamide hydrochloride–Monosodium glutamate (85:15 w/w); 2. glycinamide hydrochloride–Monopotassium glutamate–glutamic acid (92:5:3 w/w); 3. No salt.

[b] NS, nonsignificant difference between means.

also true for the broth and soup. Eggs and soup seasoned with glycinamide hydrochloride–monopotassium glutamate–glutamic acid were significantly preferred over the unseasoned products, whereas the opposite was true for bread and green beans. Differences in preference for the other foods, whether unseasoned or seasoned with the glycinamide mixtures, were nonsignificant.

Indications of possible interactions with food systems were sought from model experiments. In actual use, glycinamide hydrochloride could be sprinkled on prepared foods or be mixed in before food preparation. Complete recovery of glycinamide hydrochloride was found after autoclaving up to 30 min at 121°C of 1% water solutions adjusted to pH 5, 6, 7, and 8. When autoclaved at 150°C, less than 10% of glycinamide was lost after 10 minutes due to hydrolysis to glycine. In all cases the indicated time interval was the upper limit tested.

Heat stability of glycinamide hydrochloride solutions containing D-xylose, D-glucose, or corn starch is described in Table VIII. As expected, there was least stability and most brown color formation at pH 8.

To study stability in a protein–fat food, we selected hamburgers as a model. We expected that the surface of hamburgers, where maximum heat exposure takes place, would show more glycinamide destruction than the interior. Severe conditions of heat and low moisture prevalent on the surface of fried foods may destroy the glycinamide hydrochloride. It is, however, preserved in the interior of the fried food as evidenced not only by analytical recovery of the compound but also by the salty taste perceived on chewing the food.

The fate of ingested glycinamide hydrochloride has not yet been determined. On examination of the compound's structure, one would expect biological deamidation and conversion into glycine, a common amino acid, whose behavior

TABLE VIII

Stability of Glycinamide Hydrochloride in Mixtures with Carbohydrates[a]

Carbohydrate	pH	Percentage glycinamide recovered	Brown color
D-Xylose	5.0	98.2	+
D-Xylose	6.0	98.4	++
D-Xylose	7.0	91.3	+++
D-Xylose	8.0	79.9	++++
D-Glucose	5.0	99.1	−
D-Glucose	6.0	100.0	+
D-Glucose	7.0	98.8	++
D-Glucose	8.0	95.3	+++
Corn starch	5.0	95.2	−
Corn starch	6.0	96.4	−
Corn starch	7.0	85.9	−
Corn starch	8.0	86.9	−

[a] 1% solution—121°C, 30 min.

in laboratory animals and humans has been documented (Harper *et al.*, 1970). Early work by Waldschmidt-Leitz *et al.* (1927) and Levene *et al.* (1927) showed that a mixture of human intestinal enzymes is capable of hydrolyzing glycinamide hydrochloride. Later, Crosby *et al.* (1964) fed synthetic amino acid amides to mice and showed their ability to replace the corresponding essential amino acids in nutrition. Valine, phenylalanine, leucine, methionine, and to a lesser extent, isoleucine could be replaced by the corresponding DL-amides or amide salts. The nutritional equivalency of amides and amino acids can be explained only by very close if not similar metabolism of the two groups of substances, most likely through deamidation of amides into the corresponding amino acids. Our results, observed after incubating glycinamide hydrochloride with commercial enzyme preparations (Table IX) showed that kidney amino peptidase hydrolyzed glycinamide hydrochloride with formation of glycine. Pancreatin, a commercial mixture of pancreatic enzymes, also hydrolyzed glycinamide but to a much lesser extent. Incubation of glycinamide hydrochloride with freshly prepared rat microsomal enzymes gave an average of 17.5% decomposition.

The results of incubation with enzymes indicate hydrolysis of glycinamide in the intestine, liver, and kidneys with formation of glycine. Chances are probably good that the toxicity of glycinamide will not be different from that of glycine, the ammonium and chloride ions.

TABLE IX

Hydrolysis of Glycinamide Hydrochloride by Commercial Enzyme Preparations

	Percentage glycinamide recovered		Glycine spot shown on TLC	
Enzyme	24 hr	48 hr	24 hr	48 hr
L-Glutaminase (*E. coli*)	97.9	96.9	None	None
L-Asparaginase (*E. coli*)	98.3	97.0	None	Trace
Pancreatin 5 × (Hog pancreas)	100.0	92.4	Trace	Moderate
Aminopeptidase M (Hog kidneys)	74.3	59.4	Considerable	Considerable

V. SUMMARY

Considering the relatively simple synthetic methods reported in the literature for the preparation of glycinamide hydrochloride, the cost to the user of this prospective salt substitute seems not to be prohibitive. The tasting work reported here gives us reason to believe that glycinamide hydrochloride will be able to replace sodium chloride in the flavoring of many foods with the advantage of being a metabolizable compound free of the objectionable taste and physiological disadvantages of potassium chloride.

REFERENCES

Bergell, P., and von Wülfing, H. (1910). Über Verbindungen von Aminosauren and Ammoniak. *Hoppe-Sayler's Z. Physiol. Chem.* **64,** 348.

Crosby, D. G., Thomson, J. R., and Johnson, H. E. (1964). A dietary evaluation of synthetic amino acid amides. *J. Food Sci.* **29,** 686–689.

Encyclopaedia Britannica (1941). Vol. 19, p. 899.

Fries, E. D. (1976). Salt, volume and the prevention of hypertension. *Circulation* **53,** 589.

Harper, A. E., Benevenga, N. J., and Wohlhueter, R. M. (1970). Effect of ingestion of disproportionate amounts of amino acids. *Physiol. Rev.* **50,** 428.

Levene, P. A., Simms, H. S., and Pfaltz, M. H. (1927). Enzyme hydrolysis of dipeptides and tripeptides. *J. Biol. Chem.* **70,** 253.

Meneely, G. R., and Battarbee, H. D. (1976). Sodium and potassium. *Nutr. Rev.* **38,** 225.

Talbott, J. H. (1950). Use of lithium salts as a substitute for sodium chloride. *Arch. Intern. Med.* **85,** 1.

Thorpe, J. F., and Whiteley, M. A. (1941). "Thorpe's Dictionary of Applied Chemistry," Vol. X, p. 843.

Till, H. P., Leegwater, D. C., Slump, P., and Beens, R. B. (1976). Report to Miles Laboratories from TNO Central Institute for Nutrition and Food Research (unpublished).

Waldschmidt-Leitz, E., Grassman, W., and Schaffner, A. (1927). Spaltbarkeit Substituierter Aminosaure-Amide. *Ber. Dtsch. Chem. Ges.* **60,** 359.

Weinsier, R. L. (1976). Overview: Salt and the development of essential hypertension. *Prev. Med.* **5,** 7.

Yap, V., Patel, A., and Thomsen, J. (1976). Hyperkalemia with cardiac arrhythmia. *J. Am. Med. Assoc.* **236,** 2775.

Chapter 23

Brain Lesions and Sodium Appetite: An Approach to the Neurological Analysis of Homeostatic Behavior

GEORGE WOLF and JAY SCHULKIN

I. INTRODUCTION

Our aim in this chapter is to describe and illustrate an approach to research on the brain mechanisms of homeostatic behavior which utilizes sodium appetite in the rat as a model drive system and employs the lesion method as the principal technique of neurological analysis. The general format will be that of a research report including sections on Methods, Results, and Discussion. However, the substance will be a general summary of our research program and its findings and implications. In the Methods section we will present the rationale for our approach which is based primarily on considerations of efficiency and simplicity. We will discuss our methods of procedure, the ultimate aims and expectations of a systematic research program, and the considerations underlying our choices of specific brain regions for investigation and of questions regarding their functions. In the Results section we will summarize what we consider to be our most

BIOLOGICAL AND BEHAVIORAL
ASPECTS OF SALT INTAKE

ISBN 0-12-397750-9

interesting and generally relevant findings in the context of a comparison of the functions of two critical brain regions. In the Discussion section we will interpret our findings in terms of the functions of drive and gustation in sodium appetite and in terms of the effects of learning upon the functioning of the innate system.

II. METHODS

We selected sodium appetite as a model system because it offers several unique advantages for experimental investigation of the central control of homeostatic drives. These advantages have been detailed elsewhere (Wolf *et al.*, 1974) so that we will simply summarize the most outstanding ones here. It should be noted that to facilitate exposition we often use the term "sodium appetite" in lieu of "regulatory sodium intake." Instances where it refers specifically to the craving for sodium will be clear from the context.

The rat's ability to regulate its sodium intake is largely innate (Nachman, 1962; Schulkin, 1978). Its appetite for sodium constitutes a highly specific and powerful drive which is reliably elicited by deficits in body sodium as well as by specific hormonal changes. It seems likely that the rat's brain contains an integrated system for monitoring alterations in body sodium metabolism, eliciting a specific craving for sodium, identifying sodium in the environment, and controlling amounts and patterns of ingestion.

This innate system can be readily studied in adult rats prior to input from specific appetitive learning experiences. Since ordinary rat chows contain superabundant amounts of sodium we assume that laboratory rats raised under standard dietary conditions have had essentially no experience with sodium deficiency and alimentary repletion. Thus, sodium appetite in the rat offers ready access to a specific and innately organized neural system unmodified by repeated experiences of sodium drive, consummatory behavior, and reinforcement.

The facts that sodium salts may be given in solutions affording easy and accurate means of measuring intake, that the palatability of sodium solutions can be readily controlled by altering the concentration or the anion, and that specificity of the appetite can be studied simply by offering varieties of nonsodium as well as sodium salts greatly facilitate experimentation in this system. Finally, there are several simple procedures for reliably eliciting acute or chronic increases in sodium appetite, allowing relatively precise control over the intensity of the craving.

We chose the lesion method as our principal brain research technique in full appreciation of the many limitations upon the interpretation of lesion data. Within the scope of our aims and interests the conceptual and technical simplicity of the method clearly outweighed its disadvantages. Furthermore, many of the interpretative problems are significant only in the restricted context of isolated findings. In our experience when diverse lesion data are coherent, and when they are interpreted in conjunction with data from experiments using different research techniques and in the context of a systematic research program they yield no exceptional problems of interpretation which render them generally less informative than other types of data.

Our long-range experimental program has been to identify all brain structures in which lesions impair the ability to regulate sodium intake and to determine for each of these structures the characteristics of the lesion-induced impairment. The aim of the program is to attain ultimately an image of the functional characteristics and interconnections of all "lesion sensitive" structures relevant to sodium appetite to be envisioned within an overall schema of the functioning brain. It seems likely that such a conceptualization can reveal the neural systems mediating the various components of homeostatic behavior and provide a basis for the elaboration of a general theory. Furthermore, though this research program has a definite aim and terminus, it should yield informative data throughout the course of experimentation.

Two types of studies have been employed in our program. The first type is aimed at identification of relevant structures and the second at detailed analysis of their functions. In the structural studies we use a simple standardized test of sodium appetite. Briefly, lesioned and intact rats are given a strong saline solution in addition to water and food ad libitum in their home cages. After a few days they are treated with drugs which induce sodium appetite, and changes in saline ingestion are observed. This basic screening procedure provides an efficient means of identifying gross impairments in sodium appetite, but more subtle and specific effects such as impairments in taste sensitivity, general arousal, and relevant learning processes may not be manifested under these conditions. At the present stage in our research we are limiting our studies to lesion sites which produce clear impairments in the screening tests. Our subsequent functional studies on such effective lesion sites vary in design depending on hypotheses as to the nature of the deficit, but in general our interests have been to study the involvement of motivational and sensory functions and the effects of pre- and postoperative learning experiences.

We initiated the program by choosing as our first lesion sites the lateral hypothalamic area (LHA) and ventral posterior medial (VPM) region of the thalamus. These two regions are implicated in homeostatic drives and gustatory discrimination, respectively (Teitelbaum and Epstein, 1962; Oakley and Pfaffmann, 1962). Behavioral research had shown very convincingly that these two functions are critical components of the innate sodium appetite system (Nachman, 1962) so that it seemed likely that lesions in these brain regions would disrupt the normal functioning of this system. Concomitant with the analysis of the function of these areas we proceeded to identify and disjoin the pathways to and from these regions as the first step toward tracing the relevant systems through the brain.

III. RESULTS

Extensive damage to LHA uniformly produced a severe, persistent, and apparently irreversible loss of sodium appetite (Wolf, 1964; Wolf and Quartermain, 1967). But when we disjoined singly each of the known or hypothesized extrinsic hypothalamic pathways we found no impairment of sodium appetite under our standard testing conditions (Wolf, 1971). It is necessary that the LHA communicate its critical information to extrahypothalamic structures to activate the final common pathways for appetitive behavior. Apparently the information is not conveyed uniquely through any one of the major LHA projection pathways, and several alternative hypotheses have been suggested, including direct chemical secretion (Wolf, 1971). A recent study by Walsh and Grossman (1977) found deficits in sodium appetite after lesions dorsal to the LHA in apparent contradiction to our findings. This difference may be due to differences in preoperative conditions. The rats in their study apparently had no preoperative experience of saline ingestion while ours did. As will be shown below, preoperative experience of saline ingestion may protect rats against extrahypothalamic lesion deficits.

We have also studied the effects of lesions in various nuclei and pathways surrounding the VPM and, in contrast to the LHA, evidence of individual critical pathways was found. Lesions in the mesencephalic tegmentum immediately caudal to VPM which disjoin the cranial sensory input from the lower brainstem produced a decrement in sodium appetite which resembled that following VPM lesions (Wolf, 1968). Disruption of sodium appetite has also been observed after lesions involving cranial sensory pathways more caudally in the tegmentum (Chiaraviglio, 1972). Furthermore, there is evidence that destruction of rostral VPM projections at the striatal (Neill and Linn, 1975) though not at the cortical level (Wolf *et al.*, 1970) also produces a substantially impairment. Also, the deficits observed by Walsh and Grossman (1977) following zona incerta lesions may be due to the section of gustatory pathways between VPM and amygdala (Norgen, 1976). However, the above data are only suggestive with regard to attribution of effects to VPM pathways since other pathways and cell groups were conjointly destroyed.

Comparisons of the characteristics of the deficits after LHA and VPM lesions support the idea that these regions generate different kinds of information as well as transmit the information in different ways. As noted above, in the LHA sufficiently large lesions uniformly produce a total loss of sodium appetite, and our most recent studies indicate a correlation between the amount of LHA damage and intensity of the deficit (Ruger and Schulkin, 1979). In contrast, extensive VPM lesions do not uniformly produce a deficit (Wolf, 1968; Neill and Kaufman, 1977; Walsh and Grossman, 1977). Our studies revealed a tendency for VPM lesions to either produce a total and persistent loss or they have no observable effect at all. This difference in LHA and VPM lesion effects can be characterized as "graded" versus "all or none."

A particularly informative finding is that with regard to sodium intake LHA-lesioned rats are unresponsive not only to deficits in body sodium but also to excesses. Not only do they fail to ingest sodium when they are deficient even to the point of fatal circulatory collapse, but under certain experimental conditions they ingest grossly excessive quantities producing a pathological overloading of sodium (Wolf and Quartermain, 1967). Our studies agree with the large body of research on LHA function indicating that the deficit in sodium appetite represents a more general impairment of homeostatic behavior. For example, we regularly find deficits in thirst accompanying the sodium appetite deficits in LHA-lesioned rats, although the thirst deficit seems somewhat less severe. On the other hand, LHA damage does not seem to diminish need-free hedonic responses to palatable saline solutions since LHA rats appear to manifest a normal or even supernormal preference-aversion function (Wolf, 1964; Wolf and Quartermain, 1967).

We have not yet fully analyzed the extent of the regulatory deficit of VPM-lesioned rats. Though it is clear that, like LHA-lesioned rats, they generally manifest no ingestive response to body sodium deficiency, we do not know whether the inhibition of sodium intake by body sodium overloads is similarly disrupted. With regard to the specificity of the deficit, our studies suggest that, unlike the general alimentary deficit following LHA lesions, it is limited to sodium appetite with no corresponding impairment in thirst. However, other workers have found a broader spectrum of alimentary deficits after VPM lesions (Neill and Kaufman, 1977), and this requires further investigation. Also in contrast to LHA effects there is clear evidence of a pronounced flattening of the saline preference-aversion function (Oakley and Pfaffman, 1962). But it is important to note that with increased concentrations normal aversion is still manifested.

We have been particularly interested in the effects of preoperative and postoperative experiences of sodium appetite and saline ingestion upon the lesion-induced impairments. With regard to postoperative experiences we found no evidence of substantial effects upon recovery of function in either LHA or VPM lesioned rats (Wolf and Quartermain, 1967; Ahern *et al.*, 1978). On the other hand, specific preoperative experiences of sodium need and/or ingestion appear to have pronounced ameliorative effects upon subsequent lesion-induced deficits in both LHA and VPM, and our initial findings suggest that the critical preoperative experiential variables differ for these two brain regions. In an early study conducted for a different purpose (Wolf, 1971), rats which were allowed to ingest saline under need-free conditions prior to LHA lesioning showed a complete loss of sodium appetite postoperatively just like totally naive LHA-lesioned rats studied in our other experiments. In contrast, saline ingestion in the absence of need, uniformly protects rats from the disruptive affects of VPM lesions (Ahern *et al.*, 1978). To investigate further this difference in the effects of preoperative experience, we allowed rats to ingest saline in the presence of sodium need prior to the induction of LHA lesions (Ruger and Schulkin, 1979). In this case the preoperative experience substantially reduced the intensity of impairment in comparison to LHA-lesioned rats with no preoperative experience. Apparently the mere experience of tasting saline preoperatively is sufficient to protect the rat against VPM lesion deficits, while in the case of LHA lesions our preliminary findings suggest that effective protection depends on preoperative experience of sodium drive reduction (although it is possible that the critical variable may be simply the experience of the drive alone).

IV. DISCUSSION

The findings of our brain lesion studies are consistent with the notion of an innately organized system which mediates sodium appetite so that the sodium-deficient rat experiences a specific craving for sodium salts, actively searches for sodium, and immediately recognizes sodium by taste (Wolf, 1969). The neural system includes the LHA which presumably mediates responses to sodium need and the VPM which mediates responses to sodium taste.

Our observations on rats with LHA lesions support the conclusion that LHA function is necessary for the elicitation of an enhanced appetite for sodium in response to sodium need. This implies that the LHA must directly monitor or indirectly be apprised of conditions of body sodium metabolism. Thus, it is to be expected that neither deficits nor excesses of body sodium are experienced in the absence of LHA function as was evidenced in our studies. However, the above conclusion does not imply that the LHA elicits a specific sodium craving rather than simply arousing a general underlying motivational state to which the specificity is added by another brain structure. Considering our results along with diverse data from other research on LHA function we find evidence consistent with both of these alternatives, and we tentatively assume that the LHA both elicits a general motivational state and identifies specific homeostatic needs.

Motivational states such as sodium appetite affect a wide range of higher mental functions and behavioral dispositions. Thus, we hypothesize that the LHA modulates the activity of the entire forebrain in a diffuse manner, possibly by altering the general neurochemical milieu. This hypothesis is consistent with our data indicating that the arousal of sodium appetite by the LHA is not conveyed uniquely through any single hypothalamofugal pathway to a particular terminal site. Also our findings of a correlation between amount of LHA damage and decrements in sodium appetite suggest a relatively unpatterned efferent signal which functions principally by coding degree of deficit in terms of overall intensity of output. This diffuse output is, at least in part, dependent upon the number of active LHA cells so that the more extensive the LHA damage the weaker the output signal (whether axonal or secretory) and the less intense the experienced craving at any given level of sodium need.

The evidence that postoperative experience of the need-reducing effects of sodium ingestion do not affect recovery from the loss of sodium appetite following extensive LHA lesions is also consistent with the hypothesis that the LHA-lesioned rat does not experience a craving for sodium even when severely deficient in body sodium. However, this hypothesis seems inconsistent with our finding that preoperative experience of sodium drive reduction via saline ingestion does diminish the severity of the deficit. One possible explanation of this effect is that since the lesions in this study were relatively small the result might be due to a summation of preoperatively learned secondary reinforcing effects of saline ingestion with the residual drive eliciting activity of LHA neurons spared by the subtotal lesions. Our evidence that the reinforcing effects of the gustatory properties of palatable saline solutions (as opposed to their need-reducing properties) are not diminished by LHA lesions is relevant to this account, since the learned secondary reinforcing properties of saline may function via the enhancement of the experienced palatability of the saline which is apparently not critically mediated by the LHA. Accordingly the strong saline solution used in our study would taste less aversive to the rats with preoperative drive-reduction experience and they would consequently ingest larger amounts. A phenomenon relevant to this account was reported by Schwartz and Teitelbaum (1974). They found that preoperatively learned taste aversions can survive LHA lesions which block similar postoperative learning. Presumably alimentary learning which requires normal LHA activity modifies other brain functions in such a way that they can subsequently support the performance of alimentary behavior in the absence of normal LHA activity.

With regard to VPM we feel fairly confident that, despite the many diverse functions mediated by this region of the thalamus, those relevant to sodium appetite are involved in one or more aspects of gustation and that the VPM-lesioned rat experiences a normal craving for sodium under conditions of sodium need. Involvement of the specific gustatory projection system is supported by the finding that unlike the putative LHA drive system, lesions of individual VPM pathways are effective in disrupting sodium appetite. One would expect that specific sensory input would not have as diffuse and widespread representation in the brain as would motivational input from altered homeostatic states. However, it is not clear to what extent the VPM is specifically involved in discriminating the taste of sodium, recognizing the intensity of the sodium taste stimulus, or experiencing the hedonic or drive-reducing effects of sodium ingestion. All of these functions may be involved in mediating the alimentary responses to both palatability and appetite which are disrupted by VPM lesions.

We can account for our data on sodium appetite most parsimoniously by the hypothesis that the critical function which is disrupted by VPM lesions is a discriminatory one—that is, the VPM-lesioned rat is unable to recognize (or identify) sodium by taste. The inability to recognize the taste secondarily precludes the rewarding experience which normally sustains saline intake in the presence of need. There is strong evidence that sodium taste stimulation is both necessary and sufficient to maintain normal alimentary responding to alterations of body sodium (Mook, 1969; Nachman and Valentino, 1966). The all-or-none effect of VPM lesions is consistent with this hypothesis of a discriminatory deficit. Discrimination of taste stimuli involves coding by patterns of neural activity. If a lesion spares a sufficient number of neurons so that enough of the pattern is transmitted to allow the projection sites of VPM to interpret it as signifying a sodium stimulus, the remaining intact appetitive system could plausibly function normally in eliciting appropriate ingestive behavior.

The fact that VPM-lesioned rats show a normal avoidance of strong saline solutions under ad libitum choice conditions, as found by Oakley and Pfaffmann (1962) and also in all our VPM lesion studies, does not imply that they recognize the sodium stimulus but only that they can still experience a sufficiently aversive taste. The flattening of the preference–aversion curve can be accounted for by a loss of sodium recognition, but because of the low concentrations of palatable saline solutions, a general diminution of taste sensitivity can also account for this result.

Finally, the hypothesis of a deficit in sodium taste recognition can account for the finding that preoperative saline ingestion experience protects against the loss of the ingestive response to sodium need following VPM lesions. In our experiment the location of the saline in the cage was the same before and after VPM lesions. We know that rats can remember where they tasted sodium even if they did not need it at the time (Krieckhaus, 1970). According to our hypothesis, the naive VPM-lesioned rat experiences a craving for sodium when sodium deficient but cannot recognize sodium by taste, and thus does not ingest the saline available in its cage. The VPM-lesioned rat with preoperative experience remembers where it tasted sodium preoperatively and when the craving is induced it ingests the saline even though it cannot identify the sodium taste at this time.

ACKNOWLEDGMENTS

Supported by NIH Grant NS 12514. We are grateful to Drs. Harvey J. Grill and Paul Rozin for helpful comments on the manuscript.

REFERENCES

Ahern, G. L., Landin, M. L., and Wolf, G. (1978). Escape from deficits in sodium intake after thalamic lesions as a function of preoperative experience. *J. Comp. Physiol. Psychol.* **92,** 544–554.

Chiaraviglio, E. (1972). Mesencephalic influence on the intake of sodium chloride and water in the rat. *Brain Res.* **44,** 73–82.

Krieckhaus, E. E. (1970). "Innate recognition" aids rats in sodium regulation. *J. Comp. Physiol. Psychol.* **73,** 117–123.

Mook, D. G. (1969). Some determinants of preference and aversion in the rat. *Ann. N. Y. Acad. Sci.* **157,** 1158–1175.

Nachman, M. (1962). Taste preference for sodium salts by adrenalectomized rats. *J. Comp. Physiol. Psychol.* **55,** 1124–1129.

Nachman, M., and Valentino, D. A. (1966). The role of taste and postingestional factors in the satiation of sodium appetite in rats. *J. Comp. Physiol. Psychol.* **62,** 280–283.

Neill, D. B., and Kaufman, J. T. (1977). Deficits in behavioral responding to regulatory challenges after lesions of ventrobasal thalamus in rats. *Physiol. Behav.* **19,** 47–52.

Neill, D. B., and Linn, C. L. (1975). Deficits in consummatory responses to regulatory challenge following basal ganglia lesions in rats. *Physiol. Behav.* **14,** 617–624.

Norgren, R. (1976). Taste pathways to hypothalamus and amygdala. *J. Comp. Neurol.* **166,** 17–30.

Oakley, B., and Pfaffmann, C. (1962). Electrophysiologically monitored lesions in the gustatory thalamic relay of the albino rat. *J. Comp. Physiol. Psychol.* **55,** 155–160.

Ruger, J., and Schulkin, J. (1979). Relation of tissue damage and preoperative experience to deficits in sodium appetite following lateral hypothalamic lesions. Unpublished manuscript.

Schulkin, J. (1978). Mineralocorticoids, dietary conditions, and sodium appetite. *Behav. Biol.* **23,** 197–205.

Schwartz, M., and Teitelbaum, P. (1974). Dissociation between learning and remembering in rats with lesions in the lateral hypothalamus. *J. Comp. Physiol. Psychol.* **87,** 384–39-.

Teitelbaum, P., and Epstein, A. N. (1962). The lateral hypothalamic syndrome: Recovery of feeding and drinking after lateral hypothalamic lesions. *Psychol. Rev.* **69,** 74–90.

Walsh, L. L., and Grossman, S. P. (1977). Electrolytic lesions and knife cuts in the region of the zona incerta impair sodium appetite. *Physiol. Behav.* **18,** 587–596.

Wolf, G. (1964). Effect of dorsolateral hypothalamic lesions on sodium appetite elicited by deoxycorticosterone and by acute hyponatremia. *J. Comp. Physiol. Psychol.* **58,** 396–402.

Wolf, G. (1968). Thalamic and tegmental mechanisms for sodium intake: Anatomical and functional relations to lateral hypothalamus. *Physiol. Behav.* **3,** 997–1002.

Wolf, G. (1969). Innate mechanism for regulation of sodium intake. *Olfaction Taste, Proc. Int. Symp., 3rd, 1968* pp. 548–553.

Wolf, G. (1971). Neural mechanisms for sodium appetite: Hypothalamus positive—hypothalamofugal pathways negative. *Physiol. Behav.* **6,** 381–389.

Wolf, G., and Quartermain, D. (1967). Sodium chloride intake of adrenalectomized rats with lateral hypothalamic lesions. *Am. J. Physiol.* **212,** 113–118.

Wolf, G., DiCara, L. V., and Braun, J. J. (1970). Sodium appetite in rats after neocortical ablation. *Physiol. Behav.* **5,** 1265–1269.

Wolf, G., McGovern, J. F., and DiCara, L. V. (1974). Sodium appetite: Some conceptual and methodologic aspects of a model drive system. *Behav. Biol.* **10,** 27–42.

Chapter 24

On the Role of Sodium in Human Hypertension

FREDERIC C. BARTTER, TOSHIRO FUJITA, CATHERINE S. DELEA, and TERUKAZU KAWASAKI

I. INTRODUCTION

Despite the wealth of information relating salt intake to blood pressure in animal models, we know little about this relationship in man. We have studied (Bartter *et al.*, 1976) patients with idiopathic hypertension (mesor hypertension) during salt loading by mouth lasting 6 days. We measured blood pressure, overall retention of sodium, and the concomitant changes in the renin-angiotensin-aldosterone system, hematocrit ratio, cardiac output, and peripheral resistance. In some patients, plasma bradykinin, prostaglandin E_2 and norepinephrine were also measured. The results strongly support and partially explain a relatively short-term effect of dietary sodium on blood pressure.

II. METHODS

One group of 19 patients and a second group of 15 were admitted to the Clinical Center of the National Institutes of Health with a diagnosis of high blood

BIOLOGICAL AND BEHAVIORAL
ASPECTS OF SALT INTAKE

ISBN 0-12-397750-9

pressure. Studies of the known causes of hypertension revealed normal plasma values for renin activity, aldosterone, norepinephrine, and epinephrine; in this way aldosteronism, pheochromocytoma, and "malignant" nephrosclerotic hypertension and the hypertension of renal artery stenosis were ruled out. On balance regimen, each subject was studied on a low-sodium diet (9 mEq/day) and on high-sodium diet (249 mEq/day) each for 6 days. Sodium balance was measured throughout. Blood pressure was determined in all subjects every 4 hours. On day 6 of each regimen, plasma renin activity, aldosterone concentration, and hematocrit ratio were determined every 4 hours and blood pressure was determined by Arteriosonde (Roche) every ½ hour. In the second group of patients, cardiac output by echocardiography and peripheral resistance were calculated on day 6 of the low- and the high-salt regimen. Body weight was determined daily.

The average values from equally spaced intervals in the 24-hour span provide valid estimates of the mesor of the values. Mesors, acrophases, and amplitudes of the best-fitting cosine curves calculated for all data will be the subject of another publication (Kawasaki *et al.*, 1979). Averages of 24-hour values are given here.

III. RESULTS

As shown in Table I, blood pressure rose in almost all subjects with the 6 days of high-salt intake (Kawasaki *et al.*, 1978). In 9 of the 19 patients in the first study and in 8 of the 15 in the second, the mean blood pressure rose by 10% or more of that patient's mean value for the low-sodium diet. These patients were termed "salt-sensitive," the remainder "nonsalt-sensitive."

The group sodium balance data showed significant differences: the salt-sensitive subjects retained more sodium ($p < 0.05$), gained more weight ($p < 0.02$), and "escaped" (urinary sodium exceeding sodium intake) later (day 5 as opposed to day 3) than the nonsalt-sensitive subjects. On the low-salt diet, the nonsalt-sensitive patients showed higher values for plasma renin activity and plasma aldosterone than the salt-sensitive ones ($p < 0.05$ and $p < 0.05$, respectively). With the high-salt diet, the plasma renin activity and plasma aldosterone concentration of the 2 groups did not differ ($p = 0.5$). Thus, the nonsalt-sensitive patients showed a greater lowering of plasma renin activity ($p < 0.05$) and plasma aldosterone concentration ($p < 0.02$) with the salt loading. The decrease of hematocrit ratio (taken as an index of plasma volume expansion) with the high-salt diet was the same ($p = 0.5$) in the salt-sensitive and the nonsalt-sensitive patients.

In the second group of 15 patients, cardiac output, estimated from echocardiograms on the morning of day 6, showed an increase with the high-salt diet ($p < 0.01$) in the salt-sensitive patients but not in the nonsalt-sensitive ones. Total peripheral resistance, calculated from cardiac output and simultaneous blood pressure, actually decreased ($p < 0.01$) in the salt-sensitive patients.

TABLE I

Acute Changes with Sodium-Loading in Hypertensive Patients[a]

Variable	Salt-sensitive (n = 9)	Nonsalt-sensitive (n = 10)	p value
Mean blood pressure (mm HG)	+ 17.6 ± 2.1	+ 4.1 ± 1.0	< 0.001
Body weight (kg)	+ 0.9 ± 0.2	+ 0.2 ± 0.1	< 0.02
Cumulative urinary Na (6 days) (mEq)	+440	+180	<0.05
Hematocrit (%)	− 9.5 ± 2.0	− 6.7 ± 1.4	n.s.
Plasma renin activity	S − 1.3	− 5.3	< 0.05
(ng/ml/hr)	U − 19.8	− 20.5	n.s.
Plasma aldosterone conc. (ng/dl)	− 20	− 32	< 0.02
	(n = 8)	(n = 7)	
Prostaglandin E_2 (immunoreactive- ng/day)	−197 ± 290	+ 62 ± 384	n.s.
Prostaglandin $F_{2\alpha}$ (immunoreactive- ng/day)	−256 ± 269	−233 ± 394	n.s.
Norepinephrine (basal- ng/dl)	−42	− 2	n.s.
Bradykinin (n = 4) (ng/dl)	− 9.7	− 2.6	< 0.001
Cardiac output (liters/min)	+ 0.8 ± 0.4	− 0.3 ± 0.3	< 0.001
Peripheral resistance	− 3.91	+ 3.73	< 0.01

[a] Each number is the *change* in value from low to high-salt diet. The p value reflects the significance of the changes as between salt-sensitive and nonsalt-sensitive patients.

IV. DISCUSSION

The results suggest that cardiac output may be an important variable in the acute (i.e., 6-day) effect of salt loading on blood pressure in these patients with salt-sensitive mesor hypertension (Fujita *et al.*, 1979). This, in turn, suggests that an increase in blood volume leading to an increase in venous return to the heart had been produced in these patients (Guyton *et al.*, 1972). The hematocrit values which decreased equally with salt-loading in salt-sensitive and nonsalt-sensitive patients do not support the suggestion.

The alternative possibility, that the salt loading produced a greater rise in peripheral resistance in the salt-sensitive patients (who retained more sodium and gained more weight), appears unlikely in view of the calculated "decrease" in peripheral resistance with the blood pressure rise in the salt-sensitive patients. A further resolution of the mechanisms for the blood pressure rise must await complete values for pressors, (e.g., norepinephrine) and depressors (e.g., bradykinin) in these patients, now under study.

Whether continued ingestion of high-salt diets by the salt-sensitive patients would lead eventually to increases in peripheral resistance and lowering of cardiac output cannot, of course, be known from short-term studies such as these.

Tuck and associates (1976) infused 2 liters of physiologic saline into patients with idiopathic hypertension and observed that some of them showed a delayed decrease of plasma renin activity and a further rise of blood pressure. Those studies suggest an effect of salt loading even more acute than that described here. Cardiac output and peripheral resistance were not measured.

Weinberger and associates (1979) reported a greater increase in blood pressure with massive salt-loading in black hypertensive subjects than in white ones. The mechanism for the difference is still obscure.

V. SUMMARY

Approximately one-half of the patients with idiopathic hypertension studied without selection showed significant further rise of blood pressure with oral salt loading. The salt-sensitive subjects showed greater sodium retention, greater weight gain, and later urinary sodium "escape" than the nonsalt-sensitive ones. Increase of cardiac output was greater with salt loading, without rise in peripheral resistance, in the salt-sensitive patients.

REFERENCES

Bartter, F. C., Delea, C. S., Baker, W., Halberg, F., and Lee, J. K. (1976). Chronobiology in the diagnosis and treatment of mesor-hypertension. *Chronobiologia* **3**, 199–213.

Fujita, T., Henry, W., Bartter, F. C., and Delea, C. S. (1979). Hemodynamic factors in salt-sensitive hypertension. In preparation.

Guyton, A. C., Coleman, T. G., Cowley, A. W., *et al.* (1972). Arterial pressure regulation. Overriding dominance of the kidneys in long-term regulation and in hypertension. *Am. J. Med.* **52**, 584–592.

Kawasaki, T., Delea, C. S., Bartter, F. C., and Smith, H. (1978). The effect of high-sodium and low-sodium intakes on blood pressure and other related variables in human subjects with idiopathic hypertension. *Am. J. Med.* **64**, 193–198.

Kawasaki, T., Delea, C. S., Bartter, F. C., and Halberg, H. F. (1979). Circadian aspects of the variables involved in the development of hypertension. In preparation.

Tuck, M. L., Williams, G. H., Dluhy, R. G., Greenfield, M., and Moore, T. J. (1976). A delayed suppression of the renin-aldosterone axis following saline infusion in human hypertension. *Circ. Res.* **39**, 711–716.

Weinberger, M. *et al.* (1979). Hypertension in various racial groups. *Proc. Soc. Exp. Biol. Med.* (in press).

Chapter 25

Salt Intake and Hypertension in Rats

KUNIO TORII

I. INTRODUCTION

Several factors are considered to be important in the development and maintenance of essential hypertension: general renal function (Goldblatt *et al.*, 1934; Guyton *et al.*, 1972), operation of the renin–angiotensin–aldosterone system (Coghlan *et al.*, 1972; Ferrario *et al.*, 1972), catecholamines (DeQuattro *et al.*, 1975), response of blood vessels to angiotensin II and norepinephrine (Doyle and Fraser, 1961; Folkow, 1972; Gitlow *et al.*, 1964; Sato *et al.*, 1972), dietary sodium (Na) intake (Dahl and Love, 1954, 1957; Dahl, 1958, 1960a,b; Freis, 1976), Na and water balance (Cranston and Brown, 1963; Freis, 1976), and genetic predisposition to essential hypertension (Swaye *et al.*, 1972; Thomas, 1973; Zinner *et al.*, 1971). Page (1960) summarized these factors as "the mosaic theory of essential hypertension." Nevertheless the central mechanism of development and maintenance of essential hypertension is still unclear, although patients with this disease are reported to have some failure of Na metabolism.

Epidemiological studies (Dahl and Love, 1954, 1957; Dahl, 1958, 1960a; Freis, 1976; Issacson *et al.*, 1963; Page, 1976) suggest that incidence of hypertension in different countries is dependent upon the level of dietary salt consumption. Particularly acute examples of this phenomenon exist in South America

BIOLOGICAL AND BEHAVIORAL
ASPECTS OF SALT INTAKE

ISBN 0-12-397750-9

(Oliver *et al.*, 1975), some Pacific islands (Maddocks, 1961, 1967; Page *et al.*, 1974; Prior *et al.*, 1968), and northern Japan (Dahl, 1960b; Hatano, 1974; Sasaki, 1964). It has also been reported (Fallis *et al.*, 1962; Henkin, 1974; Schechter *et al.*, 1973, 1974; Thomas, 1973; Wotman *et al.*, 1967) that individuals with hypertension generally display elevated threshold or greater preference for salty taste than do normotensives. However, one important fact often overlooked is that the tendency to develop hypertension may have a strong genetic component (Swaye *et al.*, 1972; Thomas, 1973; Zinner *et al.*, 1971). The family of an individual with essential hypertension is likely to have a high incidence of this disease regardless of salt intake levels.

This chapter describes correlations among essential hypertension, the susceptibility to hypertension and salt intake, genetic predisposition to hypertension, the preference for salty taste, nursing on a hypertensive parent, and aging. We used three strains of rats as models for these observations in human populations (Ebihara and Martz, 1970, 1971; Ebihara, 1972).

Meneely *et al.* (1952, 1953), Meneely and Ball (1958), Tucker *et al.* (1957), Dahl (1958, 1960a,b, 1961, 1968), Dahl and Love (1954, 1957), Dahl and Schackow (1964), and Dahl *et al.* (1962, 1970, 1972), reported that chronic ingestion of excessive salt leads to the development of a pathological process in Sprague-Dawley strain (SD) rats that mimics human hypertension. These SD rats showed increased systolic blood pressure in accordance with dietary sodium concentration. This hypertensive condition was sustained even after dietary Na levels were lowered toward normal dietary ranges (Dahl, 1961). However, by substituting a diet in which potassium (K) intake equaled Na intake, hypertension in these SD rats was ameliorated when compared with the absence of K or a low K supply (Dahl *et al.*, 1972; Meneely and Ball, 1958). Some SD rats displayed hypertension as a result of excessive salt ingestion; others did not. The differences appeared to be genetically controlled. Two substrains of SD rats were segregated by selective mating (Dahl *et al.*, 1962; Iwai *et al.*, 1973). One was salt-sensitive and exhibited a high incidence of renovascular hypertension (Dahl, 1968; Dahl *et al.*, 1970). The other was resistant to a salt-induced hypertension. The latter displayed a greater preference for sodium chloride (NaCl) solution than did the former (Wolf *et al.*, 1965).

Dahl (1958) emphasized that the present average levels of salt ingestion are unnecessarily high and that a low intake of dietary sodium, 1–2 g per day or less, may aid in prevention of hypertension. He also emphasized that excessive Na in the diet is a crucial etiologic factor in the development of essential hypertension.

A second strain of rats has also been used to study hypertension. Spontaneously hypertensive rats (SHR) (Okamoto and Aoki, 1963; Okamoto *et al.*, 1966), segregated from Wistar strain rats, develop and maintain hypertension independent of Na intake (Aoki *et al.*, 1972; Louis *et al.*, 1971). SHR have been increasingly employed as a typical model of essential hypertension (Aoki, 1963;

Dahl and Tuthill, 1974; Ebihara and Martz, 1971; Folkow, 1972; Louis *et al.*, 1969; Okamoto *et al.*, 1966, 1967; Sjoerdsma, 1972; Yamori, 1972). One reason for this is that SHR (like human hypertensives) show an increased preference for salty taste compared to normotensive Wistar strain rats (Catalanotto *et al.*, 1972; McConnell and Henkin, 1973).

To evaluate further various factors influencing the development and maintenance of hypertension, I studied the effect of restricted or excessive Na intake, Na balance, the preference for salty taste, and the result of various treatments on blood pressure of adult rats. Three strains of rats were used: the SD, the SHR, and the Wistar/SLC strain (Wistar).

II. METHOD AND RESULTS

Unlike the case for SD rats, hypertension resulting from dietary salt intake could not be produced in the Wistar rats which were supplied with diets containing 0.28% (as control), 2% or 4% (w/w) Na (0, 4.8% and 9.6% NaCl (w/w) added in basal diet, respectively). The diets were introduced from 24 days, 3 and 7 months of age and continued to approximately 2 years of age. Each group was composed of ten male animals. Systolic blood pressure in individual animals was measured monthly by the tail-plethysmograph method without anesthesia. Moribund or dead animals were autopsied. Uremia, leukemia, and tumors were frequently observed among all the groups of animals over one and a half years of age. Systolic blood pressure and survival rate of each of the excessive sodium diet group were essentially the same as controls, although body weight gain and weight maintenance levels were suppressed slightly in accordance with Na concentration in diet. Data at 13 months of age are shown in Table I. Measurements of hematological (red and white cell count, packed cell volume, hemoglobin concentration) and blood chemicals (serum enzyme activities; glutamic oxaloacetic transaminase, glutamic pyruvic transaminase and alkaline phosphatase, serum concentration of total cholesterol, glucose, urea nitrogen, total protein, and albumin, and albumin to globulin ratio), including electrolytes (serum concentration of Na, K, Ca, Mg, and Cl), in survivors at the end of the experimental period (1½ years) showed no statistically significant difference among groups given 0.28 (controls), 2, and 4% Na in their diet.

Whole brain, pituitary, heart, liver, spleen, kidneys, and adrenals were weighed and analyzed histopathologically. The absolute and relative (per body weight) organ weights (except heart and kidneys) were likewise equal. However, weights of both heart and kidneys increased significantly with dietary Na ingestion. This may reflect a compensatory hypertrophy in order to enhance the excretion of excessive body Na to urine. Morphological changes of kidney included chronic glomerulonephritis and/or nephrosclerosis in the control, 2% and

TABLE I

Survivor Rate, Body Weight, and Systolic Blood Pressure of Male Wistar Rats at 13 Months of Age under Long-Term, Excessive NaCl Intake

Duration of Na loading (age)	Na content in diet (%, w/w)	Ratio of survivors[d]	Body weight (g)[d,e]	Systolic blood pressure (mm Hg)[d]
24 days to 13 months	0.28[a]	10/10	398 ± 22	127 ± 8
	2.0[b]	10/10	374 ± 15*	123 ± 10
	4.0[c]	10/10	356 ± 16**	131 ± 9
3 months to 13 months	0.28	10/10	398 ± 22	127 ± 8
	2.0	10/10	376 ± 16*	124 ± 8
	4.0	10/10	351 ± 21**	128 ± 9
7 months to 13 months	0.28	9/9 [f]	403 ± 19	129 ± 14
	2.0	10/10	394 ± 24	129 ± 9
	4.0	10/10	367 ± 10**	126 ± 11

[a] Basal diet contained 0.28% sodium as established by atomic absorption.
[b] Both diets were prepared by addition of 2.0 and 4.0% (w/w) NaCl to the basal diet [4.8 and 9.6% NaCl (w/w) in diet, respectively].
[c] See footnote *b* above.
[d] Ratio of survivors was expressed as total survivors at 13 months of age per number of animals at the beginning of experiments. Body weight and systolic blood pressure were expressed as mean ± standard deviations.
[e] * and ** indicates statistical significance between 0.28% Na diet group and 2.0 or 4.0% Na diet groups. *, $p < 0.05$; **, $p < 0.01$.
[f] An animal was dead prior to experimental period.

4% Na diet groups. As to the severity of these changes, animals of the 2% Na diet group were similar to the control group, but kidneys of the 4% Na diet group were excessively deteriorated. Considering the relationship between dietary Na and water intakes, Wistar rats were able to maintain normal functioning up to one and a half years of age in spite of excessive dietary NaCl loading (Table II). After 2 years of age, however, the animals consumed much larger amounts of water per Na intake than before. These results demonstrate that despite kidney dysfunction due to excessive dietary salt intake, the Wistar rats remained normotensive.

Additional sodium and water metabolism studies were conducted under the same experimental conditions mentioned above except that an additional group was supplied with a 0.78% Na diet [1.2% NaCl (w/w) in basal diet]. Wistar rats were used from 10 weeks of age for 4 weeks. The following results were obtained: (a) the body weight was suppressed and the relative food intake increased with the incremental increase of Na level in the diet. (b) The relationship between water consumption and urine volume and between the excretion of osmotic substances and sodium in urine paralleled the dietary Na consumption. (c) Most of the Na and K which was consumed in the diet was absorbed from the intestine, and a large proportion of the Na and K was excreted in urine. These

TABLE II

Relationship between Na and Water Intake[a]

Experiment	Dietary NaCl loading (age)		Number of animals	Regression curve $Y^b = AX^c + B$		
	Onset	Duration		A	B	r^d
I	7 Months	1 Week	29	0.107	16.3	0.963
II	3 Months	4 Months	29	0.112	13.2	0.995
III	24 Days	7 Months	30	0.118	11.5	0.989
I	7 Months	1 Year	30	0.109	17.9	0.954
I	7 Months	1.5 Years	21	0.140	22.8	0.960

[a] Na and water intake in male Wistar rats which were supplied with a diet containing 0.28, 2, or 4% Na (w/w) were measured over 24-hour periods. Na intake was calculated from food consumption.

[b] X = Na intake mg/rat/day.

[c] Y = water intake, ml/rat/day.

[d] r = correlation coefficient.

effects were noted despite the fact that the level of dietary Na varied from 0.28 (as control) to 4%. The total amount of K absorbed from intestine was not affected by excessive Na in the intestinal tract. However, the total amount of calcium and magnesium absorbed from the intestine increased in parallel with Na concentration in diet. (d) As sodium excretion in the urine increased, urine volume, osmolality clearance (C_{osm}) and free water clearance (C_{H_2O}) were all markedly increased in contrast with the decrease in urine osmolality resulting from natriuresis. Consequently, renal weight was enlarged by excessive Na intake.

In summary, Wistar rats are able to adapt to excessive Na intake and maintain the ECF homeostasis by incrementally changing factors which could contribute to the development and maintenance of essential hypertension: Na absorption, serum Na concentration, serum osmolality, ECF volume, and kidney weight. By altering these factors, these animals remained normotensive without edema regardless of the age of onset of Na loading. This result contrasts with that found with SD rats exposed to long-term NaCl loading.

Sapirstein *et al.* (1950) reported that rats (strain not described) exhibited an increased systolic blood pressure (from 101 to 131 mm Hg) when a hypertonic sodium chloride [2% NaCl (w/w)] solution was introduced as the sole source of drinking water. Additionally, they found that the relative heart weight per body weight increased significantly after the 6-week exposure to hypertonic saline. However, in this condition, it is very difficult for rats to procure free water to excrete excessive body sodium in urine by natriuresis. Figure 2 shows that the upper limit of NaCl concentration as the sole source of drinking water is approximately 0.5 *M* (2.9%). Greater concentrations lead to dehydration due to excessive NaCl loading.

TABLE III

Comparison of Na Balance, Serum Na, Protein Concentration, and Ratio of Kidney Weight per Extracellular Fluid Volume in Young Male Wistar Rats Which Were Fed a Diet Containing Varied Amounts of Na for Short Periods.

Na content in diet (%, w/w)	Dietary Na intake (mg/rat/day)	Na balance (% of dietary intake)			Serum		Kidney/ECF volume (mg/ml × 100)
		Fecal excretion	Intestinal absorption	Urinary excretion	Na (mEq/liter)	Total protein (g/day)	
0.28	53	6.1	93.9	76.1	138±1	5.9±0.2	13.8±0.9
2.0	430	14.4	85.6	77.3	142±3*	5.7±0.3	14.7±0.8
4.0	910	9.2	90.7	84.1	145±4**	5.3±0.2**	13.7±1.8
0.28	56	6.5	93.5	76.7	139±2	—	—
0.78	166	2.5	97.5	85.6	139±3	—	—

[a] Animals 10 weeks of age were supplied the diets containing 0.28, 0.78, 2.0, or 4.0% Na (w/w) for 4 weeks. Food intake, urine volume, and feces weight (dry mater) were recorded. Na contents of these samples and serum were determined using an atomic absorption photoscopy method. Extracellular fluid volume was estimated using the NaSCN dilution method (SCN space). These data are expressed as means ± standard deviations.

* and ** refer to statistical significance between 0.28% (control) and other diet groups: *, $p < 0.05$; **, $p < 0.01$.

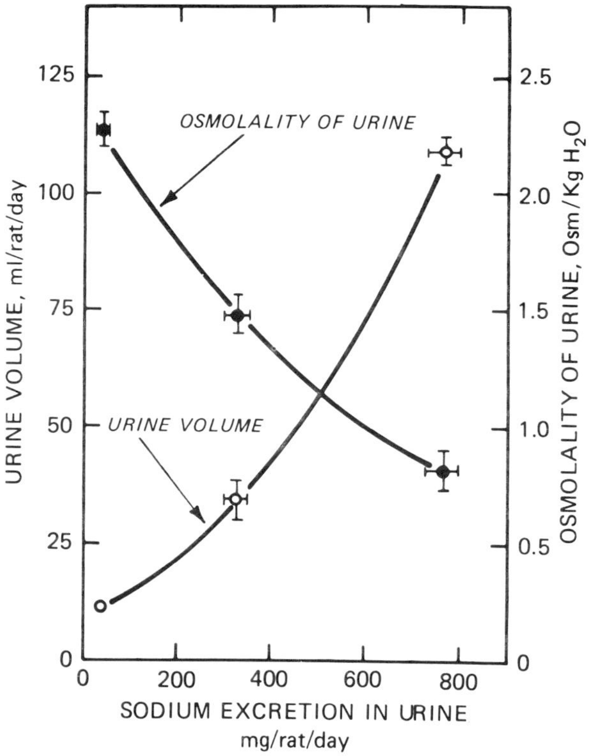

Fig. 1. Correlation between Na excretion in urine and volume or osmolality of urine. Male Wistar rats, 10 weeks of age, were supplied with the diet containing 0.28, 2.0, or 4.0% Na (w/w) for 4 weeks. Na excretion in urine, urine volume (○) for 24 hours, and osmolality of urine (●) were determined. Na content in urine was measured using the atomic absorption method. Each value is plotted as the mean ± standard deviation.

In further studies, Wistar rats were given either 0.17 *M* NaCl solution or deionized water (control) as the sole source of drinking water for three generations starting at 3 months of age for the normotensive parent to 4 months of age for the third generation (Table IV). There was no difference in reproductive function or systolic blood pressure between the groups. This difference from the Sapirstein *et al.* results may be due to the different concentrations of salt solutions used.

In liquid preference tests, the Wistar rats showed no preference for 0.17 *M* NaCl solution when they were fed diets containing 0.28, 2.0, or 4.0% Na. On a diet containing 0.03% Na, a small preference for NaCl solution was observed, reflecting the amount required for physiological needs.

In conclusion, the Wistar rat appears to tolerate excessive NaCl loading,

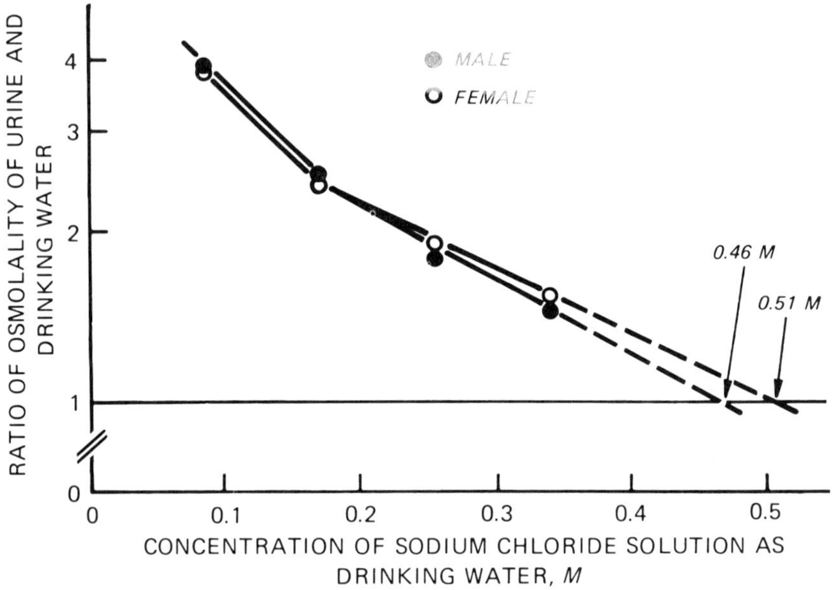

Fig. 2. Effect of concentration of NaCl solution (provided as sole source of drinking water) on urine concentration in Wistar rats. Male and female Wistar rats (littermates), 4 months of age, were kept in metabolic cages and were supplied with a diet containing 0.28% (w/w) Na. NaCl solutions ranged from 0.085 to 0.34 *M*. Osmolality of urine (pooled for 24 hours) and drinking solution were measured by the freezing point depression method. When the ratio of osmolality of urine and drinking solution becomes less than 1.0, dehydration will occur. The maximal concentrations of NaCl solution are estimated at 0.46 *M* for males and 0.51 *M* for females.

maintaining normal sodium and water metabolism. Thus, it fails to display hypertension as a result of excessive Na in the diet or drinking water.

Next, the SHR was investigated as a model of essential hypertension. Unlike the Wistar rats, the SHR showed a strong preference for 0.17 *M* NaCl solution across a dietary Na level from 0.03 to 4%, and displayed a maximal preference for NaCl in solution at 145 mEq/liter, a value equal to the plasma Na concentrations.

Fregly *et al.* (1965) also reported that the level of dietary NaCl failed to influence spontaneous intake of NaCl solutions but increased water intake in proportion to the concentration of NaCl in the food. They also found that intraperitoneal injections of saline failed to alter the pattern of spontaneous NaCl intake of Holtzman rats. When rats were injected with formalin, which causes a strong preference for salty taste, they failed to regulate the total amount of Na intake (Morrison and Young, 1972). These data suggest that the preference for NaCl solutions is not controlled by dietary intake, but that water intake could be regulated by NaCl dietary intake reflecting volume and osmolality changes in extracellular fluid (ECF). The data also suggest that the optimal concentration of

TABLE IV

Effect of 0.17 *M* NaCl Solution (as the Sole Source of Drinking Water) for Three Generations on the Systolic Blood Pressure of Wistar Rats[a]

		Systolic blood pressure (mm Hg)			
Generation	Sex	Deionized water[a]		0.17 *M* NaCl solution[a]	
Parent	Male	126	(N = 1)	124	(N = 1)
	Female	120	(N = 1)	118	(N = 1)
F_1 Generation	Male	122 ± 4	(N = 4)	122 ± 3	(N = 4)
	Female	120 ± 2	(N = 4)	118 ± 4	(N = 6)
F_2 Generation	Male	123 ± 6	(N = 19)	121 ± 4	(N = 29)
	Female	121 ± 4	(N = 20)	118 ± 3	(N = 29)

[a] A pair of normotensive Wistar rats (parent) were supplied ad libitum. Two generations of offspring of this pair were used. The male which showed the highest level of systolic blood pressure was selected as the sire. He was bred with female littermates. The systolic blood pressure of each individual at each generation was measured at 4 months of age. These data are expressed as mean or mean ± standard deviation. N = the number of animals in each group. There were no statistically significant differences between groups supplied with deionized water and a 0.17 *M* NaCl solution as drinking water.

NaCl in spontaneous intake was probably regulated by oral factors including salivary glands.

Aoki *et al.* (1972) and Louis *et al.* (1971) reported that the growth of weanling SHR was suppressed under a restricted Na diet. Therefore, an experiment to measure the growth of SHR placed on restricted Na diets from birth was conducted in order to estimate the minimal requirement of Na for normal growth and to examine the dietary effects on systolic blood pressure with age. Four groups were studied. Group A rats served as the control group. Group B rats comprised the Na-restricted group. The last two groups were nursed by either hypertensive (SHR) (Group Cs) or normotensive (Wistar) (Group Cw) foster-dam immediately after birth. There were approximately ten animals in each of these groups (see Tables V and VI and Fig. 3).

Animals of Groups B, Cs and Cw were supplied with 0.03% Na diet from birth until weaning at 21 days of age. This level is the minimal requirement of Na for lactation in albino rats (Ganguli *et al.*, 1969a,b; Kirksey and Pike, 1962). The body weights of these SHR pups were similar to control at 21 days of age (weaning). Growth of weanling SHR was severely depressed during Na restriction when the SHR dams were given a Na-restricted diet after delivery.

Following weaning, animals of Groups Cs and Cw were supplied with diets of increasing Na content chronologically as they matured. The plateau level of body weight increased step-wise with the increments of Na in diet (Fig. 3 and Table V).

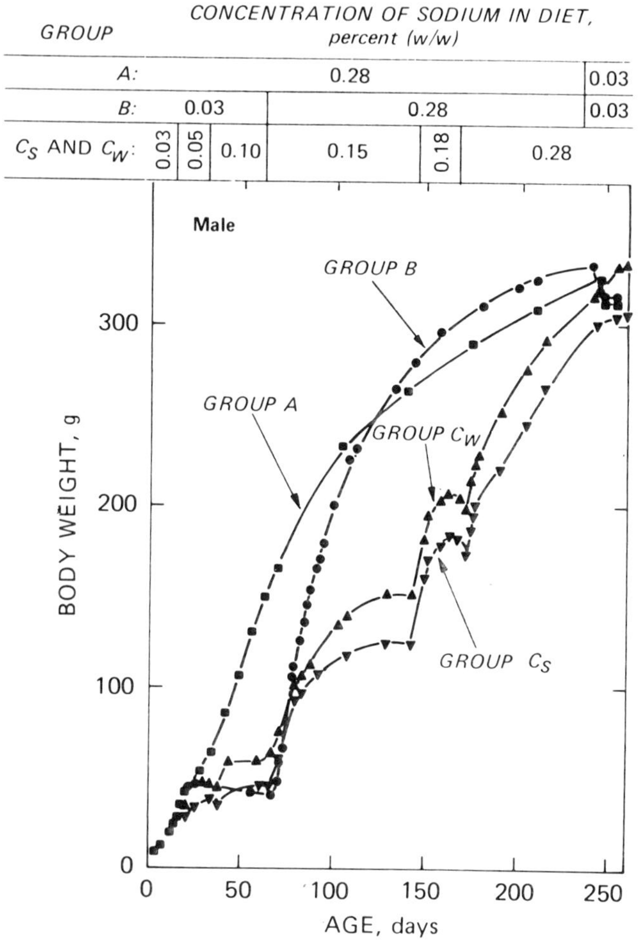

Fig. 3. Pattern of weanling SHR growth under dietary Na restriction. Sib-mated male SHR (F_2 generation) were used. Animals of Group A (■) (control) ($N = 10$), B (●) ($N = 11$), Cs (▼) ($N = 6$), and Cw (▲) ($N = 6$) were supplied ad libitum with deionized water as the sole source of drinking water and diets containing varying quantities of sodium. The exact amount of Na in the diet at any particular time for any particular group of animals can be found by referring to the display above the actual figure. Refer also to Tables V and VI. Animals of Group Cs were nursed by a foster SHR (hypertensive) dam and Group Cw by a foster Wistar (normotensive) dam. Animals in Groups A and B were nursed by their own SHR mother. At 8 months of age, Group A and B were provided with dietary Na restriction (0.03% Na diet) for 10 days, but the magnitude of body weight decreases on both groups was essentially the same. Body weight of Group Cw was significantly higher than that of Group Cs from weaning to the conclusion of the experiment.

TABLE V

Effect of Na Restriction and Nursing by Either Normotensive or Hypertensive Foster-dams on Weanling SHR[a]

Group	Strain of animals	Strain of foster-dam	Sex	Number of animals	Plateau level of body weight (g)					
					0.03[b]	0.05[b]	0.10[b]	0.15[b]	0.18[b]	0.28[b]
Cs	SHR	SHR	Male	6	28±6	38±8	55±10	124±6	184±10	307±17
Cw	SHR	Wistar	Male	6	34±1*	46±2*	63±5	151±6**	206±7**	334±6**
Cs	SHR	SHR	Female	4	34±3	48±6	63±9	116±12	149±10	186±5
Cw	SHR	Wistar	Female	4	33±1	43±4	63±2	119±7	157±5	195±3**

[a] SHR were nursed with normotensive (Wistar) (Group Cw) or hypertensive (SHR) (Group Cs) foster-dams from birth. They were supplied with Na-restricted diets containing 0.03 (birth–21 days of age), 0.05 (22–37), 0.10 (38–67), 0.15 (68–149), 0.18 (150–171), and 0.28% (172–260). These data show body weight (mean with standard deviation) at the point when it plateaus under each Na-restricted diet. Statistical significance is as follows: *, $p < 0.05$; **, $p < 0.01$ between SHR-nursed with SHR and Wistar foster-dam.

[b] Na content in diet (% w/w).

The minimal Na requirement for normal growth of SHR was estimated to be 0.27% (male) and 0.23% (female). These values are close to the amounts found in commercial chow (0.26–0.31% in diet) and they are much higher than those reported for normal albino rats (0.05%) (Grunert *et al.*, 1950).

These observations suggested that SHR may have some dysfunction of Na metabolism. To investigate this possibility, Na balance and urinary Na excretion patterns were determined for these animals. Under a 0.28% Na diet, ad libitum, the intestinal absorption of Na in SHR is 32% of intake while that for Wistar rats is 85% under the same level of relative Na consumption (per body weight). The 24-hour pattern of Na excretion in urine in SHR was quite low and constant in contrast to that of the Wistar rats which displayed a change of amount and concentration of urinary Na dependent upon feeding behavior.

Based on these data, it is suggested that the strong preference for NaCl solution in SHR originates as a consequence of physiological need. It may be induced by a dysfunction of Na absorption or a maintenance of the antinatriuretic condition. Angiotensin II may play a role in this preference through its action on brain (Minichi, 1972) and/or extracellular fluid, since rats (Long–Evans strain) injected with angiotensin II showed enhanced intake of sodium and water (Buggy and Fisher, 1974). It is also possible that intestinal Na absorption is unable to respond to mineralocorticoids.

Systolic blood pressure of these SHR was measured by the tail-microphone method (Friedman and Freed, 1949). Na restriction in SHR of groups B, Cs, and Cw from birth onward suppressed the usual increase in systolic blood pressure with age. Animals of Group Cs and Cw, which were chronologically supplied with diets of increasing Na content up to a 0.28%, grew to a normal size, and displayed significantly lower systolic blood pressure than Group B. Furthermore, the systolic blood pressure of Group Cw was significantly lower than that of Group Cs. Introduction of a 0.03% Na diet (equal to minimal Na requirement for maintenance in albino rats) for 10 days to Groups A and B during adulthood led to a significant decrease in systolic blood pressure of Group B which received restricted Na dietary levels during the neonatal period. Animals in Group A (control) were not subjected to Na restriction during growth and did not respond to this dietary treatment as adults (Table VI) (for a similar result, see Grollman and Harrison, 1945). Thus, at least two factors are involved in control of blood pressure in SHR: a variable factor and Na intake during growth. Nursing by a normotensive (Wistar) foster-dam combined with Na restriction during growth ameliorated the minimal Na requirement and the increase in systolic blood pressure of SHR to an extent greater than Na restriction alone (Table VI). These results suggest that the neonatal period may be particularly important for SHR in determining adult systolic blood pressure.

Dahl *et al.* (1972) and Meneely and Ball (1958) reported that the increase in systolic blood pressure was reduced by adding equimolar KCl to the NaCl-loaded

TABLE VI

Effect of Na Restriction from Birth on Systolic Blood Pressure of SHR as Adults[a]

Group	Sex	Systolic blood pressure at 6 months of age (mm Hg)		Change of systolic blood pressure following introduction of 0.03% Na diet at 8 months of age (mm Hg)
A	Male	187±4	($N=10$)	−0.8
B	Male	173±15*	($N=11$)	−26.0**
Cs	Male	167±3**	($N=6$)	—
Cw	Male	153±9*	($N=6$)	—
A	Female	176±3	($N=10$)	−0.4
B	Female	150±11**	($N=11$)	−24.0**

[a] Sib-mated SHR (F_2 generation) were used. Animals of Group A (control) were supplied with the diet containing 0.28% Na (w/w) from birth to 8 months of age. Animals of Group B were supplied with the diet containing 0.03% Na from birth to 67 days of age, then 0.28% Na up to 8 months of age. Subsequently both groups were provided with a 0.03% Na diet (equal to minimal requirements for maintenance of albino rats) for 10 days. From birth to 21 days of age, group Cs was nursed by SHR (hypertensive) dams and group Cw was nursed by Wistar (normotensive). Both groups were supplied with Na-restricted diets containing 0.3% (birth–21 days of age), 0.05% (22–37), 0.10% (38–67), 0.15% (68–149), 0.18% (150–171), and 0.28% (172–260). Systolic blood pressure of these animals was measured first at 6 months of age (0.28% Na diet supply) and again at 8 months of age (prior to and following Na restriction of Groups A and B). These data are expressed as means ± standard deviation. Statistical significance is as follows: *, $p < 0.05$ and **, $p < 0.01$ for B compared with A, Cs compared with A, or Cw compared with Cs.

diet. Louis *et al.* (1971) reported a similar result in SHR. We monitored the growth of neonatal SHR while substituting NaCl (0.17 *M*) or NaCl (0.17 *M*) plus equimolar KCl solution for drinking water of the lactating females. The SHR dams were also tested for preference for these solutions versus deionized water in a three-bottle test.

When SHR dams were supplied with a solution containing 0.17 *M* NaCl plus equimolar KCl as the sole source of drinking water, they failed to nurse their pups, although the Wistar dams given the same solution nursed adequately. When both SHR and Wistar dams were given either 0.17 *M* NaCl solution or deionized water as drinking water, both nursed normally. Death of neonatal SHR was observed only with the group supplied with NaCl plus equimolar KCl solution. The death rate of this group was 44% (11/25) up to 20 days of age. Half of the survivors of this group did not open their eyes before 20 days of age (Fig. 4). Normal SHR dams, 5 months of age, showed a strong preference for the NaCl solution but none for NaCl plus KCl. After removal of the NaCl solution from individual cages, SHR dams preferred deionized water as a drinking solution

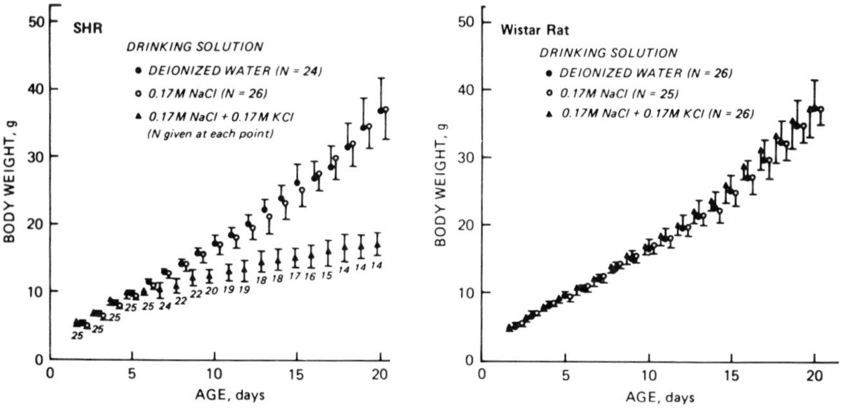

Fig. 4. Effect of NaCl alone or with KCl solution (as the sole source of drinking water) on SHR and Wistar rat growth. SHR and Wistar dams, 5 months of age, were supplied with the normal diet containing 0.28% Na (w/w) and deionized water as control, 0.17 *M* NaCl or 0.17 *M* NaCl plus equimolar KCl solution as drinking water ad libitum. Each experimental group was composed of three SHR or Wistar dams which nursed 7–10 pups. Number and body weight of pups were measured every day from 2 days to 20 days of age. Each symbol represents mean body weight and the standard deviation.

when tested against NaCl plus KCl. Potassium ion in the SHR might inhibit Na^+ ion absorption from the intestine, while K^+ ion in the SD rats apparently moderates the blood pressure increase with excessive Na intake. When a Wistar dam was given 0.17 *M* NaCl solution as drinking water from birth to 80 days of age, then given deionized water ad libitum, she subsequently (at 5 months of age) preferred a 0.17 *M* NaCl solution but did not prefer 0.17 *M* NaCl plus equimolar KCl solution (Fig. 5). These results are similar to those obtained using the SHR dam, yet the Wistar rat was normotensive. This is an indication that the Wistar rat can be "imprinted" to prefer a NaCl solution by providing it with NaCl drinking solution during its first 80 days of life.

These data suggest that dysfunction in Na absorption and a maternal factor (expressed during nursing) are possible causal agents in the development and maintenance of salt preference and hypertension in SHR. Even though Na intake with K suppressed the blood pressure increase in the SD rat, the same treatment was not clearly effective for the SHR (Louis *et al.*, 1971). Also it is interesting that salt preference is "imprintable" even if the subject is a normotensive Wistar rat.

Finally, SD rats which respond to excessive salt intake by increased systolic blood pressure (Dahl, 1961), were used to investigate the relationship between susceptibility to hypertension and treatments begun at the neonatal age. Male SD rats of an F_2 generation ($N = 42$) derived from a normotensive pair were separated into seven groups. SD rats that were fed a normal diet ad libitum were

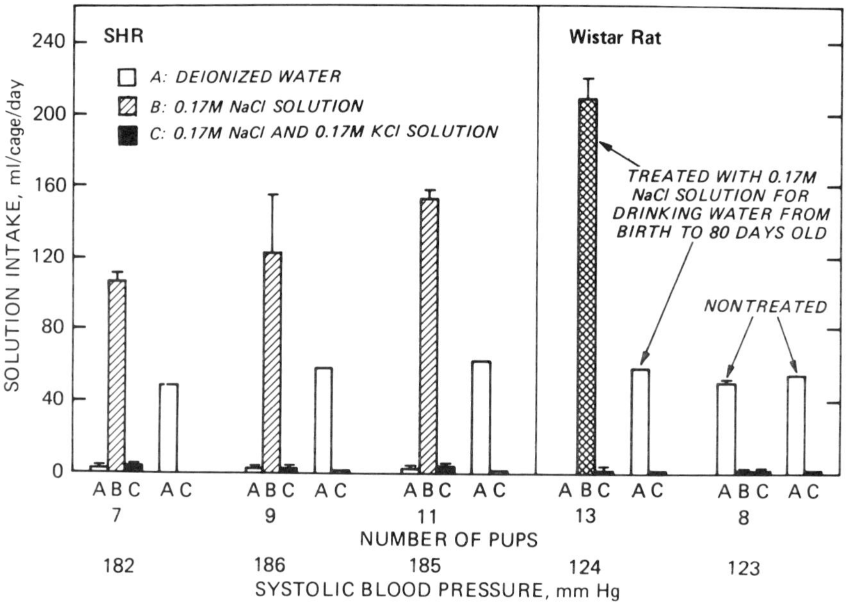

Fig. 5. Preference for NaCl alone or with KCl solutions in SHR and Wistar dams during lactation. Intake of deionized water (A), 0.17 *M* NaCl (B), and 0.17 *M* NaCl plus equimolar KCl (C) solution was determined for SHR and Wistar dams, 5 months of age after delivery of pups. The pups remained in the cage with the mothers. From day 2 after delivery to day 4 intakes of solutions A, B, and C were recorded. On day 5, only solutions A and C were offered. A Wistar dam, 5 months of age, given 0.17 *M* NaCl solution as the sole source of drinking water from birth to 80 days was given a choice, using the same time paradigm as the SHR, among solutions A, B, and C, then between A and C. These data are compared with a control ("nontreated") animal given deionized water as a fluid source from birth to 80 days. After the preference tests, systolic blood pressure and number of pups were determined (day 7). Column sets showing comparisons among solutions A, B, and C are expressed as intake per cage per 24 hours and include one standard deviation.

injected with either isotonic or hypertonic saline (300 and 600 mOsm/kg H_2O, respectively) intraperitoneally (1.25 g NaCl/kg body weight) at 10, 20, and 30 days of age. At 6 and 12 months of age, the systolic blood pressure was observed to be significantly increased for those SD rats injected with either the isotonic or hypertonic saline on days 20 or 30, but no change in blood pressure was observed for those animals injected when they were 10 days of age. There were no differences between isotonic and hypertonic saline administration. Figure 6 shows results of the systolic blood pressure in these SD rats at 6 months of age. Also those SD rats that were fostered by SHR dams immediately after delivery and given a "normal" Na diet and deionized water as the sole source of drinking water ad libitum displayed an increased systolic blood pressure as adults. On the other hand, Wistar rats similarly treated or allowed to nurse with normal Wistar

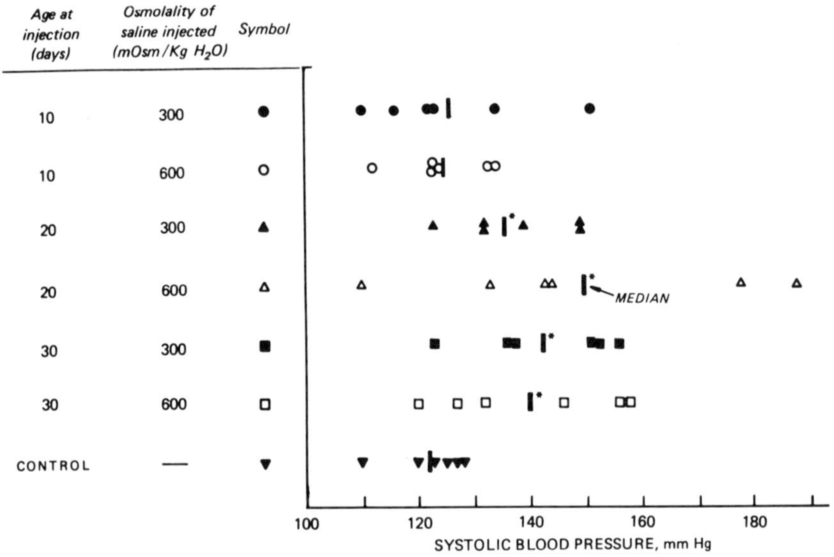

Fig. 6. The effect of single injections of iso- or hypertonic saline at various ages on the adult systolic blood pressure of SD rat. Animals which were sib-mated (F_2 generation) were injected either with iso- (closed marks) or hypertonic (open marks) saline intraperitoneally, 1.25g NaCl per kg body weight, at 10, 20, or 30 days of age. Control animals sham-operated. All animals were supplied with the normal diet [0.28% Na (w/w)] and tap water as drinking water ad libitum. Systolic blood pressure was measured at 6 months of age. Individual data are shown with the median for each group. Statistical significance ($p < 0.05$), shown as an * mark, was achieved between some sham-operated control and treated groups.

dams supplied with 0.17 *M* NaCl solution as drinking water remained normotensive (Fig. 7). It is interesting that pregnancy in SHR is associated with a marked and significant decline in blood pressure toward the normal range before and after delivery (Aoi *et al.*, 1976). These data raise the possibility that milk in the SHR dam may contain a factor which is potent in "setting" or "resetting" sodium and water metabolism and regulating subsequent blood pressure. The neonatal SD rat is susceptible to this factor but the neonatal Wistar is not.

III. CONCLUSIONS

This observation led to the following hypotheses: (a) the Wistar rat is a "nonresponder" to excessive dietary Na intake from weaning and during life. Yet this strain is "imprintable" for salt preference if given 0.17 *M* NaCl solution during its growth stage but does not develop high blood pressure; (b) the SD rat is a "responder" either to an excessive dietary Na loading or to treatment at neonatal

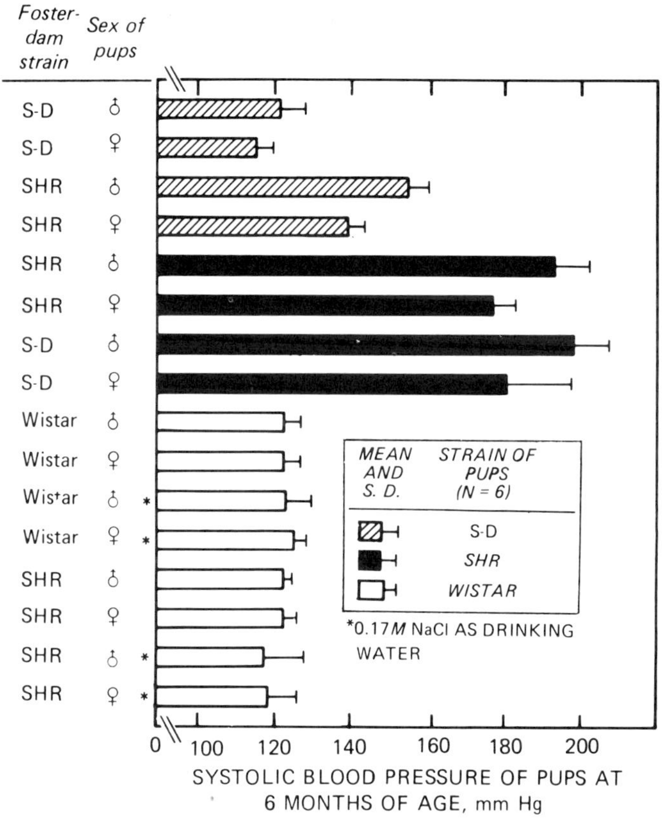

Fig. 7. Effect of hypertensive or normotensive foster-dam nursing on systolic blood pressure of SD, SHR, and Wistar rats. Pups were nursed with normotensive (Wistar or SD) or hypertensive (SHR) females from birth to weaning, and supplied with normal diet containing 0.28% Na (w/w) and deionized water. Pups of Wistar rats were nursed and/or supplied with 0.17 *M* NaCl solution as drinking water from birth to 6 months of age. Systolic blood pressure was measured at 6 months of age. Each column shows strain of pups and systolic blood pressure with standard deviation (refer to inset in this Figure). Statistical significance between pups nursed with the foster-dam of the same and another strain was observed in male and female SD rats only ($p < 0.01$).

age, and will develop high blood pressure as an adult; (c) the SHR is an "inherited nonresponder" to restricted or excessive dietary Na treatment. Under all conditions of dietary Na, it will develop hypertension. Also the SHR is unable to grow under very restricted Na intake (equal to minimal Na requirement for growth and maintenance in albino rats). SHR failed to nurse their pups under loading of NaCl plus equimolar KCl probably because of dysfunctions in intestinal Na absorption and/or renal Na regulation; (d) the SHR is able to respond to a low Na diet at adult age providing it had consumed a low Na regimen during growth. Systolic blood pressure in these adult SHR is much lower than normal SHR not subjected to this treatment. In addition to this treatment the minimal Na requirement for normal growth and the incremental change of systolic blood pressure with age could be lowered if the SHR pups were nursed by a normotensive Wistar female.

While it may be controversial to extrapolate this hypothesis to human populations, several intriguing parallels make such an extension warranted. In Northern Japan where people consume high levels of NaCl (used as preservatives and taste stimuli)—similar to usage of sugar in the United States—a high incidence of essential hypertension is found in some but not in all individuals. Apparently some are "responders" to high salt intake but others are "nonresponders" maintaining normal blood pressure. Since there is a large supply of NaCl in the diet, both the "responder" and "nonresponder" are able to reproduce, thus maintaining their percentage within the population. In South America where some Indian populations have a "no-salt" culture, individuals show a normal blood pressure range, and exhibit no increases of blood pressure with age. Since there is little salt in the diet, the "inherited nonresponders" (analogous to the SHR) fail to reach sexual maturity and are naturally selected out of the population. The "responders" (analogous to SD rats) never express their predisposition to hypertension since they are never exposed to "normal" or "high" salt diets. Consequently, it may be hypothesized that the human population contains individuals of at least three types: those who will not develop hypertension regardless of salt intake, those who have a genetic predisposition to high salt intake and who will, as a consequence of diet, develop this disease, and those who are unable to grow normally under "low" salt diets and will develop hypertension with or without high salt intake over their requirement for growth. Only those individuals who develop hypertension due to excessive salt intake can be treated by a diet programmed to lower salt intake. It does not follow, of course, that all individuals will profit by an "ideal" salt diet. The most important problem is how to confirm and classify these different types of people before that portion of the human population becomes hypertensive.

ACKNOWLEDGMENTS

The constructive criticisms and editorial advice of Drs. Joseph G. Brand, Gary Beauchamp, Carol Christensen, and Morley R. Kare are appreciated.

REFERENCES

Aoi, W., Gable, D., Cleary, R. E., Young, P. C. M., and Weinberger, M. H. (1976). The antihypertensive effect of pregnancy in spontaneously hypertensive rats. *Proc. Soc. Exp. Biol. Med.* **153,** 13-15.

Aoki, K. (1963). Experimental studies on the relationship between endocrine organs and hypertension in spontaneously hypertensive rats. I. Effect of hypophysectomy, adrenalectomy, thyroidectomy, nephrectomy and sympathectomy on blood pressure. *Jpn. Heart J.* **4,** 443–461.

Aoki, K., Yamori, Y., Ooshima, A., and Okamoto, K. (1972). Effects of high or low sodium intake in spontaneously hypertensive rats. *Jpn. Circ. J.* **36,** 539–545.

Buggy, J., and Fisher, A. E. (1974). Evidence for a dual central role for angiotensin in water and sodium intake. *Nature (London)* **250,** 733–735.

Catalanotto, F. C., Schechter, P. J., and Henkin, R. I. (1972). Preference for NaCl in the spontaneously hypertensive rats. *Life Sci.* **11,** 557–564.

Coghlan, J. P., Doyle, A. E., Jerums, G., and Scoggins, B. A. (1972). The effects of sodium loading and deprivation on plasma renin and plasma and urinary aldosterone in hypertension. *Clin. Sci.* **42,** 15–23.

Cranston, W. I., and Brown, W. (1963). Diurnal variation in plasma volume in normal and hypertensive subjects. *Clin. Sci.* **25,** 107–114.

Dahl, L. K. (1958). Salt intake and salt need. *N. Engl. J. Med.* **258,** 1152–1157.

Dahl, L. K. (1960a). Possible role of salt intake in the development of essential hypertension. *In* "Essential Hypertension. An International Symposium" (K. D. Bock and P. T. Cottier, eds.), pp. 53–65. Springer-Verlag, Berlin and New York.

Dahl, L. K. (1960b). Salt, fat and hypertension. The Japanese experience. *Nutr. Rev.* **18,** 97–99.

Dahl, L. K. (1961). Effects of chronic excess salt feeding. Induction of self-sustaining hypertension in rats. *J. Exp. Med.* **114,** 231–236.

Dahl, L. K. (1968). Salt in processed baby foods. *Am. J. Clin. Nutr.* **21,** 787–792.

Dahl, L. K., and Love, R. A. (1954). Evidence for relationship between sodium (chloride) intake and human essential hypertension. *Arch. Intern. Med.* **94,** 525–531.

Dahl, L. K., and Love, R. A. (1957). Etiological role of sodium chloride intake in essential hypertension in humans. *J. Am. Med. Assoc.* **164,** 397–400.

Dahl, L. K., and Schackow, E. (1964). Effects of chronic excess salt ingestion: Experimental hypertension in the rat. *Can. Med. Assoc. J.* **90,** 153–160.

Dahl, L. K., and Tuthill, R. (1974). Further evidence of the toxicity of NaCl, increased blood pressure and mortality in the spontaneously hypertensive rat. *J. Exp. Med.* **139,** 617–626.

Dahl, L. K., Heine, M., and Tassinari, L. (1962). Effect of chronic salt ingestion: Evidence that genetic factors play an important role in susceptibility to experimental hypertension. *J. Exp. Med.* **115,** 1173–1190.

Dahl, L. K., Heine, M., Leitl, G., and Tassinari, L. (1970). Hypertension and death from consumption of processed baby foods by rats. *Proc. Soc. Exp. Biol. Med.* **133,** 1405–1408.

Dahl, L. K., Leitl, G., and Heine, M. (1972). Influence of dietary potassium and sodium/potassium molar ratios on the development of salt hypertension. *J. Exp. Med.* **136,** 318–330.

DeQuattro, V., Miura, Y., Lurvey, A., Cosgrove, M., and Mendez, R. (1975). Increased plasma catecholamine concentrations and vas deferens norepinephrine biosynthesis in men with elevated blood pressure. *Circ. Res.* **36,** 118–126.

Doyle, A. E., and Fraser, J. R. E. (1961). Essential hypertension and inheritance of vascular reactivity. *Lancet*, Part 2, 509–511.

Ebihara, A. (1972). Studies on the pathogenesis of experimental hypertension in rats. *Jpn. Circ. J.* **36,** 603–605.

Ebihara, A., and Martz, B. L. (1970). Comparative effects of currently available antihypertensive agents on spontaneously and renal hypertensive rats. *Am. J. Med. Sci.* **259,** 257–261.

Ebihara, A., and Martz, B. L. (1971). Observations on several experimental models of hypertension in mice. *Jpn. Heart J.* **12,** 275–280.

Fallis, N., Lasagna, L., and Tetréault, L. (1962). Gustatory thresholds in patients with hypertension. *Nature (London)* **196,** 74–75.

Ferrario, C. M., Gildenberg, P. L., and McCubbin, J. W. (1972). Cardiovascular effects of angiotensin mediated by the central nervous system. *Circ. Res.* **30,** 257–262.

Folkow, B. (1972). The importance of adaptive changes in vascular design for the establishment and maintenance of primary hypertension, as studied in man and spontaneously hypertensive rats. *In* "Spontaneous Hypertension. Its Pathogenesis and Complications" (K. Okamoto, ed.), p. 103. Igakushoin Ltd., Tokyo.

Fregly, M. J., Harper, J. M., and Radford, E. P. (1965). Regulation of sodium chloride intake by rats. *Am. J. Physiol.* **209,** 287–292.

Freis, E. D. (1976). Salt, volume and the prevention of hypertension. *Circulation* **53,** 589–595.

Friedman, A., and Freed, S. C. (1949). Microphonic manometer for indirect determination of systolic blood pressure in the rat. *Proc. Soc. Exp. Biol. Med.* **70,** 670–672.

Ganguli, M. C., Smith, J. D., and Hanson, L. E. (1969a). Sodium metabolism and its requirement during reproduction in female rats. *J. Nutr.* **99,** 225–234.

Ganguli, M. C., Smith, J. D., and Hanson, L. E. (1969b). Sodium metabolism in lactating rats. *J. Nutr.* **99,** 395–400.

Gitlow, S. E., Mendlowitz, M., Wilk, E. K., Wilk, S., Wolf, R. L., and Naftchi, N. E. (1964). Plasma clearance of DL-β-^{3}H-norephinephrine in normal human subjects and patients with essential hypertension. *J. Clin. Invest.* **43,** 2009–2015.

Goldblatt, H., Lynch, J., Hanzal, R. F., and Summerville, W. W. (1934). Studies on experimental hypertension. I. Production of persistent elevation of systolic blood pressure by means of renal ischemia. *J. Exp. Med.* **59,** 347–379.

Grollman, A., and Harrison, T. R. (1945). Effect of rigid sodium restriction on blood pressure and survival of hypertensive rats. *Proc. Soc. Exp. Biol. Med.* **60,** 52–55.

Grunert, R. R., Meyer, J. H., and Phillips, P. H. (1950). The sodium and potassium requirements of the rat for growth. *J. Nutr.* **42,** 609–618.

Guyton, A. C., Coleman, T. C., Cowley, A. W., Scheel, K. W., Manning, R. D., and Norman, R. A. (1972). Arterial pressure regulation. Overriding dominance of the kidneys in long-term regulation and in hypertension. *Am. J. Med.* **52,** 584–594.

Hatano, S. (1974). Hypertension in Japan: A review. *In* "Epidemiology and Control of Hypertension" (O. Paul, ed.), pp. 63–99. Continental Medical Book Corp., New York.

Henkin, R. I. (1974). Salt preference in patients with essential hypertension and with hypertension due to primary hyperaldosteronism. *J. Chronic Dis.* **27,** 235–244.

Issacson, L. C., Modlin, M., and Jackson, W. P. U. (1963). Sodium intake and hypertension. *Lancet*, Part 1, 946.

Iwai, J., Dahl, L. K., and Knudsen, K. D. (1973). Genetic influence on the renin angiotensin system. Low renin activity in hypertension-prone rats. *Circ. Res.* **32,** 678–684.

Kirksey, A., and Pike, R. L. (1962). Some effects of high and low sodium intakes during pregnancy in the rat. I. Food consumption, weight gain, reproductive performance, electrolyte balances, plasma total protein and protein fractions in normal pregnancy. *J. Nutr.* **77,** 33–42.

Louis, W. J., Spector, S., Tabei, R., and Sjoerdsma, A. (1969). Synthesis and turnover of norepinephrine in the heart of the spontaneously hypertensive rat. *Circ. Res.* **24,** 85–91.

Louis, W. J., Tabei, R., and Spector, S. (1971). Effects of sodium intake on inherited hypertension in the rat. *Lancet*, Part 2, 1283–1286.

McConnell, S. D., and Henkin, R. I. (1973). Increased preference for Na^+ and K^+ salts in spontaneously hypertensive (SH) rats. *Proc. Soc. Exp. Biol. Med.* **143,** 185–188.

Maddocks, I. (1961). Possible absence of essential hypertension in two complete Pacific island populations. *Lancet* **2,** 396–399.

Maddocks, I. (1967). Blood pressures in Melanesians. *Med. J. Aust.* **1,** 1123–1126.

Meneely, G. R., and Ball, C. O. T. (1958). Experimental epidemiology of chronic sodium chloride toxicity and protective effect of potassium chloride. *Am. J. Med.* **25,** 713–725.

Meneely, G. R., Tucker, R. G., and Darby, W. J. (1952). Chronic sodium chloride toxicity in the albino rat. I. Growth on a purified diet containing various levels of sodium chloride. *J. Nutr.* **48**, 489–498.

Meneely, G. R., Tucker, R. G., Darby, W. J., and Auerbach, Sh.H. (1953). Chronic sodium chloride toxicity in the albino rat. II. Occurrence of hypertension and of a syndrome of edema and renal failure. *J. Exp. Med.* **98**, 71–80.

Minichi, J. L. (1972). Subcellular localization of cerebral reninlike activity. *In* "Hypertension '72" (J. Genest, ed.), p. 432. Springer-Verlag, Berlin and New York.

Morrison, G. R., and Young, J. C. (1972). Taste control over sodium intake in sodium-deficient rats. *Physiol. Behav.* **8**, 29–32.

Okamoto, K., and Aoki, K. (1963). Development of a strain of spontaneously hypertensive rats. *Jpn. Circ. J.* **27**, 282–293.

Okamoto, K., Tabei, R., Fukushima, M., Nosaka, S., Yamori, Y., Ichijima, K., Haebara, H., Matsumoto, M., Maruyama, T., Suzuki, Y., and Tamegai, M. (1966). Further observations of the development of strain of spontaneously hypertensive rats. *Jpn. Circ. J.* **30**, 703–716.

Okamoto, K., Nosaka, S., Yamori, Y., and Matsumoto, M. (1967). Participation of neural factor in the pathogenesis of hypertension in the spontaneously hypertensive rats. *Jpn. Circ. J.* **8**, 168–180.

Oliver, W. J., Cohen, E. L., and Neel, J. V. (1975). Blood pressure, sodium intake, and sodium related hormones in the Yanomamo Indians, a "no-salt" culture. *Circulation* **52**, 146–151.

Page, I. H. (1960). The mosaic theory of hypertension. *In* "Essential Hypertension. An International Symposium" (K. D. Bock and P. T. Cottier, eds.), pp. 3–15. Springer-Verlag, Berlin and New York.

Page, L. B. (1976). Epidemiologic evidence on the etiology of human hypertension and its possible prevention. *Am. Heart J.* **91**, 527–534.

Page, L. B., Damon, A., and Moellering, R. C. (1974). Antecedent of cardiovascular disease in six Solomon Islands societies. *Circulation* **49**, 1132–1146.

Prior, L. A., Evans, J. G., Harvey, H. P. B., Davidson, F., and Lindsey, M. (1968). Sodium intake and blood pressure in two Polynesian populations. *N. Engl. J. Med.* **279**, 515–520.

Sapirstein, L. A., Brandt, W. L., and Drury, D. R. (1950). Production of arterial hypertension in the rat by substitution of hypertonic sodium chloride solution for drinking water. *Am. J. Med.* **8**, 525–526.

Sasaki, N. (1964). The relationship of salt intake to hypertension in the Japanese. *Geriatrics* **19**, 735–744.

Sato, R., Masuyama, Y., Tanaka, S., Nishio, I., and Yoshitoshi, Y. (1972). Preventing effect of salt loading on pressor responses and tachyphylaxis of angiotensin infusion in the rats. *Jpn. Circ. J.* **36**, 995.

Schechter, P. J., Horwitz, D., and Henkin, R. I. (1973). Sodium chloride preference in essential hypertension. *J. Am. Med. Assoc.* **225**, 1311–1315.

Schechter, P. J., Horwitz, D., and Henkin, R. I. (1974). Salt preference in patients with untreated and treated essential hypertension. *Am. J. Med. Sci.* **267**, 320–326.

[illegible], S. (1972). Catecholamine metabolism in spontaneously hypertensive rats. *In* "Spontaneous Hypertension: Its Pathogenesis and Complications" (K. Okamoto, ed.), p. 39. Igaku-shoin Ltd., Tokyo.

Swaye, P. S., Gifford, R. W., and Berrettoni, J. N. (1972). Dietary salt and essential hypertension. *Am. J. Cardiol.* **29**, 33–38.

Thomas, C. B. (1973). Genetic patterns of hypertension in man. *In* "Hypertension: Mechanisms and Management" (G. Onesti, K. E. Kim, and J. D. Moyer, eds.), pp. 67–73. Grune & Stratton, New York.

Tucker, R. G., Ball, C. O. T., Darby, W. J., Early, W. R., Kory, R. C., Youmans, J. B., and

Meneely, G. R. (1957). Chronic sodium chloride toxicity in the albino rat. III. Maturity characteristics, survivorship, and organ weights. *J. Gerontol.* **12,** 182–189.

Wolf, G., Dahl, L. K., and Miller, N. E. (1965). Voluntary sodium chloride intake of two strains of rats with opposite genetic susceptibility to experimental hypertension. *Proc. Soc. Exp. Biol. Med.* **120,** 301–305.

Wotman, S., Mandel, I. D., Thompson, R. H., and Laragh, J. H. (1967). Salivary electrolytes and salt taste thresholds in hypertension. *J. Chronic Dis.* **20,** 833–840.

Yamori, Y. (1972). Organ difference of catecholamine metabolism in spontaneously hypertensive rats. *In* "Spontaneous Hypertension. Its Pathogenesis and Complications." (K. Okamoto, ed.), pp. 59–73. Igakushoin Ltd., Tokyo.

Zinner, S. H., Levy, P. S., and Kass, E. H. (1971). Familial aggregation of blood pressure in childhood. *N. Engl. J. Med.* **284,** 401–404.

Chapter 26

Salt Taste and Salt Preference in Normal and Hypertensive Rats and Humans

ROBERT I. HENKIN

I. SALT TASTE STUDIES

It is widely believed that excessive salt intake plays a role in the development of hypertension in man (Ambard and Beaujard, 1905; Allen, 1920; Dahl and Love, 1954; Meneely and Dahl, 1961). Conversely, it has been clearly demonstrated that deprivation of salt and water is efficacious in the treatment of hypertension (Ambard and Beaujard, 1905; Allen, 1920; Dahl and Love, 1954; Meneely and Dahl, 1961; Perera and Blood, 1947; Dole *et al.*, 1951). Since salt

BIOLOGICAL AND BEHAVIORAL
ASPECTS OF SALT INTAKE

ISBN 0-12-397750-9

intake in man is under voluntary control, several investigators in the past have measured salt taste acuity in patients with hypertension (Fallis *et al.*, 1962; Wotman *et al.*, 1967) in an attempt to evaluate the possible role this variable might play in the development of this disease. Their results suggested that, as a group, patients with hypertension exhibited lower than normal salt taste acuity. From this observation one group reasoned that these patients used excessive amounts of salt on their food to achieve the preferred salty taste and thereby unmasked whatever genetic propensity they might have had to develop hypertension.

Although this reasoning is quite attractive, critical studies of salt taste acuity in patients with hypertension were not carried out by previous investigators. In an effort to do this, specific measurements of salt taste acuity, i.e., detection and recognition thresholds for NaCl, were evaluated in 50 patients with well-documented essential hypertension and in 10 patients with hypertension due to primary hyperaldosteronism. In some patients thresholds were measured before and after therapy which was efficacious in lowering blood pressure to or toward normal. Results of these studies indicate that, as a group, taste thresholds for NaCl in patients with either essential hypertension or hypertension due to primary hyperaldosteronism do not differ from normal.

A. Patients with Essential Hypertension

Fifty patients (27 men, 23 women) aged 16–63 years, mean 44 years, were studied. Each patient exhibited a diastolic blood pressure $\geq$100 mm Hg without any antihypertensive therapy on at least two separate occasions prior to study. Eleven patients were studied as outpatients of the Hypertension Clinic of the National Heart and Lung Institute; these patients represented eleven consecutive admissions to this clinic over a period of 2 months. Thirty-nine patients were studied while hospitalized in a semiprivate room at the Clinical Center, NIH, for periods ranging from 1 to 35 days, mean 6 days; these patients represented thirty-nine consecutive admissions to the ward of the Experimental Therapeutics Branch, National Heart and Lung Institute at two intervals separated by 6 years.

Forty-nine of the 50 patients were taken off all antihypertensive therapy or salt restriction for 10 days to 7 weeks prior to study. Ten patients had never been treated previously; 8 of 11 outpatients were studied while receiving therapy which was efficacious in returning their blood pressure to or toward normal in each case. This therapy included hydrochlorothiazide, α-methyl dopa, guanethidine, or some combination of these drugs.

The following diagnostic tests were performed to establish the diagnosis of essential hypertension: intravenous pyelogram (normal in all 50 patients); ^{131}I hippuran/renogram or ^{203}Hg chlormerodrin renal scan (normal in 38 patients, abnormal in 5, indicative of decreased unilateral renal tubular function, not performed in 7 patients); transfemoral renal arteriogram (normal in 27 patients, abnormal in 2, one with scarring of one kidney, one with nephrosclerosis, not performed in 21 patients); estimation of vanilmandelic acid (VMA) by the method of Pisano *et al.* (1962) from a sample of a 24-hour urine excretion (normal in 45 patients, not performed in 5 patients); urinalysis, and if indicated, urine culture (normal in 49 patients, *E. coli* found in one patient); blood urea nitrogen by the method of Annino (1967) and creatinine by the method of Chasson *et al.* (1961) (normal in 47 patients, slightly elevated, BUN$>20<50$, creatinine$>1.2<1.8$, in 3 patients); creatinine clearance (normal in 46 patients, decreased, $<70>50$ ml/min in 4 patients).

Careful evaluation of the results of these tests failed to reveal any specific etiology for the elevation in blood pressure in any patient studied.

In all patients blood pressure was measured in the reclining position with a cuff and sphygmomanometer by auscultation of the Karotkoff sounds at the antecubital fossa 15 min after the patient had reclined and rested. Without treatment and just prior to measurement of salt taste acuity in the afternoon (after 13:00) the mean reclining blood pressure was 174/116 (range 120–240/80–180); without treatment and just prior to measurement of salt taste acuity in the morning (before 12:00) the mean reclining blood pressure was 161/111 (range 130–206/76–138). During drug treatment and just prior to measurement of salt taste acuity in the afternoon the mean reclining blood pressure was 156/107 (range 94–200/60–128) and during drug treatment just prior to measurement of salt taste acuity, in the morning, mean blood pressure was 156/104 (range, 116–186/80–120).

B. Patients with Primary Hyperaldosteronism

Ten patients (6 men, 4 women) aged 39–57 years, mean 49 years, were studied. These patients represented ten consecutive admissions to the metabolic ward of the Endocrinology Branch, National Heart and Lung Institute, for evaluation of hyperaldosteronism. Each patient was placed in a semiprivate, air-conditioned room for periods ranging from 1 week to 9 months.

Eight of the patients were studied after all antihypertensive agents or salt restriction had been discontinued for 3–10 weeks. Due to their sustained hypertension, 1 patient was studied while receiving α-methyldopa, 1 while receiving reserpine. Each patient took a metabolic diet containing 9 mEq NaCl with 100 mEq NaCl added daily by means of a salt shaker during which time aldosterone secretion rates were carried out by a double isotope dilution technique (Kliman and Peterson, 1960). Six patients were also placed on an intake of both 9 and 249 mEq of NaCl, and aldosterone secretion rates were measured.

The following diagnostic tests were performed in each patient to establish the diagnosis of primary hyperaldosteronism: aldosterone secretion rate (elevated above normal in each patient with a daily intake of 109 mEq Na^+); significant fall in serum potassium with a daily intake of 249 mEq Na^+ (present in each patient); intravenous pyelogram (normal in each patient), ^{131}I hippuran renogram (normal in 9 patients, loss of tubular function bilaterally in 1 patient); transfemoral renal arteriogram (normal in each patient although 1 patient had an abdominal aortic aneurysm discovered incidentally above the exit point of the renal artery); urinary VMA (normal in each patient); BUN and creatinine (normal in 8 patients, slightly elevated, BUN>20<30, creatinine>1.2<1.5, in 2 patients); creatinine clearance (normal in 8 patients, slightly decreased, >70<50 ml/min in 2 patients).

Each patient underwent an exploratory laparotomy. At operation, 5 patients had a unilateral adrenalectomy performed to remove a unilateral adrenal adenoma and 5 patients had a subtotal adrenalectomy as treatment for bilateral nodular adrenocortical hyperplasia. Postsurgery 4 patients required no medication of any type, 4 patients required adrenocortical hormone replacement therapy alone, while 2 patients required both adrenocortical hormone replacement therapy and antihypertensive agents. After surgery, patients were once again placed on a metabolic diet containing 9 mEq NaCl with 100 mEq NaCl added daily by means of a salt shaker and salt taste acuity was measured. In some, aldosterone secretion rates were measured again.

Each patient exhibited diastolic blood pressure >90 mm Hg off all antihypertensive agents on at least two separate occasions prior to surgery. At the time of measurement of salt taste acuity with a daily intake of 109 mEq Na^+ the mean reclining blood pressure for the patients was 190/111 (range, 150-250/90-130); when measured with a daily intake of 9 mEq Na^+, mean reclining blood pressure was 152/98 (range, 130-188/82-110) and when measured with a daily intake of 249 mEq Na^+ mean reclining blood pressure was 194/115 (range, 170-220/110-130). Mean blood pressure after surgery with a daily intake of 109 mEq Na^+ and with adrenocortical replacement and/or antihypertensive therapy in those patients who required it was 133/88 (range, 118-154/76-100).

C. Measurements of Taste Thresholds

Detection and recognition thresholds for the taste of NaCl were determined in each patient by a forced-choice three stimulus drop technique previously described (Henkin *et al.*, 1971). In addition, thresholds for sucrose (sweet), HCl (sour), and urea (bitter) were obtained in 24 patients with essential hypertension and in 6 patients with primary hyperaldosteronism. These additional thresholds were always measured if any abnormality in detection or recognition threshold for NaCl was observed. In patients with primary hyperaldosteronism, all measurements were made in the afternoon at least 1 hour after the patient had eaten, drunk, or smoked. In 32 patients with essential hypertension, detection and recognition thresholds for NaCl were determined off treatment in both the morning (prior to 12:00), and in the afternoon (after 13:00); thresholds were also determined in 12 patients with essential hypertension on treatment with various antihypertensive agents in both the morning and in the afternoon. Testing was always carried out by the same investigator on at least one occasion. If thresholds for NaCl were elevated at the first testing session, at least one additional testing session was carried out. If thresholds for NaCl were within normal limits at the first testing session and additional tests performed, thresholds for NaCl always remained within normal limits. Thresholds for NaCl in 22 patients with essential hypertension were measured at least twice as were thresholds for NaCl in each patient with primary hyperaldosteronism. The last or lowest threshold values for each patient are reported. Comparison of thresholds is always made with measurements taken at similar times during the day under similar conditions.

Median detection and recognition thresholds for NaCl for each group of patients under each condition studied were calculated. Median detection and recognition thresholds for 150 normal volunteers and patients with various diseases in which taste was not affected have been reported previously (Henkin and Solomon, 1962; Pittman and Beschi, 1967; Henkin *et al.*, 1972; Schechter *et al.*, 1972). Measurements of central tendency between taste thresholds of hypertensive patients and normals and between the various patient groups under the conditions studied were also calculated by the Wilcoxon Rank Sum Statistic (Schechter *et al.*, 1972) as previously described. Significance of differences was calculated using this test.

Median detection and recognition thresholds for NaCl in patients with essential hypertension or hypertension due to primary hyperaldosteronism were not different from normal (Table I). Of the 50 patients with essential hypertension studied, only 4 (8%) exhibited elevations of either detection or recognition thresholds for NaCl above the upper limits of the normal range while only 1 of 10 (10%) patients with primary hyperaldosteronism exhibited an elevation in taste thresholds for NaCl. Of the 4 patients with essential hypertension in whom elevations in NaCl thresholds were observed, each exhibited elevated thresholds for at least one other taste quality always including bitter (Table I) as did the one patient with primary hyperaldosteronism (Table I).

No characteristic of patients with hypertension studied could be correlated with their salt taste acuity. Blood pressure measurements in hypertensive patients with elevated taste thresholds for NaCl and in hypertensive patients with normal taste thresholds were not different (Table I). Patients with essential hypertension exhibited no differences in NaCl taste thresholds with or without treatment with antihypertensive agents which significantly ($p < 0.01$) lowered their blood pressure (Table II). Salt taste acuity was not related to differences in the age, sex, race, or diastolic blood pressure of the patients studied nor to whether they were studied in hospital or as outpatients (Table II). However, salt taste thresholds in patients with essential hypertension decreased significantly ($p < 0.001$) in the

TABLE I

Taste Thresholds in Patients with Essential Hypertension and Hyperaldosteronism

Patient groups		Taste threshold Detection threshold/recognition threshold NaCl	Sucrose	HCl	Urea	Age	Race	Sex	Blood pressure at time of taste test systolic/diastolic mm Hg[c]
Patients with normal thresholds									
Diagnosis									
Essential									
Hypertension		12/30[a]	30/30	3/6	150/150				170±8/113±4
(EH) range: 24[b]		(3–60/6–60)	(0.8–60/6–60)	(0.5–6/0.5–6)	(60–150/60–150)				
Hyperaldosteronism		30/30[a]	30/30	3/6	150/150				195±12/107±3
(HA) range: 6[b]		(12–30/12–30)	(30–60/30–60)	(0.8–6/0.8–6)	120–150/120–150)				
Patients with elevated thresholds									
Diagnosis									
R.R.	EH	90/90	60/60	30/30	1K/1K	50	B	M	180/120
J.J.	EH	60/500	90/90	6/30	800/800	52	C	M	150/122
R.T.	EH	12/150	12/60	6/6	500/500	40	C	M	160/100
B.W.	EH	300/300	500/500	500/500	800/800	35	B	F	140/80
L.O.	HA	300/300	150/300	15/150	300/800	51	C	M	150/90
Median	—	90/300	90/90	15/30	500/800	—	—	—	156±7/102±8
Normal thresholds									
Detection/recognition		12/30	12/30	3/6	120/150	—	—	—	—
(Range)		(0.8–60/6–60)	(0.8–60/6–60)	(0.5–6/0.5–6)	(60–150/60–150)	—	—	—	—

[a] Median (in m*M*).
[b] Detection and recognition thresholds were obtained for four qualities in each patient tested and were within the normal range.
[c] Mean ± SEM.
B, Black; C, Caucasian
K, × 1000

TABLE II

NaCl Taste Thresholds in Patients with Essential Hypertension in Relationship to Various Conditions and Blood Pressure

Condition[a]	Number of patients tested	NaCl thresholds (mM/liter)	Blood pressure systolic/diastolic (mm Hg)	Condition[a]	Number of patients tested	NaCl thresholds (mM/liter)	Blood pressure systolic/diastolic (mm Hg)
Inpatients	39	12/30[e]	171±6/114±4[f]	Outpatients	11	12/30	179±8/120±5
Male	27	12/30	172±16/118±4	Female	23	6/30	179±7/114±4
Black	27	12/30	173±6/116±3	Caucasian	23	12/30	176±6/115±5
All untreated or on placebo	49	12/30	174±4/116±2	All treated	14	12/30	143±15/98±10
Patients untreated	14	12/30	172±5/115±11	Same patients treated	14	12/30	143±15/98±10
AM (pre 12:00)	32	30/60	167±4/111±2	PM (Same patients after 13:00)	32	12/30[d]	183±5[b]/122±3[c]
Diastolic blood pressure (mm Hg)				Age (Yr)			
≦100	17	30/30		≦40	12	12/30	164±7/113±4
>100≦120	17	12/30		>40≦50	19	12/30	178±6/122±4
>120	16	12/30		>50≦70	11	12/30	175±12/106±6

[a] All patients were tested without treatment in afternoon except where indicated.
[b] $p < 0.02$ with respect to AM value.
[c] $p < 0.01$ with respect to AM value.
[d] < 0.001 with respect to AM value.
[e] Numerator of fraction is median detection threshold; denominator of fraction is median recognition threshold.
[f] mean ± SEM.

afternoon at the time that systolic and diastolic blood pressures were significantly elevated ($p < 0.01$) above those measured in the morning (Table II), consistent with the circadian pattern of variation previously observed for both of these parameters (Henkin *et al.*, 1963; Henkin, 1973; Cranston and Brown, 1963).

The degree of aldosterone hypersecretion in patients with hypertension and primary hyperaldosteronism did not influence salt taste acuity nor did the degree of dietary sodium restriction or addition to which they were subjected. Although sodium restriction significantly lowered systolic and diastolic blood pressure in these patients, this did not affect salt taste acuity. Differences in the type of adrenal tumor which produced the hyperaldosteronism did not influence salt taste acuity. There was no difference in salt taste acuity in patients studied before operation, when hypertensive, or postoperatively, after systolic and diastolic blood pressure had decreased significantly (Table III). Although blood pressure increased significantly ($p < 0.01$) in these patients after increases in sodium intake (Table III) and fell significantly ($p < 0.01$) after sodium restriction or surgical removal of their tumors (Table III), no change in salt taste acuity could be measured.

Although NaCl thresholds were elevated in approximately 10% of the patients with hypertension, as a group, patients with either essential hypertension or with hypertension due to primary hyperaldosteronism exhibited normal detection and recognition thresholds for NaCl. In addition, among those patients who exhibited elevated NaCl thresholds, thresholds for other taste qualities were also elevated, indicating that their taste abnormality was not specific for NaCl but rather a generalized hypogeusia. These data are in disagreement with previous reports in which salt taste acuity was indicated to be depressed in most patients with hypertension (Fallis *et al.*, 1962).

A generalized decrease in taste acuity (hypogeusia) is not an uncommon occurrence. Indeed, estimates from our clinic suggest that as many as 1 in 500 persons may exhibit hypogeusia secondary to a variety of not uncommon etiological factors, e.g., influenzalike illnesses or surgical procedures not involving the head or neck regions (Henkin *et al.*, 1971; Schechter *et al.*, 1972). As did the patients with hypertension in this study, previous patients with hypogeusia exhibited abnormalities of detection and recognition of the taste of bitter and in most cases other thresholds as well. Since taste qualities other than NaCl were not systematically investigated in previous studies of hypertensive patients, it is not possible to determine the specificity of their taste abnormality for NaCl or to relate their hypertension simply to addition of more salt to food in an effort to produce a desired salty taste. Whether any of the hypertensive patients studied by others had reasons for their depressed NaCl taste acuity other than their hypertension is not known.

In addition, several procedural details may relate to the differences noted between results of the present study and those of previous workers. If thresholds

TABLE III

NaCl Taste Thresholds in Patients with Primary Hyperaldosteronism in Relationship to Various Conditions and Blood Pressure

Condition	Number of patients tested	NaCl thresholds (mM/liter)	Blood pressure systolic/diastolic (mm Hg)	Condition	Number of patients tested	NaCl thresholds (mM/liter)	Blood pressure systolic/diastolic (mm Hg)
ASR≦500 (Na^+, 109 mEq) intake daily	3	30/30 [a]	187±16/103±10	ASR>500 (Na^+, 109mEq) intake daily	7	30/30 [a]	173±9/108±6
Diastolic blood pressure (mm Hg) ≦110	4	30/30	—	Diastolic blood pressure (mm Hg) >110≦130	6	30/30	—
Na^+ intake daily (mEq)							
109	10	30/30	190±9/111±4 [a]				
9	6	30/30	152±9 [b]/98±4				
249	6	30/30	194±9/115±3				
Preoperation (Na^+, 109 mEq) intake daily	10	30/30	190±10/110±4	Postoperation (Na^+, 109 mEq) intake daily	10	30/30	133±4 [d]/88±4 [d]
Unilateral adenoma at operation (Preoperation test (Na^+, intake daily 109 mEq)	5	30/30	190±10/112±4	Bilateral cortical hyperplasia at operation (Preoperation test (Na^+, intake daily 109 mEq)	5	30/30	189±8/108±7

[a] Numerator of fraction is median detection threshold; denominator of fraction is median recognition threshold. ASR, aldosterone secretion rate.
[b] $p < 0.01$ with respect to value on 109 or 249 mEq Na^+ intake.
[c] $p < 0.05$ with respect to value on 109 mEq Na^+ intake; $p < 0.01$ with respect to value on 249 mEq Na^+ intake.
[d] $p < 0.01$ with respect to preoperation value.

are measured only in the early morning hours, results will reflect the higher values obatined in the AM consistent with the circadian variation previously demonstrated for the detection of NaCl (Henkin, 1973). If abnormally elevated thresholds are obtained, taste acuity must be retested to ensure that the abnormalities observed are not a function of lack of patient understanding of the test procedure. Ensuring an adequate time span between the last meal or usage of tobacco is also an important aspect to achieve uniform test results. Failure to observe these precautions generally results in the finding of higher than normal thresholds.

It is of interest that of the patients who were classified as having idiopathic hypogeusia and who exhibited abnormalities of taste for more than one taste quality (including the addition of excessive quantities of salt to their food to obtain the desired salty taste), approximately 15% were first discovered to have hypertension at the time they were initially evaluated for their taste loss (Henkin *et al.*, 1971); over 25% of the total number of patients with this syndrome exhibited hypertension, a figure somewhat higher than published values for the prevalence of hypertension in American adults (Henkin *et al.*, 1974). Whether some factor(s) which influences taste acuity also influences changes in blood pressure is not known. Although excessive salt intake may play some role in the etiology of hypertension, an abnormality of salt taste acuity per se is not a constituent factor of established hypertension.

II. RAT PREFERENCE STUDIES

Since it is clear that salt taste per se is not a constituent factor of established hypertension we wondered if other aspects of salt appetite might influence salt intake in humans. These thoughts were activated by results in a group of rats in which spontaneous hypertension was discovered and perpetuated on a genetic basis. In these rats, called spontaneously hypertensive (SH), preference for NaCl was found to be significantly higher than that of control normotensive rats (Catalanotto *et al.*, 1972). In these studies, SH rats and normotensive controls were housed individually and given free choice between two solutions, one containing NaCl of variable concentration, the other containing water in a paradigm previously described in detail (Kare, 1961), and preference and volume intake measured.

Preference responses of control and SH rats are shown in Figs. 1 and 2, each point representing the mean $\pm$ 1 SEM of each group on each day of the study. Preference in percentage is reported as

$$(\text{ml test solution consumed/ml total fluid consumed}) \times 100$$

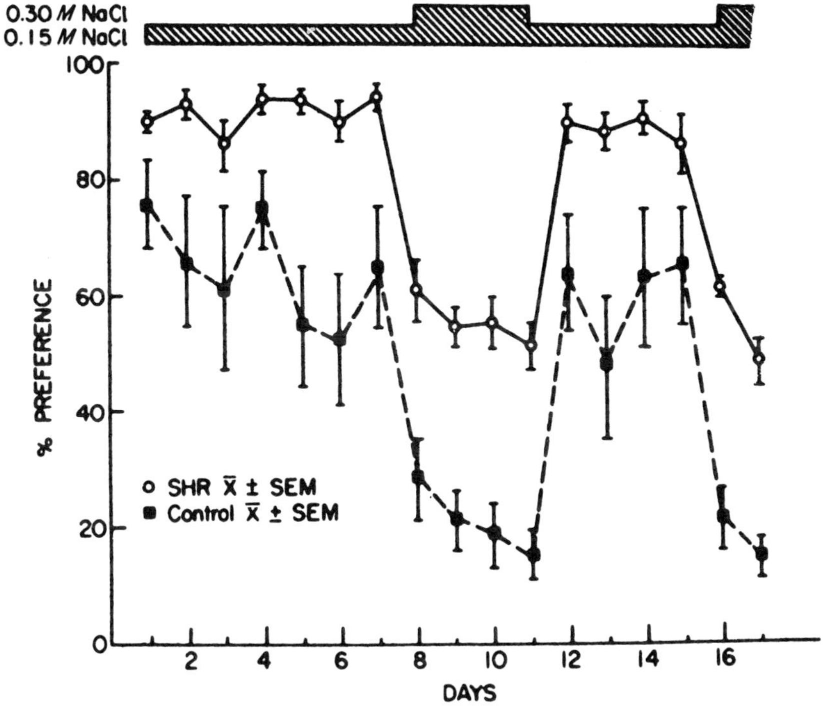

Fig. 1. Comparison of preference for NaCl between Holtzman controls and spontaneously hypertensive (SH) rats. Each symbol represents the mean ± 1 SEM of seven Holtzman and eight SH rats. SH rats used in this and all other studies were of a Wistar strain. Percentage preference is plotted on the abscissa; time in days on the ordinate.

When presented with either 0.15, 0.30, or 0.45 *M* NaCl solution, control rats (closed circles) preferred significantly less NaCl than did the SH rats. Volume intake (ml total fluid/g body weight) in the SH rats was usually, but not always, greater than in controls (Figs. 3 and 4). However, when Wistar controls were compared with the SH rats (a Wistar variant), volume intake for NaCl was uniformly increased for 0.15, 0.30, or 0.45 *M* NaCl.

These results, first reported in 1972, were the first demonstration of persistent increased NaCl preference in a hypertensive rat given a free choice between NaCl and water.

Rats made hypertensive through administration of deoxycorticosterone acetate exhibited only a transient increase in salt preference (Tosteson *et al.*, 1951) while rats made hypertensive subsequent to adrenal regeneration exhibited an increased salt appetite, but only saline was offered to them (Takeda *et al.*, 1964).

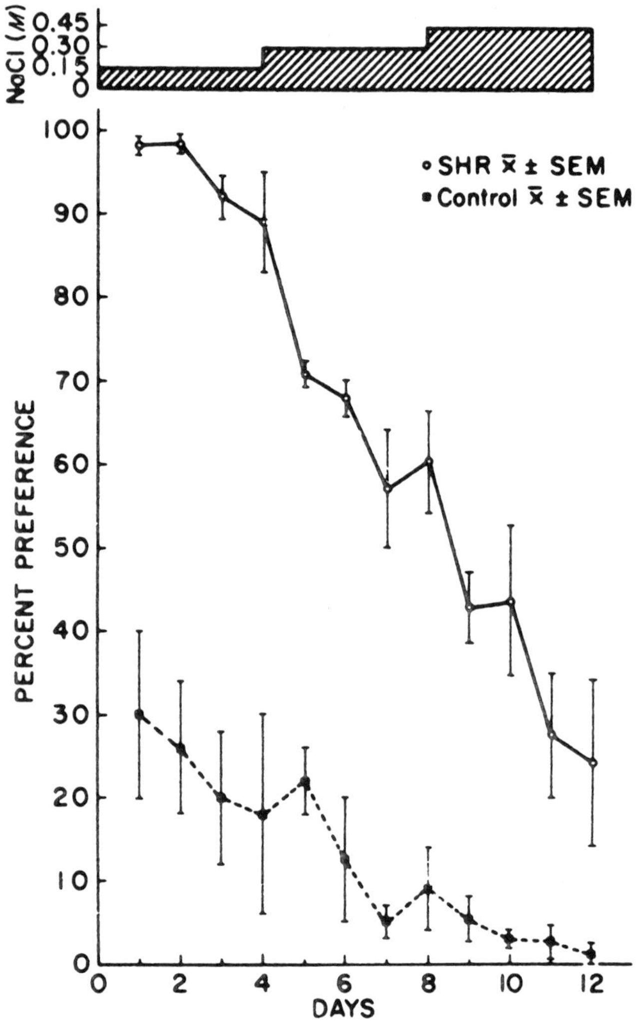

Fig. 2. Comparison of preference for NaCl between six Wistar controls and six SH rats. Preference for NaCl among the SH rats was greater than that of either control group.

Indeed, most previous studies demonstrated that rats with experimentally induced hypertension of several etiologies exhibited a decreased rather than an increased preference for salt (Abrams *et al.*, 1969; Fregly, 1956; Green *et al.*, 1952a; Wolf *et al.*, 1965). Aversive behavior toward NaCl has been previously demonstrated in a genetic strain of hypertensive rats. These animals were predisposed to develop hypertension by administration of large quantities of NaCl and

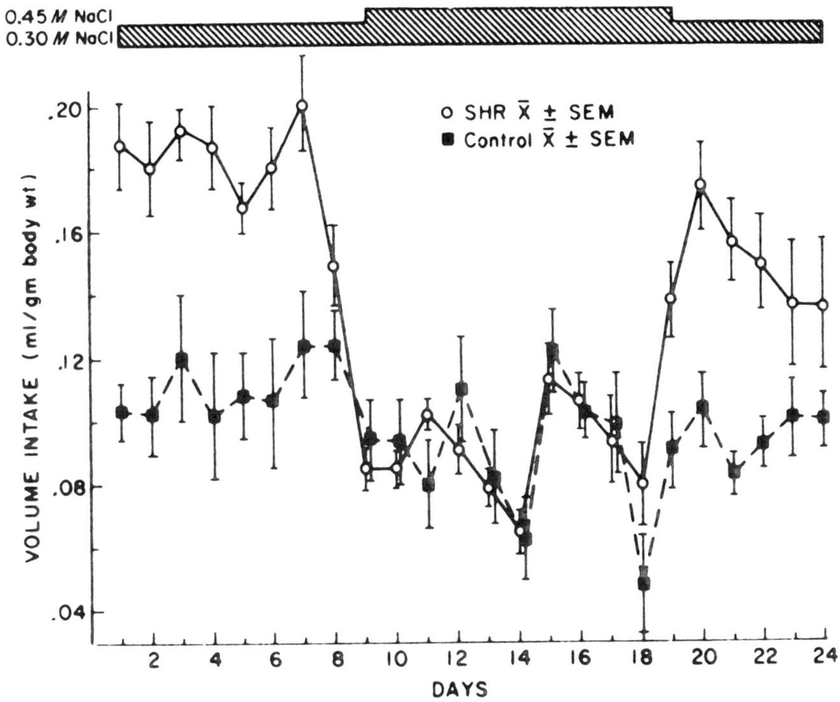

Fig. 3. Comparison of volume intake (NaCl plus water) between Holtzman control and SH rats. Each symbol represents the mean ± 1 SEM of seven control rats and eight SH rats. Volume intake is plotted on the abscissa, time in days on the ordinate.

were usually compared to another genetic strain of rats who remained normotensive following administration of similar quantities of NaCl (Wolf *et al.*, 1965). These hypertensive rats also did not exhibit increased fluid intake (Wolf *et al.*, 1965). The results suggested to these investigators, as well as to us, that the preference behavior and fluid intake responses of these hypertensive rats were not typical of the behavior of the majority of hypertensive animals or of man.

In the present studies responses of two control groups of rats were compared with those of SH rats. SH rats exhibited a consistent and significant increase in preference for 0.15 and 0.30 *M* NaCl solution with respect to either control group. However, as the concentration of NaCl was increased, the preference of the SH rats decreased, suggesting that they maintain an ability to distinguish increasing concentrations of NaCl, responding to them in the same manner as do the controls but at significantly higher levels of preference.

Previous investigators demonstrated that rats made hypertensive by several means exhibited an increased volume intake (Tosteson *et al.*, 1951; Abrams *et al.*, 1969; Fregly, 1956; Green *et al.*, 1952a). Although the SH rat did not

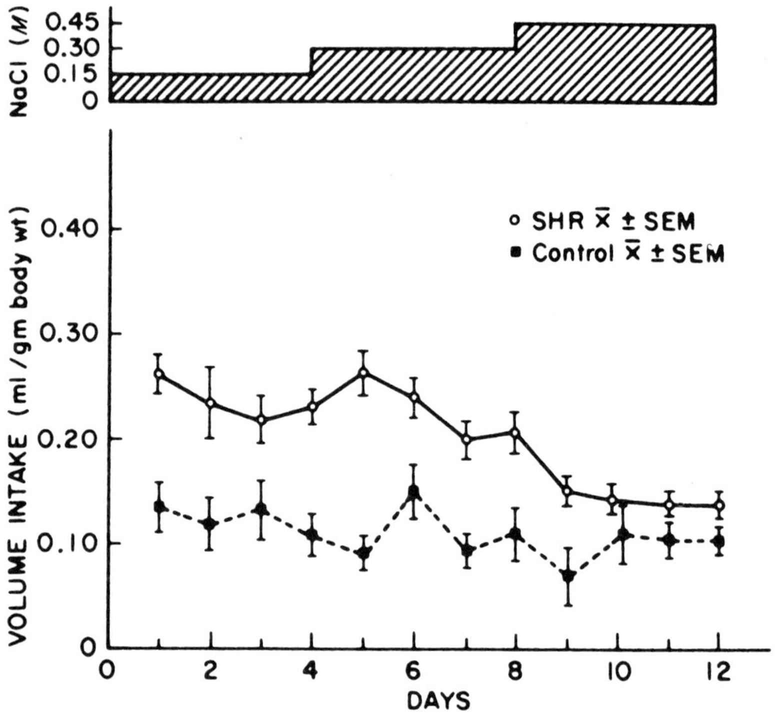

Fig. 4. Comparison of volume intake between six Wistar control and six SH rats. During the time when preference for NaCl was greater in the SH rats compared to either control group (either Wistar/NIH or Holtzman rats) there was a concomitant significant increase in volume intake.

consistently exhibit this phenomenon, increased volume intake occurred when NaCl preference was significantly elevated above controls, especially during exposure to 0.30 *M* NaCl.

Further studies with the SH rat revealed that these animals not only preferred more NaCl solution than Wistar control rats but they also preferred more KCl, $NaHCO_3$, and $NaC_2H_3O_2$ than controls (Fig. 5). As the concentration of $NaHCO_3$ increased to 0.45 *M*, preference responsiveness between SH and normotensive control rats was not significantly different (McConnell and Henkin, 1973a). These results indicate that SH rats prefer Na as well as K salts and that the counterion (Cl, HCO_3, $C_2H_3O_2$) is not critically important in this increased preference responsiveness. Also SH rats did not differ from controls with respect to preference for bitter (quinine) or sour (HCl) solutions (Fig. 5).

Total fluid intake in the SH rats was again tested and compared with appropriate normotensive Wistar control rats (Fig. 6). Fluid intake was greater in the SH rats for all NaCl solutions presented, for KCl, 0.15 *M* $NaHCO_3$ and

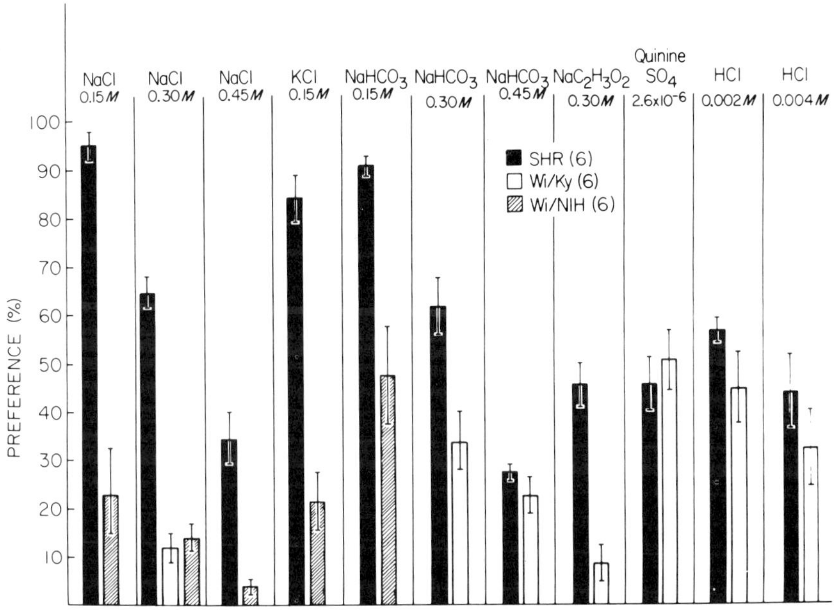

Fig. 5. Preference for various salt solutions, HCl, and quinine in SH rats and in two groups of normotensive control rats [Wistar/Kyoto (Wi/Ky) and Wistar/NIH (Wi/NIH)]. Vertical bars represent the mean daily preference for a 4-day test period in each group of rats for each substance tested. Lines through the bars represent ± 1 SEM.

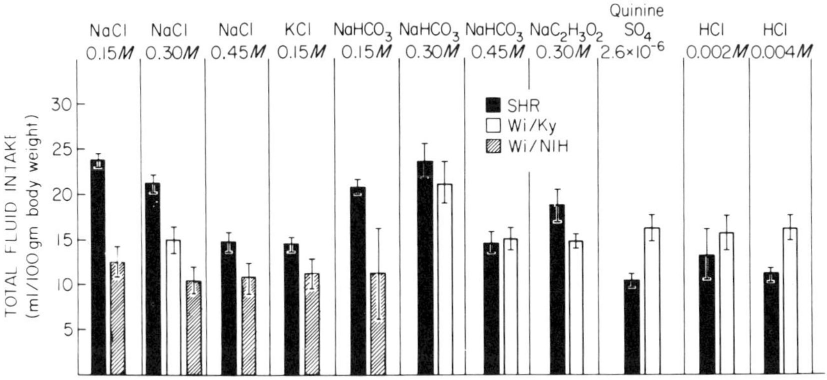

Fig. 6. Total fluid intake (water plus test solution) imbibed by SH, Wi/Ky, and Wi/NIH rats during each 4-day test period. Vertical bars represent the mean daily intake calculated per 100 g body weight for each group of rats for each substance tested. Lines through the bars represent ± 1 SEM.

$NaC_2H_3O_2$. For quinine and HCl (0.004 *M*) the control rats imbibed significantly greater amounts of total fluid.

When given a choice between 0.30 *M* NaCl and water, SH rats imbibed 2-5 times the amount of Na^+ imbibed by normotensive, control rats (McConnell and Henkin, 1973a). And, as noted above, SH rats imbibed significantly more total fluid (salt and water) than did controls as long as salts were presented. However, as soon as water alone was presented, total fluid intake returned to control levels (McConnell and Henkin, 1973a). Preference for NaCl in SH rats increased both as blood pressure increased to the hypertensive range and as the animals increased in age (McConnell and Henkin, 1973b). Both increased preference for NaCl solution and hypertension reached maximal levels at 14 weeks of age and remained at these levels thereafter (McConnell and Henkin, 1973b).

III. HUMAN PREFERENCE STUDIES

The studies in the SH rat suggested that perhaps salt preference could play some role in the development of hypertension since it was clear that salt taste, per se, did not. In an effort to evaluate this hypothesis systematically in hypertensive subjects, 10 patients with a history of sustained essential hypertension of a mild to moderate degree and 12 nonhypertensive volunteers were studied (Schechter *et al.*, 1973). The patients were 10 consecutive inpatients admitted to the Experimental Therapeutics Branch, National Heart and Lung Institute for study of their hypertension. The 12 volunteers were consecutively admitted to the normal volunteer study program designated to the Experimental Therapeutics Branch. Assignment to the hypertensive or nonhypertensive group was based on diastolic blood pressure at admission. Blood pressure was always measured by the arm cuff method after the subject had remained supine at rest for 15 minutes. If diastolic blood pressure was greater than or equal to 100 mm Hg, the subject was assigned to the hypertensive patient group; if less than or equal to 90 mm Hg, the subject was assigned to the normotensive volunteer group.

A. Hypertensive Patients

The patients were 4 whites and 6 blacks, 7 men and 3 women, and had a mean age of 45 years (range, 25-56 years). On admission, the mean blood pressure, measured while supine, was 163/109 mm Hg (range, 140-190/100-130). Each patient underwent diagnostic studies, which included intravenous pyelography, urinalyses, urine culture, creatinine clearance, and determination as follows: renogram with iodohippurate sodium I^{131} or chlormerodrin Hg^{203} (6 patients), transfemoral renal arteriogram (3 patients), determination of 24-hour urinary excretion of vanilmandelic acid or metanephrine (8 patients). Results of these tests failed to reveal any specific cause for the elevation in blood pressure in any patient. Three of the 10 patients had never been treated for their hypertension. The remaining 7 had been taking no antihypertensive agents for 10 days to 2 months prior to the study. Six patients had received relatively short-acting antihypertensive agents (methyldopa in 2 patients, spironolactone and hydrochlorothiazide in 3, chlorthalidone in 1, and trichlormethiazide in 1). One patient received pargyline hydrochloride therapy, which was discontinued 1 month prior to the study. None of the patients had dietary salt restriction prior to study. None of the patients exhibited any clinical signs of congestive heart failure, and none were being treated with any digitalis preparations. All patients had serum creatinine levels below 1.5 mg/100 ml, normal liver function, and no evidence of glycosuria. The present study began 1 to 24 days after each patient was hospitalized. At the time of study, the mean blood pressure of the patients was 135/93 mm Hg (range, 112–170/74–120 mm Hg).

Detection and recognition thresholds for the taste of NaCl were determined in each patient by a forced-choice three-stimulus drop technique by at least one investigator and found to be normal in each patient (range for detection and recognition thresholds, 6–60 m*M*). These thresholds were measured in 2 patients at least twice. Only the lowest thresholds are reported here.

B. Normotensive Volunteers

The volunteers were 12 whites, 9 men and 3 women, mean age 22 years (range, 19–43 years). At the time of admission, their mean blood pressure, measured while supine, was 121/74 mm Hg (range 100–136/60–84 mm Hg). Volunteers began the present study 2 days to 3 months after their hospitalization began. At this time, their mean blood pressure was 107/65 mm Hg (range, 90–120/60–84 mm Hg). Each volunteer had serum creatinine levels below 1.5 mg/100 ml, normal liver function, and no evidence of glycosuria. Each demonstrated detection and recognition thresholds that were within the normal range for the taste of NaCl (range for detection and recognition thresholds, 6–60 m*M*). Thresholds were measured by at least one investigator. Thresholds in 3 volunteers were measured at least twice and only the lowest thresholds are reported.

C. Study Protocol

All subjects were housed in semiprivate rooms, restricted to an air-conditioned environment for the entire course of the study, and their activity was limited to normal walking without strenuous exertion. For this study, each patient or volunteer was placed on a constant diet containing 9 mEq of Na^+ for 4 to 7 days. The diet contained no fluids other than the natural fluid content of the foods chosen; fruit juice, milk, coffee, tea, soft drinks, and soups were excluded. The diet was served at normal mealtimes. The only source of fluids available to either the patients or volunteers was the contents of two 2-liter Erlenmeyer flasks, one filled with distilled water, the other filled with a solution of 0.15 *M* NaCl made with reagent grade NaCl and distilled water. The flasks were kept at room temperature, covered at all times with plastic laboratory film, and opened only for decantation of fluid into a 150-ml beaker for immediate drinking. Fluids were aerated prior to presenting them to the subjects.

Each flask was coded and the code changed daily, so that the subjects were visually unaware of which one contained salt. Flasks were changed daily at 8 AM. Each subject was required to sample the contents of each flask daily.

Each subject was instructed to drink as little or as much of each fluid as he desired. The subject was encouraged to mix different amounts of each test fluid, if he so desired, until a preferred mixture was obtained. Fluids could be added to foods but had to be consumed in their entirety if this were done.

The amount of fluid taken from each flask was calculated daily from the difference between initial and final volumes. Urine was collected for 24 hours each day, and total volume, and sodium, potassium, and creatinine contents were measured. Body weight of each subject was measured daily; this allowed an external control as to salt or fluid intake from sources other than the diet and prescribed fluids. Data from a single additional hypertensive patient were rejected when it was found that her urinary output exceeded her ostensible total fluid intake by an average of 450% without any appreciable change in body weight.

Several aspects of the data were analyzed. Preference for NaCl was calculated as follows:

$$\% \text{ pref} = (\text{ml } 0.15\ M \text{ NaCl/ml total volume}) \times 100$$

In addition, median detection and recognition thresholds for the taste of NaCl, the average daily sodium intake (in milliequivalents), the average daily sodium intake per kilogram of body weight, and the daily total fluid intake (salt and water) were compared in each patient in the two groups, and between the two groups. Statistical significance of differences for sodium and total fluid intake was determined by the Student t test. Significance of differences between median detection and recognition thresholds was determined by the Wilcoxson rank sum statistic as previously described (Schechter *et al.*, 1972).

D. Results

The mean daily preference of NaCl for the hypertensive patients was significantly greater than that of the normal volunteers for each of the first 4 days of the study ($p < 0.05$ two-sided t test) (Fig. 7). On days 5 through 7, mean NaCl preference for the patients was consistently greater than for the normal volunteers

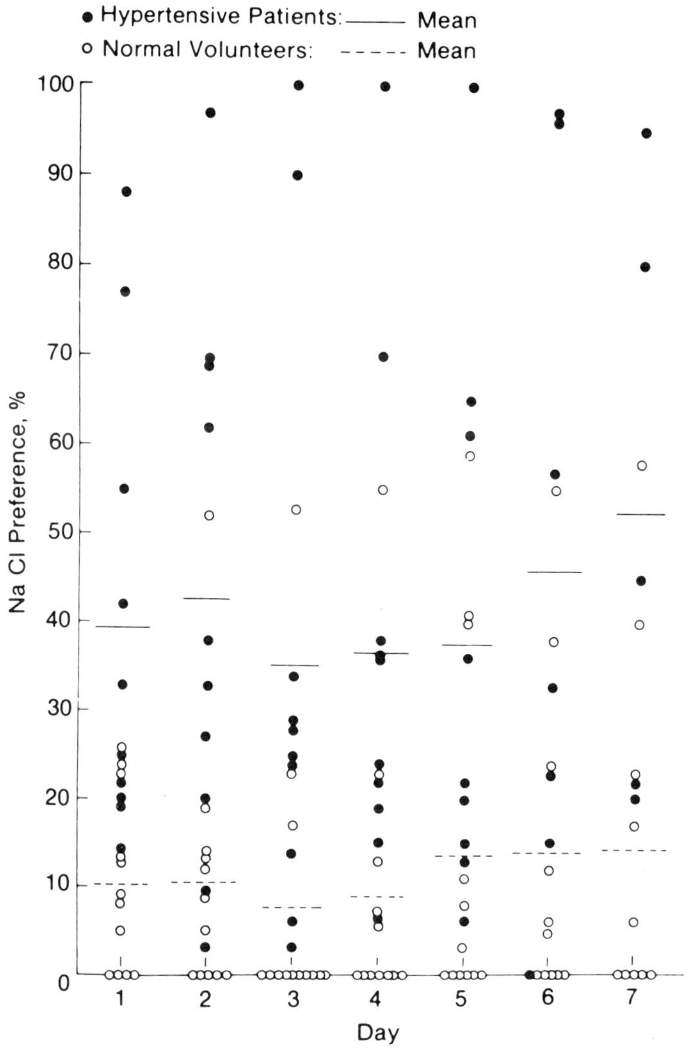

Fig. 7. Sodium chloride preference (in %) in hypertensive patients (solid circles) and normal volunteers (open circles) for each day of study. Mean value of hypertensive patients (solid line) was consistently greater than mean of normal volunteers (hatched line).

but was not statistically significant ($p > 0.05$). (This may be due, in part, to the decreased number of subjects participating in the study after day 4. Some subjects terminated the study prior to day 7 because of their unwillingness to persist in eating the low sodium diet or because of personal reasons which necessitated their leaving the hospital). The daily mean total fluid intake of the patients and the volunteers is shown in Fig. 8. The average total fluid consumption by the patients was significantly greater than that of the volunteers ($p < 0.05$, two-sided t test) for the first 6 days of the study.

The daily mean total intake of Na^+ (in milliequivalents) of the patients and the volunteers is shown in Fig. 9. The average daily intake of Na^+ by the patients was significantly greater than that of the volunteers ($p < 0.05$, two-sided t test) for each of the first 4 days of the study. On days 5 to 7, mean total intake of Na^+ for the patients was consistently greater than for the normal volunteers but was not statistically significant ($p > 0.05$). (This, too, may have been the result of the decreased number of subjects participating in the study.)

Table IV shows the mean daily intake of Na^+ (excluding the 9 mEq of constant dietary intake) in each subject. On the average, patients with hypertension consumed over four times as much Na^+ as did the volunteers. This was true whether

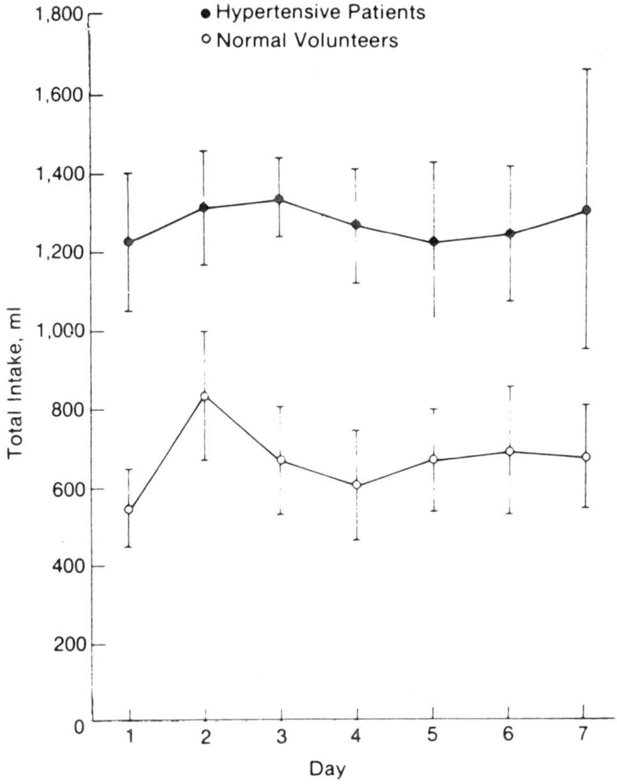

Fig. 8. Daily total fluid intake (in ml) of hypertensive patients (solid circles) and normal volunteers (open circles). Total fluid intake (0.15 *M* NaCl with distilled water) is plotted on ordinate, days of study on abscissa. Each point and vertical bars represent the group mean ± 1 SEM.

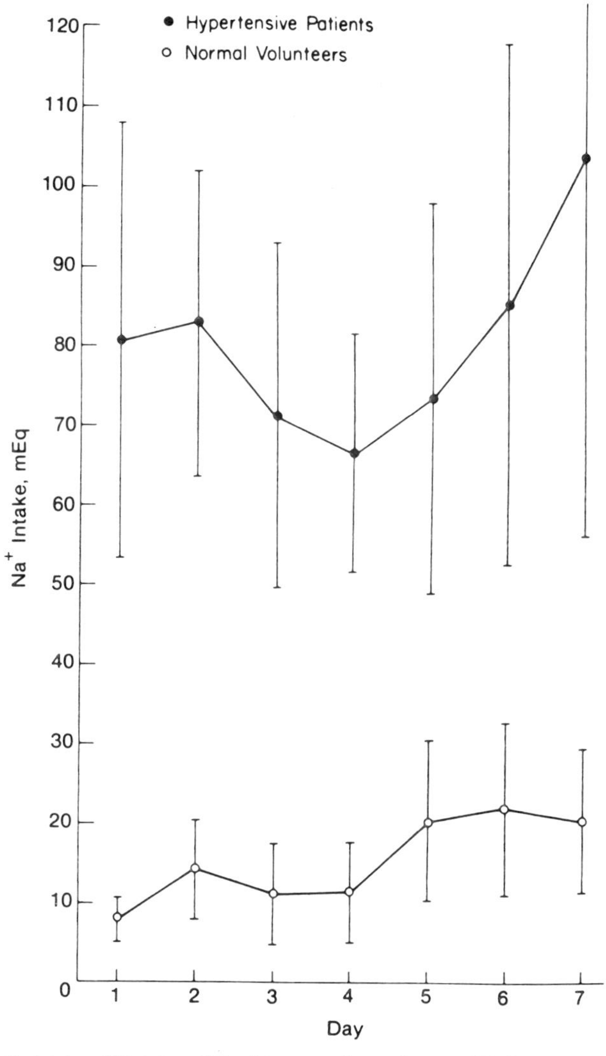

Fig. 9. Daily intake of Na^+ (in mEq) of hypertensive patients (solid circles) and normal volunteers (open circles). Na^+ intake is plotted on ordinate, days of study on abscissa. Each point and vertical bars represent group mean ± 1 SEM.

the absolute Na^+ intake (patients, 74.3 ± 21.0 mEq/day, mean ± 1 SEM; volunteers, 14.4 ± 6.5, $p < 0.02$) or the Na^+ intake per 100 kg body weight (patients, 92.1 ± 24.4 mEq/100 kg/day; volunteers, 21.3 ± 9.9 mEq/100 kg/day, $p < 0.02$) were compared.

The increased salt preference, total fluid intake, and Na^+ intake observed in

TABLE IV

Comparison of Body Weight, Blood Pressure, NaCl Taste Thresholds, and Mean Daily Intake of Na^+ of Hypertensive Subjects and Volunteers

	Comparative data					
Subject	Sex/Age/Race	Body weight (kg)	Admission blood pressure, (mm Hg)	Sodium chloride thresholds, (mM)[a,b]	Average daily Na^+ intake, (mEq)[c]	Average daily Na^+ intake/ body weight, (mEq/100 kg)
Hypertensives						
1.	F/43/C	81.00	160/100	30/30	92.8	114.6
2.	M/39/B	89.02	150/100	12/12	54.8	64.6
3.	F/25/C	73.32	170/130	30/60	51.6	70.4
4.	M/51/B	100.75	190/110	6/6	61.7	61.2
5.	F/44/C	84.44	150/108	60/60	250.8	297.0
6.	M/56/C	76.78	180/120	30/60	84.5	110.0
7.	M/50/B	56.92	170/102	60/60	34.7	60.9
8.	M/42/B	84.40	140/100	30/30	62.2	73.7
9.	M/47/B	70.42	156/112	30/30	11.0	15.7
10.	M/54/B	73.40	162/108	60/60	39.1	53.3
Mean		79.05		30/45[e]	74.3 ± 21.0[d,f]	92.1 ± 24.4[d,f]

Volunteers						
1.	M/19/C	72.20	128/72	12/60	10.2	14.2
2.	M/19/C	69.60	120/72	30/60	2.2	3.2
3.	F/43/C	54.58	130/78	12/12	0	0
4.	M/19/C	71.02	100/60	60/60	2.6	3.7
5.	M/19/C	72.04	132/70	60/60	0	0
6.	M/21/C	61.72	136/84	60/60	43.1	73.6
7.	M/23/C	80.82	124/80	30/30	45.8	56.6
8.	M/21/C	65.40	110/70	12/12	63.6	97.2
9.	M/19/C	73.46	120/80	30/30	1.8	2.4
10.	M/19/C	58.68	120/70	30/30	0	0
11.	M/21/C	78.66	118/80	30/30	3.7	4.8
12.	F/19/C	61.10	118/70	6/6	0	0
Mean		68.27		30/30[e]	14.4±6.5[d]	34.2±9.9[d]

[a] Numerator of fraction is detection threshold, denominator of fraction is recognition threshold.
[b] Normal values according to Henkin *et al*[13] 12/30 m*M* (range, 0.8 to 60/6 to 60 m*M*).
[c] Excluding daily 9 mEq of Na^+ intake in constant diet.
[d] Mean ± SE.
[e] Median values (not significant, Wilcoxson rank sum statistic).
[f] $p < 0.02$ (two-sided *t* test) compared to normal volunteers.
C, Caucasian; B, Black.

the hypertensive patients occurred even though the median detection and recognition thresholds for the taste of NaCl were similar in the two groups (Table IV).

No correlations could be made between the amount of Na^+ consumed by the patients and whether they had had prior antihypertensive drug therapy or prior diuretic therapy.

These studies indicated that salt preference was significantly greater in patients with essential hypertension than in normotensive controls and that this preference itself could be, in part, responsible for the increased intake of salt observed in some patients with hypertension.

IV. EFFECTS OF ANTIHYPERTENSIVE TREATMENT

It also seemed of interest to determine what role, if any, antihypertensive therapy might play in salt preference in patients with essential hypertension. Efforts to evaluate effects of antihypertensive medication in the SH rat proved very difficult since these drugs, to be effective as antihypertensive agents, often produced sedation of the animals to such a degree that performance of the two-bottle free choice test could not be measured reliably. Since these agents in humans are not associated with such problems, it seemed useful to carry out these studies in a paradigm similar to the one previously performed in hypertensive patients.

Four patients with essential hypertension were tested for NaCl preference in a 2-day trial on two occasions, first, off all antihypertensive medication for 10 days to 2 months and then on antihypertensive agents which included α-methyldopa, guanethidine, thiazide diuretics and spironolactone alone or in combination (Schechter *et al.*, 1974). The time interval between the two trials during which the patients were treated varied between 7 and 17 months. For the treatment studies the patients were readmitted to the hospital 1 day prior to testing and their antihypertensive therapy continued throughout a 2-day test period. At the time of admission, on treatment, their mean blood pressure was 131/87 mm Hg (range: 116–152/70–104) compared to 166/110 mm Hg (range: 140–190/100–120) at their first admission without treatment. Detection and recognition thresholds for NaCl were measured again in each patient and did not differ significantly from previous measurements which were all within the normal range. The results of studies in these patients indicated that antihypertensive agents significantly lowered their diastolic blood pressure an average of 23 mm Hg (range: 18–40 mm Hg, $p < 0.02$, paired t test). Following treatment (Fig. 10) mean NaCl preference, mEq Na^+ intake, and total fluid intake all decreased although these differences were not statistically significant.

These studies demonstrate that patients with essential hypertension show a greater preference for saline and consume a greater total volume of fluid than

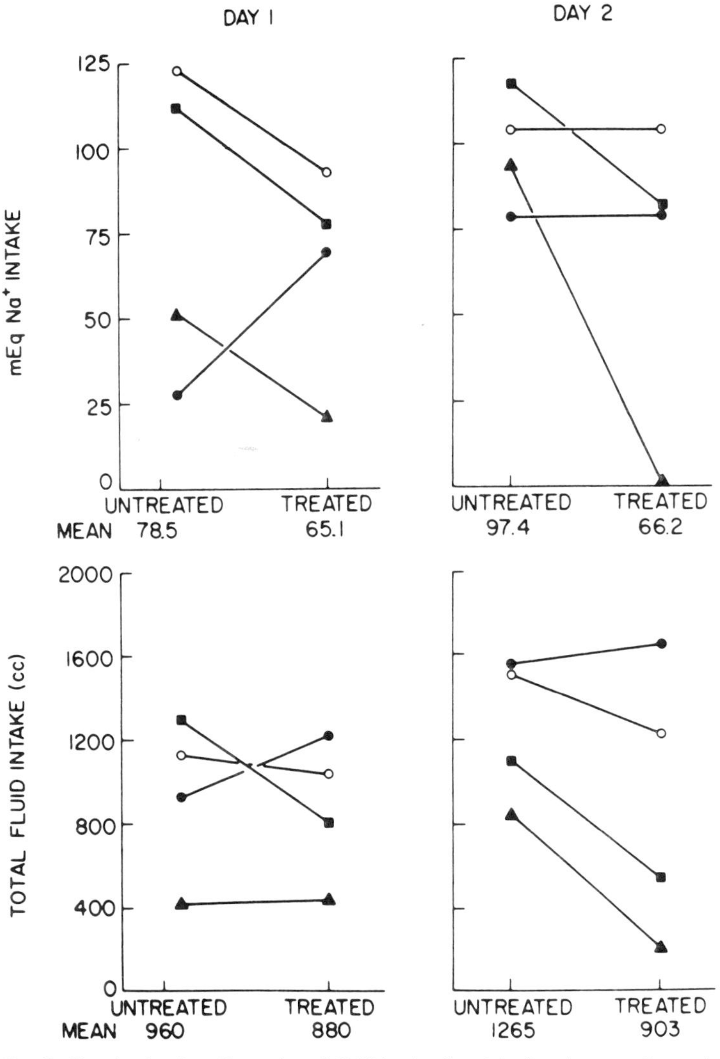

Fig. 10. Sodium intake (in mEq) and total fluid intake (in cc) in four hypertensive patients for each day of the study during untreated and treated periods. Each symbol represents an individual patient. Treatment with several antihypertensive agents resulted in a significant decrease in diastolic blood pressure ($p < 0.02$, paired t-test) and a decrease in sodium and total fluid intake, although this decrease was not significant ($p > 0.10$, paired t-test).

normotensive volunteers when given a choice between 0.15 *M* NaCl and water as their sole source of fluid.

Because of this increased preference, hypertensive patients exhibited a greater Na^+ intake than did normotensive volunteers. These differences cannot be explained on the basis of altered taste acuity for NaCl since the patients exhibited detection and recognition thresholds for the taste of NaCl similar to the volunteers.

The two study groups were assembled based only upon differences in blood pressure. However, evaluation of the data obtained from the hypertensive patients indicated no significant differences in NaCl preference, total fluid intake, or mEq Na^+ consumed when the data from 7 Caucasian and 9 Black patients were compared ($p > 0.4$) or when the data from the 11 men were compared with those from the 5 women ($p > 0.1$). Similarly, there were no differences found among any of these parameters when patients of different age groups were compared. Indeed, similar results were obtained when several volunteers, aged 50–65 years, were tested. No correlations were found between the amount of Na^+ consumed by the patients and the type of prior antihypertensive therapy or whether the patient had ever been treated with antihypertensive drugs.

Using a questionnaire technique one group of investigators concluded that there was no significant difference between dietary salt habits of normotensive subjects and hypertensive patients (Swaye *et al.*, 1972; Dawber *et al.*, 1967), whereas Dahl (1957), using a similar technique, found that hypertensive patients added more salt to their food. These differences in results indicate the difficulty in obtaining valid information about salt intake with a questionnaire technique (Dawber *et al.*, 1967). However, measurements of urinary Na^+ excretion as an index of sodium intake in normotensive subjects and hypertensive patients also indicate conflicting results. Dahl (1957), measuring 24-hour urinary Na^+ excretion in 9 hypertensive patients and 19 normotensive subjects on an ad libitum salt intake, over an average period of 9 days, found a significantly greater Na^+ excretion in the hypertensives. Schneckloth *et al.* (1962), measuring Na^+ excretion in casually collected urine samples, found no consistent differences between hypertensive patients and normotensive subjects. Ashe and Mosenthal (1937), using 24-hour urinary Na^+ output and urinary volume to reflect NaCl and fluid intake, found no differences in either NaCl or fluid intake between 563 normotensive subjects or 298 subjects who were found to have hypertension that they did not suspect. Dawber *et al.* (1967) made similar observations with respect to Na^+ excretion. It is obvious that variables such as age, race, sex, socioeconomic factors, definition of hypertension, the manner by which blood pressure is measured, and other factors which are difficult to specify contribute to the variable results previously observed.

The relationship between salt preference, as measured under the conditions of this study, and actual dietary intake of sodium, as practiced outside the hospital setting, is difficult to specify and, at present, is not well studied. Although as a group, the hypertensive patients consumed significantly more NaCl than did the controls, the NaCl intake of both groups was relatively low due to the conditions of the study. However, it may be of interest to note that only among some of the hypertensive patients was total fluid preference for NaCl noted and more than 2 liters of saline consumed daily.

Whether salt appetite in man is acquired by dietary and social customs (Dahl and Love, 1954; Meneely and Dahl, 1961) or, as in other animals, reflects a sensitive mechanism for the maintenance of sodium homeostasis (Quartermain *et al.*, 1967; Denton, 1969) is not known. However, alterations in the handling of sodium and fluid have been suggested in patients with hypertension (Farnsworth and Barker, 1943; Green *et al.*, 1952b; Brodsky and Graubarth, 1953; Weller and Hoobler, 1959). The increase in salt preference found in hypertensive patients may either reflect this altered metabolism or may be a manifestation of some other, as yet unidentified, agent of hypertension. Since increased salt intake may serve as one causal factor in the genesis of hypertension in genetically susceptible individuals (Dahl and Love, 1954, 1957; Meneely and Dahl, 1961), the increase in salt appetite shown by our patients may have contributed to the development of their hypertension.

The decreases in mean NaCl preference, sodium intake, and total fluid volume observed following treatment with antihypertensive agents is an interesting observation even though these decreases were not statistically significant. These changes which suggest some effect of treatment with antihypertensive agents on salt appetite may be important for our understanding of some of the mechanisms in hypertension.

It is obvious that many factors are important in the etiology of hypertension. The present studies lend support to the concept that two factors, one genetic, the other, increased salt intake, may be important in the genesis of essential hypertension. The role of genetic factors in essential hypertension has been recently reviewed (Editorial, 1978). It is possible that the concatenation of both genetic factors and increased salt intake, because of hedonic factors in some patients, leads to the development of hypertension. However, the possible role of antihypertensive agents in correcting both the hypertension and the increased salt preference suggests that some control mechanisms are present which may fundamentally alter these factors.

Of interest in the present studies is that the only two normotensive subjects who exhibited preference for NaCl in the range of responsiveness of the hypertensive patients had both a hypertensive mother and father. These were the only two normotensive subjects studied who gave such a family history, the others having either one or no hypertensive parent. Since these two subjects have not been subsequently followed, it is not known whether they have themselves become hypertensive. However, such studies could have predictive value in identifying an at risk population, and may prove of value in an effort to define the relationships between genetic factors and increased salt intake in the genesis of human hypertension.

REFERENCES

Abrams, M., DeFreiz, A. I. C., Tosteson, A. C., and Landis, E. M. (1969). Self-selection of salt solutions and water by normal and hypertensive rats. *Am. J. Physiol.* **156,** 233.

Allen, F. M. (1920). Arterial hypertension. *J. Am. Med. Assoc.* **74,** 652.

Ambard, L., and Beaujard, E. (1905). La Rétention chlorurée seche. *Sem. Med.* **25,** 133.

Annino, J. S. (1967). An improved automated method for the determination of urea. *Am. J. Clin. Pathol.* **48,** 147.

Ashe, B. I., and Mosenthal, H. O. (1937). Protein, salt and fluid consumption of 1000 residents of New York. *J. Am. Med. Assoc.* **108,** 1160-1163.

Brodsky, W. A., and Graubarth, H. N. (1953). Excretion of water and electrolytes in patients with essential hypertension. *J. Lab. Clin. Med.* **4,** 43-55.

Catalanotto, F. C., Schechter, P. J., and Henkin, R. I. (1972). Preference for NaCl in the spontaneously hypertensive rat. *Life Sci.* **11,** 557.

Chasson, A. L., Grady, H. J., and Stanley, M. A. (1961). Determination of creatinine by means of automatic chemical analysis. *Am. J. Clin. Pathol.* **35,** 83.

Cranston, W. I., and Brown, W. (1963). Diurnal variation in plasma volume in normal and hypertensive subjects. *Clin. Sci.* **25,** 107.

Dahl, L. K. (1957). Evidence for an increased intake of sodium in hypertension based on urinary excretion of sodium. *Proc. Soc. Exp. Biol. Med.* **94,** 23-26.

Dahl, L. K., and Love, R. A. (1954). Evidence for relationship between Na (chloride) intake and human essential hypertension. *Arch. Intern. Med.* **94,** 525-531.

Dahl, L. K., and Love, R. A. (1957). Etiological role of NaCl intake in essential hypertension in humans. *J. Am. Med. Assoc.* **164,** 397-400.

Dawber, T. R., Kannell, W. B., Kagan, A., Donabedian, R. K., McNamara, P. M. and Pearson, G. (1967). Environmental factors in hypertension. *In* "The Epidemiology of Hypertension" (J. Stamler, R. Stamler, and T. N. Pullman, eds.), pp. 255-288. Grune & Stratton, New York.

Denton, D. A. (1969). Salt appetite. *Nutr. Abstr. Rev.* **39,** 1043-1049.

Dole, V. P., Dahl, L. K., Cotzias, G. C., Dziewiatkowski, D. D., and Harris, C. (1951). Dietary treatment of hypertension. II. Sodium depletion as related to the therapeutic effect. *J. Clin. Invest.* **30,** 584.

Editorial (1978). Immunogenetic and essential hypertension. *Lancet* **2,** 409.

Fallis, N., Lasagna, L., and Tetréault, L. (1962). Gustatory thresholds in patients with hypertension. *Nature (London)* **196,** 74.

Farnsworth, E. B., and Barker, M. H. (1943). Tubular reabsorption of chloride in hypertensive and in normal individuals. *Proc. Soc. Exp. Biol. Med.* **52,** 74-75.

Fregly, M. J. (1956). Effect of renal hypertension on the preference threshold of rats for sodium chloride. *Am. J. Physiol.* **187,** 288.

Green, D. M., Saunders, F. J., Van Armen, C. G., Calvin, L. D., and Sturtevant, F. M. (1952a). Mechanisms of desoxycorticosterone action. IX. Temporal relationships of polyuria, polydipsia, sodium exchange and hypertension. *Am. J. Physiol.* **170,** 486.

Green, D. M., Wedell, H. G., Wald, M. H., and Learned, B. S. (1952b). The relation of water and sodium excretion to blood pressure in human subjects. *Circulation* **6,** 919-924.

Henkin, R. I. (1973). A study of circadian variation in taste and smell in normal man and in patients with adrenal cortical insufficiency: The role of adrenal cortical steroids. *In* "Biorhythms and Human Reproduction," pp. 397–408. Wiley, New York.

Henkin, R. I., and Solomon, D. H. (1962). Salt-taste threshold in adrenal insufficiency in man. *J. Clin. Endocrinol. Metab.* **22,** 856.

Henkin, R. I., Gill, J. R., Jr., and Bartter, F. C. (1963). Studies on taste thresholds in normal man and patients with adrenal cortical insufficiency: The effect of adrenocorticosteroids. *J. Clin. Invest.* **42,** 727.

Henkin, R. I., Schechter, P. J., Hoye, R. C., and Mattern, C. F. T. (1971). Idiopathic hypogeusia with dysgeusia, hyposmia and dysosmia: A new syndrome. *J. Am. Med. Assoc.* **217,** 434.

Henkin, R. I., Talal, N., Larson, A. L., and Mattern, C. F. T. (1972). Abnormalities of taste and smell in Sjogren's syndrome. *Ann. Intern. Med.* **76,** 375.

Henkin, R. I., Schechter, P. J., Raff, M. S., Bronzert, D. A., and Friedewald, W. T. (1974). Zinc and taste acuity: A clinical study including a laser microprobe analysis of the gustatory receptor area. *In* "Clinical Aspects of Zinc Metabolism" (W. Pories and W. Strain, eds.), pp. 204–228. Thomas, Springfield, Illinois.

Kare, M. R. (1961). *In* "Physiological and Behavior Aspects of Taste" (M. R. Kare and B. P. Halpern, eds.), p. 8–15. Univ. of Chicago Press, Chicago, Illinois.

Kliman, B., and Peterson, R. E. (1960). Double isotope derivative assay of aldosterone in biological extracts. *J. Biol. Chem.* **235,** 1639.

McConnell, S. E., and Henkin, R. I. (1973a). Increased preference for Na^+ and K^+ salts in spontaneously hypertensive (SH) rats. *Proc. Soc. Exp. Biol. Med.* **143,** 185.

McConnell, S. D., and Henkin, R. I. (1973b). NaCl preference in spontaneously hypertensive rats: Age and blood pressure effects. *Am. J. Physiol.* **225,** 624.

Meneely, G. R., and Dahl, L. K. (1961). Electrolytes in hypertension: The effects of NaCl. *Med. Clin. North Am.* **45,** 271–283.

Perera, G. A., and Blood, D. W. (1947). The relationship of sodium chloride to hypertension. *J. Clin. Invest.* **26,** 1109.

Pisano, J. J., Crout, J. R., and Abraham, D. (1962). Determination of 3-methoxy-4-hydroxymandelic acid in urine. *Clin. Chim. Acta* **7,** 285.

Pittman, J. A., and Beschi, R. J. (1967). Taste thresholds in hyper- and hypothyroidism. *J. Clin. Endocrinol. Metab.* **25,** 895.

Quartermain, D., Miller, N. E., and Wolf, G. (1967). Role of experience in relationship between sodium deficiency and rate of bar pressing for salt. *J. Comp. Physiol. Psychol.* **63,** 417–420.

Schechter, P. J., Friedewald, W. T., Bronzert, D. A., Raff, M. S., and Henkin, R. I. (1972). Idiopathic hypogeusia: A description of the syndrome and a single-blind study with zinc sulfate. *Int. Rev. Neurobiol.* **13,** 125.

Schechter, P. J., Horwitz, D., and Henkin, R. I. (1973). Sodium chloride preference in essential hypertension. *J. Am. Med. Assoc.* **225,** 1311.

Schechter, P. J., Horwitz, D., and Henkin, R. I. (1974). Salt preference in patients with untreated and treated essential hypertension. *Am. J. Med. Sci.* **267,** 320.

Schneckloth, R. E., Corcoran, A. C., Stuart, K. L., and Moore, F. E. (1962). Arterial pressure and hypertensive disease in a West Indian Negro population: Report of a survey in St. Kitts, West Indies. *Am. Heart J.* **63,** 607–628.

Swaye, P. S., Gifford, R. W., Jr., and Berrettoni, J. N. (1972). Dietary salt and essential hypertension. *Am. J. Cardiol.* **29,** 33–38.

Takeda, R., Morimoto, S., Miyabo, S., and Murakumi, M. (1964). A study of adrenal regeneration hypertension: Effect of the delayed adrenal enucleation on the development of hypertension and salt appetite. *Endocrinol. Jpn.* **11,** 19.

Tosteson, D. C., DeFreiz, A. I. C., Abrams, M., Gottschalk, C. W., and Landis, E. M. (1951).

Effects of adrnealectomy deoxycorticosterone acetate and increased fluid intake on intake of sodium chloride and bicarbonate by hypertensive and normal rats. *Am. J. Physiol.* **164,** 369.

Weller, J. M., and Hoobler, S. W. (1959). Salt metabolism in hypertension. *Ann. Intern. Med.* **50,** 106–114.

Wolf, G., Dahl, L. K., and Miller, N. E. (1965). Voluntary sodium chloride intake of two strains of rats with opposite genetic susceptibility to experimental hypertension. *Proc. Soc. Exp. Biol. Med.* **120,** 301.

Wotman, S., Mandel, I. D., Thompson, R. H., and Laragh, J. H. (1967). Salivary electrolytes and salt taste thresholds in hypertension. *J. Chronic Dis.* **20,** 833.

Chapter 27

Taste and Salt Intake in Human Hypertension

R. A. BERNARD, R. L. DOTY, K. ENGELMAN, and R. A. WEISS

I. INTRODUCTION

Essential hypertension, which accounts for approximately 90% of the estimated 24 million cases of high blood pressure in the United States, is one of our most serious public health problems (Marx, 1976). Although, by definition, no one knows what causes the condition, excessive salt (NaCl) intake is believed to be an important factor in its development (Dahl and Love, 1957). The evidence for this comes mainly from epidemiological studies, which show that, across populations, the incidence of high blood pressure is correlated with salt intake (Freis, 1976).

The problem with demonstrating a causal relationship between salt intake and hypertension is that within a population such as ours, the correlation between the two is not very high. The average salt intake in this country ranges from 6 to 18 g (100–300 mEq Na)/day. This contrasts with the 1 to 3 g (15–50 mEq Na)/day

BIOLOGICAL AND BEHAVIORAL
ASPECTS OF SALT INTAKE

ISBN 0-12-397750-9

recommended by the National Research Council (Meneely and Battarbee, 1976). In spite of this apparently unphysiologically high level of intake the majority of people do not develop hypertension. Only a minority is genetically susceptible to the hypertensive effects of salt, either alone or in combination with other factors, such as stress and life style. How these susceptible individuals can be identified before they become hypertensive, and what are the mechanisms of their susceptibility are challenging questions for which we do not yet have satisfactory answers.

An important consideration is that essential hypertension is not a homogeneous disease, but rather it is a condition that can be brought about by disorders in one or more of the various physiological mechanisms that maintain systemic arterial pressure and regulate the overall water and electrolyte balance of the body (Guyton, 1976). For the past 10–15 years much attention has been paid to the role of renin, an enzyme produced by the kidney, which is involved in the regulation of blood pressure, together with angiotensin and aldosterone. Laragh (1973) found that a high percentage of hypertensive individuals had blood plasma levels of renin that were significantly lower or higher than those of normotensives. Consequently he proposed that low- and high-renin hypertension were two distinct categories of the disease, resulting from two distinct mechanisms. Low-renin hypertension would result predominantly from increased blood volume, whereas high-renin hypertension would be due to increased vasoconstriction. Since it is well established that the level of renin activity in the blood tends to be inversely related to salt intake, low-renin hypertension would appear to be a likely candidate for a form of hypertension that would be associated with high salt intake.

The next question, which is what attracts a sensory physiologist to this field, is whether there is a physiological explanation for the elevated salt intake found in our culture, particularly as this may relate to low-renin hypertension. Is our high salt intake mainly due to a passive acquiescence to our man-made environment, with its escalating content of salt in the steadily proliferating variety of commercially prepared foods? Or, alternatively, and perhaps correspondingly, either as cause or effect, is there a biological alteration in the sense of taste which makes salt more acceptable and/or makes people less sensitive to it?

The possibility that a change in acceptability and/or sensitivity underlies elevated salt intake arises from the early work of Richter (1936, 1939), to whom this whole field of inquiry owes its existence. He showed that rats rendered deficient in NaCl through adrenalectomy made an appropriate adjustment in salt intake through a change in taste preference for NaCl through a wide concentration range. Many workers have studied this phenomenon in great detail since then, but the search for the mechanisms underlying the preference changes recently took a new and exciting turn in the work of Contreras (1977), reported earlier in this Symposium. Prior to this the behavioral changes were believed to be mediated through some unknown central mechanism, but the new data show that

peripheral taste input from the tongue is indeed modified, as Richter first postulated, although it is in the direction of lesser rather than heightened sensitivity.

The relationship of these findings to hypertension arises from the fact that spontaneously hypertensive rats (SHR) show an elevated preference for NaCl that is similar to that of salt-deficient rats (Catalanotto *et al.*, 1972; Fregly, 1975; McConnell and Henkin, 1973). However, unlike salt-deficient rats, they also show a large increase in KCl preference and intake (Fig. 1; Dalzell and Bernard, 1979). That the relationship between salt intake and hypertension is not a simple one is exemplified by the fact that it depends on the kind of hypertensive rat being studied. Where hypertension results from experimental impairment of kidney function (Abrams *et al.*, 1949; Fregly, 1956) rats show an aversion for salt. In genetically hypertensive rats, the Dahl strain shows an aversion for NaCl (Wolf *et al.*, 1965), the GHR strain (Phelan, 1968) shows no preference (R. A. Bernard and W. J. Dalzell, unpublished observations) and the Doca-salt-sensitive strain shows increased preference (Ben-Ishay *et al.*, 1976). The experimental rat data, although seemingly contradictory, underline the fact that hypertension results from many different mechanisms, only one of which may be related to elevated salt intake.

In a recent review, Contreras (1978) has shown that the question of salt taste and human hypertension has generated conflicting answers. This may be due to differences in methodology, especially with respect to threshold measurements, as well as to the heterogeneity of the disease. The goal of the experiment to be reported here was to reduce the variability within the hypertensive population by using Laragh's renin-based classification and to measure taste responsiveness at suprathreshold concentrations with the newer methods of magnitude estimation and category scaling.

II. METHODS

Experimental subjects were selected from walk-in patients at the Hypertension Clinic of the Hospital of the University of Pennsylvania. Control subjects were recruited from among staff, employees, and students of the University such that they matched the experimentals in age, sex, and race. All individuals were chosen following their agreement to participate and their signing of a consent form. Participants had to be free of any medication and be willing to return for a second visit with a 24-hour urine sample and donation of a blood specimen, for which they received ten dollars. Blood pressure was measured in the supine and upright position on both visits by the regular staff of the clinic, and systolic (S) and diastolic (D) values were expressed as a single mean blood pressure (MBP) according to the formula: $(1\ S + 2\ D)/3 = MBP$. The four single MBP's were averaged into an overall MBP and subjects were assigned to the hypertensive

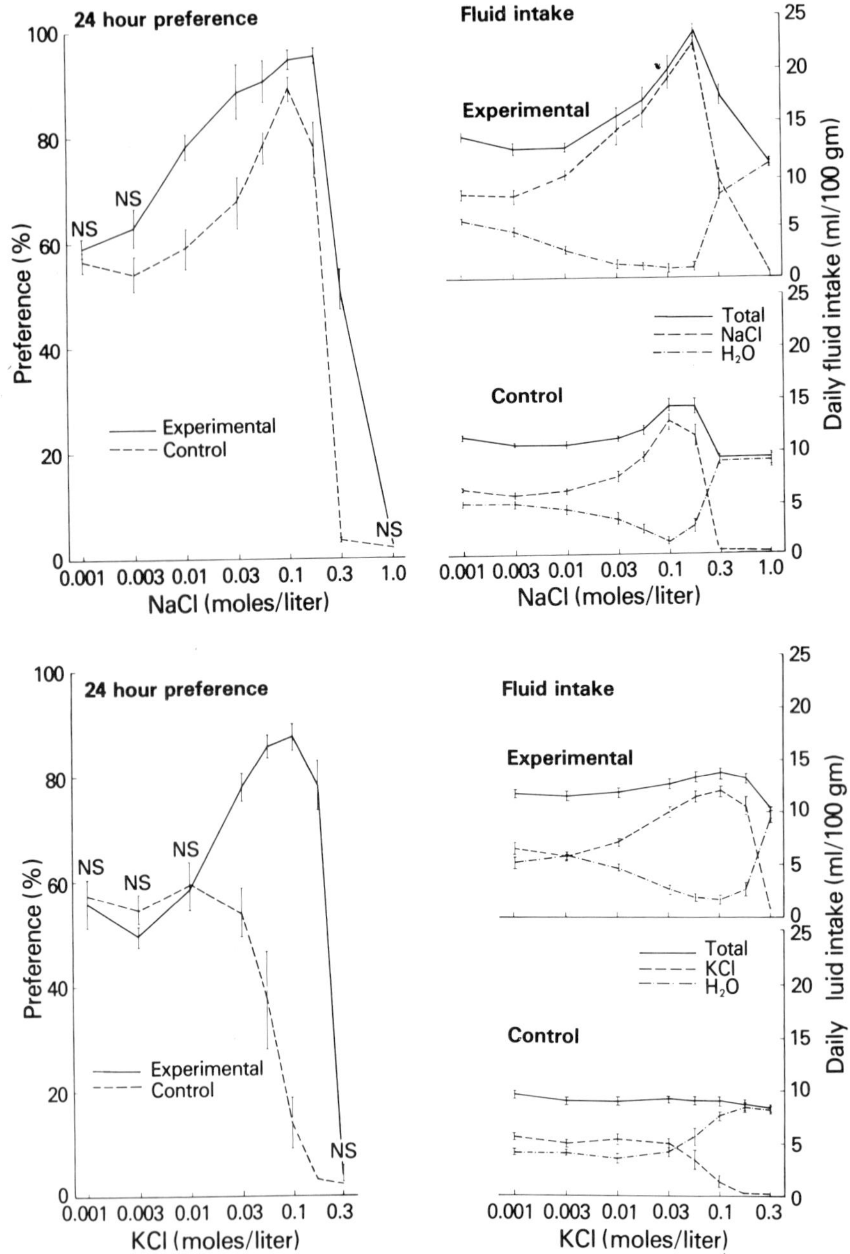

Fig. 1. (Upper) NaCl preference and fluid intake of spontaneously hypertensive (SH) rats and WKY controls. Each point represents the mean of four separate presentations ± 1 standard deviation. All preference values except those labelled NS are significantly different with p at least < 0.05. The SH rats show a significantly elevated NaCl appetite. (Lower) KCl preference and fluid intake for the same rats, which show a remarkably elevated KCl appetite.

category if the overall MBP was 107 or greater, which corresponds to the upper limits of 140/90 for normal systolic and diastolic values. The taste tests were administered on both visits but only the second series was used. Blood specimens were taken only if a 24-hour urine sample was presented and both were analyzed according to the routine procedures of the hospital laboratories. Renin assays were performed in duplicate according to the method of Haber *et al.* (1969) which measures renin activity in terms of ng/ml/hour of angiotensin I produced in incubated plasma samples. In order to normalize the effect of sodium intake on renin, the raw values were divided by the amount of sodium excreted and expressed on a per 100 mEq Na basis (% Na). Urine samples were considered complete when the total creatinine content exceeded 0.95 g and the amount of sodium excreted was taken as a sufficiently accurate measure of daily sodium intake.

The stimuli used for the taste tests were NaCl and sucrose dissolved in distilled water and presented at five concentrations ranging from 0.05 to 1.0 *M* for NaCl and 0.075 to 1.2 *M* for sucrose. Each test consisted of approximately 5 to 7 ml of solution in a small paper cup which the subject swished in his mouth for 5–10 sec and rinsed away with sufficient distilled water to remove any lingering taste. Each test in a concentration series occurred at 1 min intervals.

Two types of tests were performed: one measured the intensity of the stimulus, the other measured its pleasantness or unpleasantness, also called its hedonic value. Measurements of intensity were made with the method of magnitude estimation with a prescribed modulus, in which each subject was asked to compare each test stimulus to a reference stimulus, taken from the midpoint of the concentration range, and assigned an arbitrary value of 10. The subject was instructed to assign a number to the test stimulus that would describe how much stronger or weaker it tasted in comparison to the reference stimulus. If it tasted twice as strong it should be assigned a value of 20, with other numbers to be used depending on how much stronger it tasted; if it tasted weaker it should be assigned a value less than 10, the exact number depending on the degree of its perceived weakness. Each concentration was presented twice in a restricted random order and each series of five concentrations was preceded by the reference stimulus.

The hedonic ratings used the free-modulus variation of the method of magnitude estimation, i.e., a reference stimulus was not used. The subject was instructed to rate the pleasantness or unpleasantness of the solution with corresponding positive or negative numbers of his own choosing. The only constraint was that zero should be used for a stimulus which tasted neither pleasant nor unpleasant, and that the numbers used should be proportional to the degree of pleasantness or unpleasantness experienced. Each concentration was presented twice in a random sequence. As a check on the previous method, an additional hedonic test was performed in which a category scaling method was used. In this procedure the subject was given a scale ranging from 1 to 9 which corresponded to a verbal description ranging from very unpleasant to very pleasant, and instructed to use any number within that range to describe each solution which was presented once in the random sequence. Further details about these scaling methods and associated data analysis may be found in Engen (1972). Each testing session was made up of 54 separate tests, equally divided between NaCl and sucrose, and lasted approximately one hour. Although the status of each subject's blood pressure was either known or suspected at the time of testing, neither the renin nor the salt intake status was known, thus providing the safeguard of a double blind procedure.

III. RESULTS

A total of 53 individuals participated in all the tests, 40 of whom met the criterion for completeness of the urine sample. Of these, 24 were hypertensive and 16 were normotensive, with ages ranging from 22 to 61. Each group was

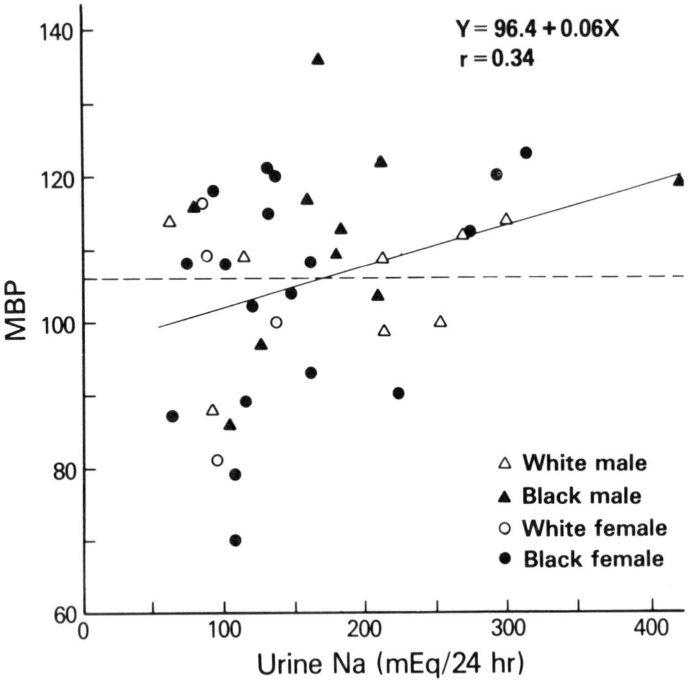

Fig. 2. Correlation between mean blood pressure (MBP) and 24-hour urinary sodium excretion. The population was 70% Black and 30% White. Below 270 mEqNa/24 hours the correlation was very small ($r = 0.14$) and not statistically significant ($p = 0.42$).

approximately 70% Black and 30% White. Urinary sodium excretion ranged from 62 to 437 mEq/24 hours and MBP ranged from 70 to 136 (Fig. 2). The correlation between blood pressure and sodium excretion was statistically significant ($p = 0.02$) but not very high ($r = 0.34$) nor very useful as a predictor of hypertension, especially at levels of excretion below 270 mEq/24 hours, where the correlation was very small ($r = 0.14$) and no longer statistically significant ($p = 0.42$).

Plasma renin activity ranged from 0.03 to 2.53 ng/ml/hr, and was inversely correlated with sodium excretion ($r = -0.31$; $p < 0.03$). These values are much lower than those reported in the literature, with over 60% of the normotensives falling below the range of normal values reported by Laragh and his colleagues (Brunner *et al.*, 1972). None of the values for the hypertensives could fit into the high-renin category. Accordingly the limits that define low-renin hypertension were adjusted to reflect the normotensive population in this study and to reduce the overlap with the hypertensives. Using the normalized renin (% Na) values, which ranged from 0.02 to 3.56 ng/ml/hour per 100 mEq Na ($r = -0.42$; $p < 0.01$), a natural cluster of low-renin hypertensives ($N = 17$) was identified, and the new limits now shifted 75% of the controls into the normal renin category (Fig. 3). Even with these new limits it is not clear whether any of the hypertensives could be placed into a high-renin category. Of the 17 low-renin hypertensives thus identified, 7 were closely matched in age, sex, and race with 7 normotensives to constitute the experimental low-renin hypertensive group and its normotensive control.

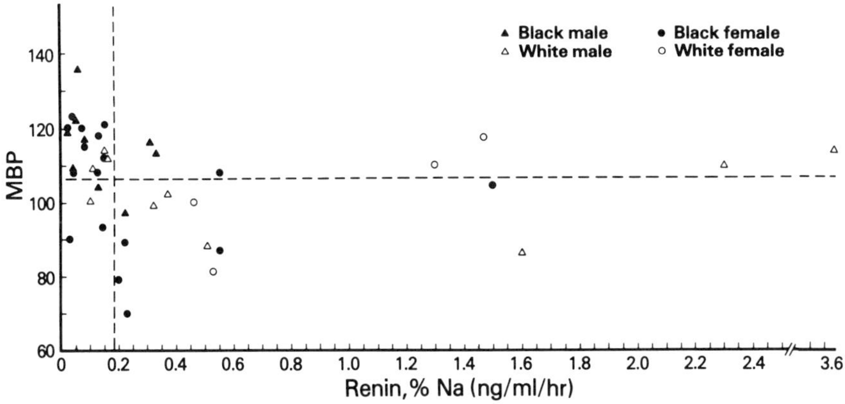

Fig. 3. Distribution of plasma renin activity, expressed on a per 100 mEq Na basis (% Na), with respect to mean blood pressure (MBP). The dashed vertical line represents the upper limit for the low-renin category and the dashed horizontal line the upper limit for normal blood pressure. The upper left quadrant represents the individuals with low-renin hypertension, whereas the lower right quadrant contains the normotensive controls. A few of the normotensives had low renin levels (lower left quadrant) and a minority of the hypertensives had normal renin levels (upper right quadrant).

TABLE I

Salt and Hypertension

		Urine		Plasma		Blood pressure	
	Age	Na (mEq/24 hours)	K (mEq/24 hours)	Renin[a] (ng/ml/hour)	Renin[a] % Na	S/D	Mean
Normotensive ($N=16$)	33	142	48	0.32	0.28	116/76	89
Hypertensive ($N=24$)	41	178	48	0.20	0.12	148/100	116

[a] Median

TABLE II

Salt and Low-Renin Hypertension

		Urine		Blood pressure	
	Age	Na (mEq/24 hours)	K (mEq/24 hours)	S/D	Mean
Normotensive ($N=7$)	31	118	47	114/74	87
LR Hypertensive ($N=7$)	33	246[a]	54	142/98	113

[a] $p < 0.01$.

Table I illustrates that when all the hypertensives were considered together, they did not differ significantly from the normotensives in the amount of sodium or potassium excreted nor in the amount of plasma renin activity. However, when the low-renin hypertensive group was compared with its normotensive control a significant difference in sodium excretion appeared (Table II).

The low-renin hypertensive group rated the NaCl solutions as a whole more acceptable than the normotensives (χ^2 test, $p < 0.01$), finding the lower concentrations more pleasant and the higher concentrations less unpleasant than the controls when using the magnitude estimation method (Fig. 4). However, this

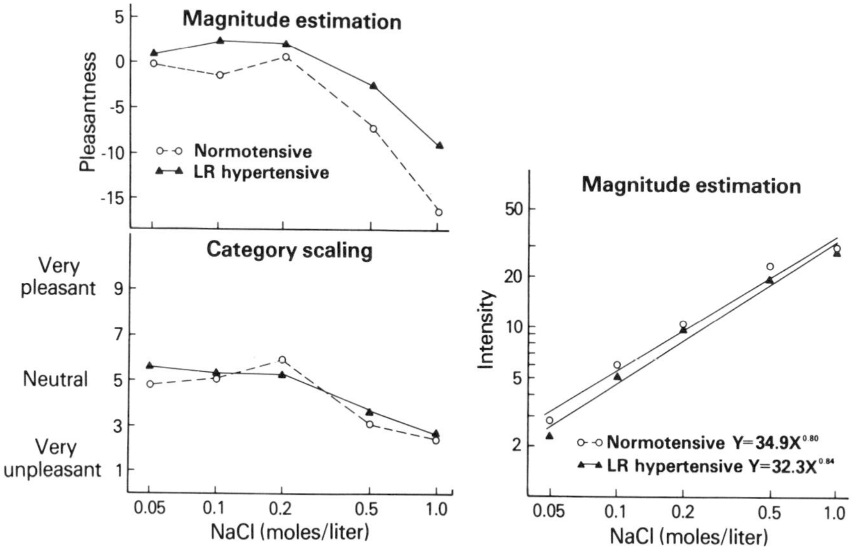

Fig. 4. Pleasantness (left panel) and intensity (right panel) ratings of NaCl solutions made by the low-renin (LR) hypertensive group ($N = 7$) and a control group ($N = 7$) closely matched in age, sex, and race. The LR hypertensives showed a significantly higher ($p < 0.01$, χ^2 test) acceptability for the salt solutions as a whole with the free-modulus variation of the magnitude estimation procedure but not with category scaling. There was no difference in the intensity ratings between the two groups using magnitude estimation with reference to a fixed standard (0.2 M NaCl = 10).

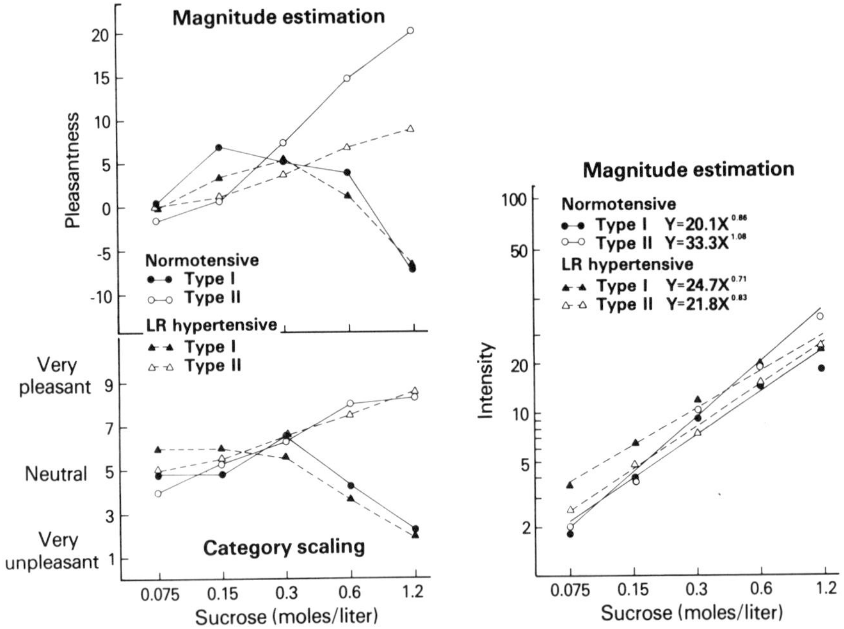

Fig. 5. Pleasantness (left panel) and intensity (right panel) ratings of sucrose solutions, as in Fig. 4. Because of the existence of Type I and Type II sugar responders, the subgroups are too small to achieve statistical significance. There is a suggestion that the Type II LR hypertensives found sucrose less pleasant and less intense than the controls.

difference did not appear with category scaling. No significant difference appeared in the ratings of the intensity of the salt solutions by the two groups.

The results with the sucrose solutions are inconclusive because the existence of Type I and Type II responses (Thompson *et al.*, 1976) made the resultant subgroups too small for satisfactory statistical analysis. However, there is a suggestion that the Type II but not the Type I low-renin hypertensives found sucrose less pleasant or acceptable than the controls (Fig. 5). No such difference is apparent with category scaling. Interestingly the Type II, but not the Type I low-renin hypertensives appear to rate the intensity of sucrose lower than the controls.

IV. DISCUSSION

The results of this experiment indicate that within the overall population of individuals with essential hypertension there is a subgroup in which the disease can be reasonably categorized by a change in the mechanisms that regulate the sodium balance of the body. In the past a great deal of attention has been paid to the excretory mechanisms of this balance, but what appears to be abnormal in these individuals are the intake mechanisms. These people find salt more acceptable to their taste and ingest significantly more of it than normal people or other types of hypertensives. According to the theory of alliesthesia proposed by Cabanac (1971), the pleasantness of gustatory as well as olfactory and thermal stimuli is related to the body's internal state, such that a change in hedonic quality leads to a change in behavior that is adapted to the body's need. Thus, in the case of salt-deficient rats, their increased need for salt is met by an increase in pleasantness of salt and a decrease in its intensity, both of which lead to a higher intake. A similar mechanism may be operating in the SH rats and the results of this study suggest that low-renin hypertension may be associated with an abnormal yet physiological need for NaCl. Although the low-renin hypertensive group did not show a lower sensitivity to NaCl in this study (Fig. 4), this may be due to use of a reference stimulus, which was given the same arbitrary value to all individuals. Thus if there had been a difference in the perceived intensity of the salt solutions between the groups, prescribed use of the same numbers would have tended to obscure it. Similarly, the category scaling method may have failed to show a change in the pleasantness of the solutions because all the subjects had to use the same numbers. It seems reasonable to suppose that the free-modulus variation of the method of magnitude estimation yielded a significant difference in pleasantness between the two groups because it allowed the subjects to use their own numbers to indicate perceived pleasantness. Thus those who found salt more pleasant tended to use larger numbers than those who found it less pleasant.

If some hypertensives ingest high amounts of salt in response to a salt "need," this may indicate that the sodium control system of the body is regulating at a higher set point than normal, in a fashion analogous to the higher set point for body temperature seen in fever. That a change in regulatory set point may be occurring in hypertension was suggested by recent evidence (Langford *et al.*, 1977) that patients on antihypertensive diuretic therapy excreted significantly more sodium than those not on therapy, and showed a decrease in salt taste threshold. As a consequence these workers suggested that the increased sodium intake was negating the antihypertensive effects of the therapy. They also compared their patients' behavior to that of classically salt-deprived rats.

The existence of an apparent salt "need" in one form of essential hypertension does not answer the question of whether the higher salt intake is a cause or an effect of the high blood pressure. Although it is more conventional to assume that high blood pressure would be a result of prolonged high salt intake, it is also possible that the latter is a consequence of the hypertensive disease. For, as Guyton (1976) points out, the kidneys of essential hypertensive patients require elevated pressure in order to function normally, and water and salt are retained so that arterial pressure rises high enough to allow normal filtration.

The use of plasma renin levels to categorize different forms of hypertension has recently been questioned (Kaplan, 1977; Rosei *et al.*, 1978). The normalized renin values used in this study increase the negative correlation with sodium excretion. The use of log–log rather than linear coordinates further increases the correlation ($r = -0.63$; $p < 0.0001$), so that our use of plasma renin levels becomes another index of sodium intake and does not correspond to the concept of suppressed renin activity, as developed by Laragh (1973).

V. SUMMARY

Urinary sodium excretion, plasma renin activity, and taste responses of hypertensive and normotensive individuals were examined. A subgroup of the hypertensive population had higher sodium excretion, lower renin activity and rated NaCl solutions more acceptable than a group of normotensive controls carefully matched for age, sex, and race. It is suggested that the combination of high salt intake, low plasma renin activity, and increased pleasantness of salt constitute a form of essential hypertension in which the biological mechanisms that regulate the sodium balance of the body are reset at a higher level.

ACKNOWLEDGMENTS

This investigation was supported in part by an NIH National Research Service Award, 1 F32 HL 5501-01, an NIH Biomedical Research Support Grant to Michigan State University and the Monell Chemical Senses Center. This work was made possible in large part by the cooperation of Paula Levine, R.N., and Jane Davis, R.N., and other staff of the Hypertension Clinic of the Hospital of the University of Pennsylvania.

REFERENCES

Abrams, M., DeFriez, A. I. C., Tosteson, D. C., and Landis, E. M. (1949). Self-selection of salt solutions and water by normal and hypertensive rats. *Am. J. Physiol.* **156,** 233–247.

Ben-Ishay, D., Dikstein, S., and Shalita, B. (1976). Sodium chloride preference in hypertensive (H) and normotensive (N) rats. *Pfluegers Arch.* **361,** 153–157.

Brunner, H. R., Laragh, J. H., Baer, L., Newton, M. A., Goodwin, F. T., Krakoff, L. R., Bard, R. H., and Bühler, F. R. (1972). Essential hypertension: Renin and aldosterone, heart attack, and stroke. *N. Engl. J. Med.* **286,** 441–449.

Cabanac, M. (1971). Physiological role of pleasure. *Science* **173,** 1103–1107.

Catalanotto, F., Schechter, P. J., and Henkin, R. I. (1972). Preference for NaCl in the spontaneously hypertensive rat. *Life Sci.* **11,** Part 1, 557–564.

Contreras, R. J. (1977). Changes in gustatory nerve discharges with sodium deficiency: A single unit analysis. *Brain Res.* **121,** 373–378.

Contreras, R. J. (1978). Salt taste and disease. *Am. J. Clin. Nutr.* **31,** 1088–1097.

Dahl, L. K., and Love, R. A. (1957). Etiological role of NaCl intake in essential hypertension in humans. *J. Am. Med. Assoc.* **164,** 397–400.

Dalzell, W. J., and Bernard, R. A. (1979). In preparation.

Engen, T. (1972). Psychophysics. II. Scaling methods. *In* "Experimental Psychology" (J. W. Kling and L. A. Riggs, eds.), 3rd ed., Chapter 3, pp. 47–86. Holt, New York.

Fregly, M. J. (1956). Effect of renal hypertension on the preference threshold of rats for sodium chloride. *Am. J. Physiol.* **187,** 288–292.

Fregly, M. J. (1975). NaCl intake and preference threshold of spontaneously hypertensive rats. *Proc. Soc. Exp. Biol. Med.* **149,** 915–920.

Freis, E. D. (1976). Salt, volume and the prevention of hypertension. *Circulation* **53,** 589–595.

Guyton, A. C. (1976). Regulation of arterial pressure. II. The renal–body fluid system for long-term pressure control mechanisms of hypertension. *In* "Textbook of Medical Physiology," 5th ed., Chapter 22, pp. 291–293. Saunders, Philadelphia, Pennsylvania.

Haber, E., Koerner, T., Page, L. B., Kliman, B., and Purnode, A. (1969). Application of a radioimmunoassay for angiotensin I to the physiologic measurements of plasma renin activity in normal human subjects. *J. Clin. Endocrinol. Metab.* **29,** 1349–1355.

Kaplan, N. M. (1977). Renin profiles. The unfilled promises. *J. Am. Med. Assoc.* **238,** 611–613.

Langford, H. G., Watson, R. L., and Thomas, J. G. (1977). Salt intake and the treatment of hypertension. *Am. Heart J.* **93,** 531–532.

Laragh, J. H. (1973). Vasoconstriction–volume analysis for understanding and treating hypertension: The use of renin and aldosterone profiles. *Am. J. Med.* **55,** 261–274.

McConnell, S. D., and Henkin, R. I. (1973). Increased preference for Na^+ and K^+ salts in spontaneously hypertensive (SH) rats. *Proc. Soc. Exp. Biol. Med.* **143,** 185–188.

Marx, J. L. (1976). Hypertension: A complex disease with complex causes. *Science* **194,** 821–825.

Meneely, G. R., and Battarbee, H. D. (1976). Sodium and potassium. *In* "Nutrition Reviews' Present Knowledge in Nutrition," 4th ed., Chapter 26, pp. 259–279. Nutr. Found., New York.

Phelan, E. L. (1968). The New Zealand strain of rats with genetic hypertension. *N. Z. Med. J.* **67,** 334–344.

Richter, C. P. (1936). Increased salt appetite in adrenalectomized rats. *Am. J. Physiol.* **115,** 155–161.

Richter, C. P. (1939). Salt taste thresholds of normal and adrenalectomized rats. *Endocrinology* **24,** 367–371.

Rosei, E. A., Brown, J. J., Cumming, A. M. M., Fraser, R., Semple, P. F., Lever, A. F., Morton, J. J., Robertson, A. S., Robertson, J. I. S., and Tree, M. (1978). Is the "sodium index" a useful way of expressing clinical plasma renin, angiotensin and aldosterone values. *Clin. Endocrinol.* **3,** 141–147.

Thompson, D. A., Moskowitz, H. R., and Campbell, R. C. (1976). Effects of body weight and food intake on pleasantness ratings for a sweet stimulus. *J. Appl. Physiol.* **41,** 77–83.

Wolf, G., Dahl, L. K., and Miller, N. E. (1965). Voluntary sodium chloride intake of two strains of rats with opposite genetic susceptibility to experimental hypertension. *Proc. Soc. Exp. Biol. Med.* **120,** 301–305.

Chapter 28

Biological and Behavioral Aspects of Salt Intake: A Summation

V. G. DETHIER

Seldom has a substance more romantic, ubiquitous, and slighted than common salt been the subject and unifying theme of a symposium. Few natural materials are so influentially intertwined with historical events, politics, economics, religion, and culture in general. Salt provides a common meeting ground for politicians, economists, historians, military strategists, theologians, ethnologists, anthropologists, chemists, psychologists, and biologists.

This symposium, the first devoted to biological and behavioral aspects of sodium chloride, could hardly explore all of these facets; however, the nexus of interests provided the theme of three presentations that served as enlightening perspectives for more cloistered laboratory colleagues. M. S. Fregly, after presenting an introduction to early speculations on the evolution of the presence of sodium chloride in the extracellular fluid of all organisms and the physiological origin and appetite for salt, outlined the social history of the compound and its impact on politics throughout history, culminating in Gandhi's treatise protesting the British salt tax in 1930. Dickinson described the world distribution of commercially available salt, the methods and extent of production in the United States, the monetary value of the product, and the uses to which it is put. The fact that 44% of all salt produced in the United States ends up spread on highways, while probably not news to environmentalists, came as a revelation. Other revelations followed later in Multhauf's address "Salt and History" in which he described the importance of salt in providing the chemical industry with an abundant source of chlorine. As he pointed out, chlorine is the staple for the

BIOLOGICAL AND BEHAVIORAL
ASPECTS OF SALT INTAKE

ISBN 0-12-397750-9

synthesis of innumerable compounds of contemporary culture not the least of which are, or were, DDT and other chlorinated hydrocarbons.

These three presentations placed salt in perspective for the studies that followed. They suggested that regardless of the biological, behavioral, or medical aspects of salt intake that may be operating at the individual level, there are significant global forces at work at all levels. Some of the influences of economics and politics were revealed in Forsythe and Miller's survey of problems associated with the developing, labeling, and marketing of processed foods. The intricacies of reconciling governmental recommendations for reduction of the salt content of processed foods with the need to effect preservation, maintain palatbility, cater to consumer whims, and realize a profit are almost dismaying.

To these nonbiological constraints on salt intake must be added the particular demands imposed by ecology. While ecological modulation was implicit in some papers as, for example, those comparing the different salt requirements of herbivores and carnivores, the subject was focused upon most clearly in a provocative presentation by Paque. This dealt with Bedouins and the salt waters of the Sahara. The contrast between American consumption of salty processed foods and Bedouin abstention from salt was striking. Since for many Bedouins the only source of water contains up to 11 mg of NaCl per liter, salt is neither eaten nor used in cooking. The salt economy of these people, regulated at low levels (if sweet water is encountered) by salt appetite, at high levels by headache stop signs, and by careful economy of water and diet, provides a striking model of salt intake.

As investigators have narrowed their sights on the many peculiar phenomena associated with salt intake, they have emphasized (1) the behavior of organisms vis-a-vis salt in normal and deficit situations, and (2) the biological mechanisms operating at many levels to mediate this behavior. These fields of study began, or at least were given their greatest impetus, by Richter's investigations of the laboratory white rat, a pale representative of a real animal. As Denton reminded us, it is not even representative of rats, of which there are many and strikingly varied species. Inroads to the laboratory have been made, however, by rabbits and sheep, representing the herbivores (Denton and Nelson), dogs, representing the carnivores (M. J. Fregly), and birds, of which Kare made a valiant defense. The value of these comparative studies of different species as well as of different human cultures (e.g., Bedouins and Americans) was proved by the different findings that emerged. Conspicuously absent from the symposium were studies of marine organisms and invertebrates.

Another comparative approach was that involving age. Weiffenbach examined "saltines" in developmental perspective from the fetus to age 1–3 years, and Chauncey and Wallace investigated salt threshold, salivary salt levels, and salt intake at the opposite end of the age spectrum, namely, at ages 33 to 83. Both studies revealed some of the vexing problems in methodology and touched upon the confounding role of saliva. Evidence on the behavior of fetuses with respect to salt is shaky, and, in the case of neonates, hedonic aspects had to be inferred from facial expressions. Facial expression suggested a ''dislike'' for salt even though intake was not inhibited. At ages 1-3 years, salt was rejected even though thresholds were comparable to adult thresholds. Since fetuses are exposed to salt *in utero,* and neonates acquire salt from cow's milk and formula, the role of experience is a confounding feature. There is also clearly a problem in distinguishing between hedonics and detection. In the aged, one problem is the inability to use each subject as his own control and the uncertainty of early experience. Because it was not possible to know antecedent characteristics, as, for example, what the threshold of a 65-year-old subject was at age 33, it is difficult to know to what extent differences in threshold before and after age 50 are due to age per se. This bears upon the interesting finding that thresholds are higher in the elderly while the salt content of saliva is lower. Since it is known that taste receptors are replaced approximately every 11 days, it would be interesting to search for a correlation between threshold and the number of taste receptors present at each age.

The particular issues that surfaced in these studies and permeated all discussions were: the relations between the taste ''saltiness,'' preference, appetite, and intake; the relative causative roles of peripheral and central neural factors; and the complexity of hormonal interactions. Of necessity, we have tended to investigate these phenomena separately simply in order to be able to handle them. It is apparent that the relationships are extremely complex and that too vigorous an employment of Occam's razor could produce lesions in our thinking. Clearly sensory, central, and hormonal events are working in concert, as are hedonic phenomena. Epstein suggested early in the conference that more rigorous application of the terms ''preference'' and ''appetite'' would have a salutary effect on our thinking. He proposed that the word ''preference'' be reserved for normal responses and the term ''appetite'' for need. Discussion did not fully resolve the issue; however, in practice the words were generally employed in the context suggested.

From the classic studies of Richter to the many behavioral studies of the present, the role of a variety of changes in an animal's physiology in evoking changes in sensitivity, preference, and appetite for salt has challenged, and is still challenging, the ingenuity of investigators. At one level, Morrison, showing that adrenalectomy reduced sensitivity and preference for salt at high concentrations, illustrated the difficulty of interpreting threshold and sensitivity data and arriving at logical deductions. At the peripheral level, the initial interface between the animal and the substance salt, Contreras demonstrated for the first time that electrophysiological responses of taste receptors changed as adrenalectomy changed behavioral salt preference. These and other studies reminded us how far we are from understanding the basic mechanisms of behavior related to the ingestion of salt.

Even the nature of primary events at the sensory level still eludes us. We are ignorant of the manner in which sodium chloride initiates the flow of information upon which preferences, appetites, and hedonic experiences depend. The theory proposed several decades ago by Beidler remains the most widely accepted model for taste stimulation by salts; yet ultimate proof is lacking. In this view the relevant constituents in the plasma membrane are proteins. Brand proposed that the important acceptors are lipids rather than proteins. He presented evidence supporting a hypothesis that the transduction of the information "salty" may involve a reduced pyridine nucleotide intermediate. He made the interesting suggestion that stimulation by salt involves a mechanism not unique to cells of taste buds. This contention is in agreement with phylogenetic studies of salt responses of many diverse organisms as well as of diverse tissues. The phylogenetic study suggested that the modern salt receptor might be the descendant of an ancient common chemical sense cell that acquired an anatomical location most favorable for subserving a taste function.

In another type of analysis, based upon monitoring summated chorda tympani activity, Mooser showed that activation of taste receptor cells, at least in rats, is consistent with the concerted transition allosteric model of Monod, Wyman, and Changeux. In this model the conformational transition following stimulus binding implicated a protein constituent of the membrane.

Much remains to be learned about stimulus/receptor interaction. We know only that receptors have evolved that transmit to the central nervous system messages essential, at least in some mammals, to the proper maintenance, via behavior, of salt balance. It is worth a reminder, however, that there are equally sensitive salt receptors in many animals that are seldom, if ever, called upon to correct inadequacies of salt intake by behavioral adjustment.

Not only do we remain in ignorance of the molecular basis of salt stimulation, we must struggle with the fact that the microenvironment in which the interaction between cell and salt occurs is a variable one. Moreover, it varies as the internal environment of the whole organism varies so that ultimately the message that the salt receptor transmits reflects not only the characteristics of the stimulus per se (chemical species, concentration, and duration) but also some of the characteristics (even if indirectly) of the internal milieu of the animal. This situation obtains because the receptors are constantly bathed in saliva and because saliva, due to its derivation and intimate relation to other body fluids, partially reflects the constituency of some of these fluids. Most especially it reflects changes in sodium content.

It is hardly surprising that some of the past difficulty in assessing stimulus activity, especially as it relates to thresholds, has arisen from ignoring the role of saliva. The influence of ambient conditions on the tongue has long been suspected, but close attention to salivary events has been of more recent origin. A number of presentations have dealt with the modulating effect of saliva in relation to threshold, preference, appetite, and hedonics. Thrasher and Fregly proposed that the concentration of sodium in saliva determines the preference threshold in rats and that the ambient concentration of sodium in saliva plays a part in regulating the intake of NaCl. A similar relation between saliva and salt threshold was also reported for humans by Chauncey and Wallace.

It follows that bodily changes, normal or experimentally manipulated, that alter the sodium concentration of saliva affect the response of the taste receptor to salt stimuli. From this it would also follow that bodily changes potentially could influence behavior toward exogenous salt via the peripheral nervous system. This was the thrust of Contreras' presentation; however, the question remains as to whether changes in peripheral neural activity are affected by changes in saliva, blood chemistry, or disadaptation. In any case it would be premature to deny the sensory system a contributing role in behavioral changes associated with deprivation by placing exclusive emphasis on central mechanisms.

Whatever else may be, there is obviously a primary relation between the sensory information passing upstream to the central nervous system and palatability in animals and hedonics in man. Attempts to relate the quality saltiness to sensory events, and indeed to relate any gustatory quality thusly, have generated two schools of thought, the so-called labeled line hypothesis and the across-fiber-pattern hypothesis. According to the first, taste qualities are based upon a number of primaries, and perception of mixtures is accomplished by an analytic process. According to the second hypothesis, there are essentially no primaries, or many primaries, and perception of compounds or mixtures generating complex tastes is a synthetic process. Bartoshuk discussed such phenomena as the sweet taste of dilute salt, qualities other than saltiness that characterize salt, and the nature of enhancement within the framework of the analytic view. She also presented evidence supporting the new view that saltiness appears to be produced by cations rather than by anions as formerly believed. In the case of invertebrates, effective stimulation by salts has always been attributed primarily to the cation.

Schiffman, espousing the synthetic view, has employed multidimensional scaling to go beyond descriptive words (e.g., salty, sour). She has presented evidence that the concept of four taste primaries is depauperate insofar as explaining taste perception in humans is concerned. The final word in the controversy is yet to be spoken. As is so often the case, both views may contain elements of truth.

The difficulties of relating taste quality to chemical structure and of trying to understand hedonics in terms of structure and receptor characteristics are not merely academic. How advances in this realm relate to practical problems became apparent in discussions of the report of Sternberg and his colleagues concerning their efforts to find a substitute for sodium chloride on the table. The report described the testing and development of glycinamide hydrochloride.

However much peripheral events and the transmission of information concerning them may be involved in perception, solution of the mechanism or mechanisms underlying appetite as distinct from preference must be sought in the central nervous system. The manner in which the brain is responsive to direct or indirect changes in the internal milieu is a mystery. A reminder of the complexity of the coupling of preference and appetite in normal and in adrenalectomized rats was revealed at the neural level by the brain lesion studies of Wolf and Schulkin. These brought some aspects of central involvement into clear focus. Even with increasingly more accurate neural road mapping within the brain the contribution of the various areas over and above that of implementing local passage of through signals remains obscure.

Equally obscure are the mechanisms by which the brain is tuned to changes in internal states leading to homeostatic behavior. Stricker explored this problem by asking whether sodium appetite was analogous to thirst. He concluded that there was no supportive evidence for volume changes in various water compartments of the body or for hormones being responsible for sodium appetite.

On the other hand, there are many observations to be explained. Falk and Tang described the development of salt appetite after interperitoneal dialysis. Bryant, Epstein, and Fluharty described results that suggested to them that angiotensin might play an important role in eliciting sodium appetite. M. J. Fregly and Newsome presented evidence that the oral contraceptive Enovid induced spontaneous salt appetite in male rats, possibly through involvement of the renin–aldosterone system. That hormones are somehow involved in sodium appetite, though not necessarily responsible for it, was also made clear by the experiments of Denton and Nelson on rabbits and sheep. During pregnancy and lactation both salt deficiency and salt appetite develop. The evidence suggests that appetite at this time is hormonally induced, the hormones being a combination of ACTH, oxytocin, and prolactin.

The basis of salt appetite is unknown even in the animal most thoroughly studied, the laboratory rat. Even if the puzzle is solved here, the question remains whether the results can be generalized to other animals, even other mammals. At the present level of knowledge the behavior of dogs, in which Fregly could detect no sodium appetite, is different from rats, rabbits and sheep; and the rat differs from all of them.

Insofar as human beings are concerned, the question of salt appetite acquires a medical importance because of the supposed link between high salt ingestion and the development of hypertension. This relationship was alluded to by several authors but was treated most fully in the final three papers of the symposium. Torii, in referring to the high incidence of essential hypertension in northern

Japan and the greater preference for salt by these individuals, pointed out the paucity of investigations of possible genetic bases. In demonstrating that a genetic component did exist in rats, he suggested that human beings may also fall into genetic "responder" and "nonresponder" categories and that the latter are "nonresponders" despite high salt preference. A general belief is that several different mechanisms may operate independently to produce essential hypertension. Henkin and Bernard and his associates explored some of the relations between taste, preference, intake, and hypertension.

The impression that emerges from this symposium is that mystery is compounded upon mystery, and yet, considering the short span of time that has elapsed since Richter first began to study behavior related to salt deficiencies, the compounding of mystery is a measure of the volume of work that has been produced by a relatively small number of investigators. The great value of this symposium lay in assembling for the first time investigators from many disciplines, seeking solutions to different immediate problems, and entertaining different philosophies, but bound by a common interest, salt.

Index

SOME people make salt by another method, from salt water which flows from hot springs that issue boiling from the earth. They set earthenware pots in a pool of the spring-water, and into them they pour water scooped up with ladles from the hot spring until they are half full. The perpetual heat of the waters of the pool evaporates the salt water just as the heat of the fire does in the cauldrons. As soon as it begins to thicken, which happens when it has been reduced by boiling to a third or more, they seize the pots with tongs and pour the contents into small rectangular iron pans, which have also been placed in the pool. The interior of these pans is usually three feet long, two feet wide, and three digits deep, and they stand on four heavy legs, so that the water flows freely all round, but not into them. Since the water flows continuously from the pool through the little canals, and the spring always provides a new and copious supply, always boiling hot, it condenses the thickened water poured into the pans into salt; this is at once taken out with shovels, and then the work begins all over again. If the salty water contains other juices, as is usually the case with hot springs, no salt should be made from them.

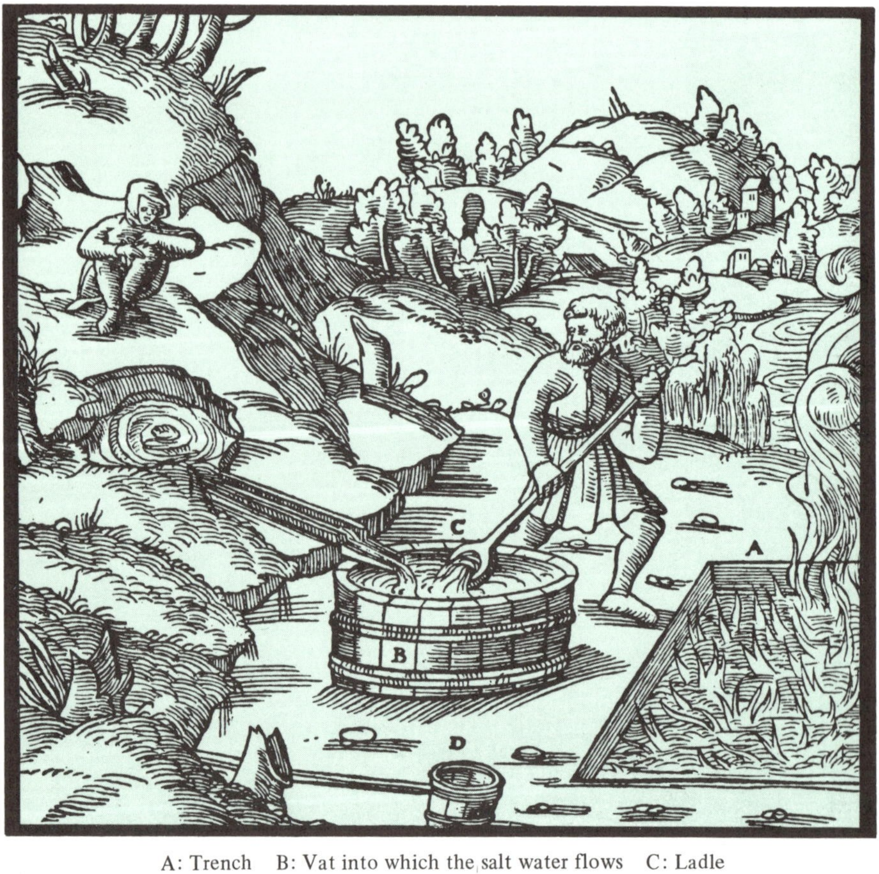

A: Trench B: Vat into which the salt water flows C: Ladle
D: Small bucket with pole fastened into it